FUNCTIONS OF THE STOMACH AND INTESTINE

FUNCTIONS OF THE STOMACH AND INTESTINE

Edited by

M. H. F. FRIEDMAN
Emeritus Professor of Physiology
Jefferson Medical College of the
Thomas Jefferson University

HM+M
MEDICAL & SCIENTIFIC PUBLISHERS

Proceedings of the J. Earl Thomas Memorial Symposium, held November 19 - 20, 1973, at the Jefferson Medical College, Philadelphia; sponsored by The Physiological Society of Philadelphia and the Department of Physiology, Jefferson Medical College of the Thomas Jefferson University

University Park Press
International Publishers in Science and Medicine
Chamber of Commerce Building
Baltimore, Maryland 21202

Printed in the United States of America

British, European, Australasia, and South African edition published by
HM+M Medical and Scientific Publishers
Milton Road
Aylesbury, Bucks., England

ISBN 0-85602-048-6

CONTENTS

Preface vii

In Memorium — J. Earl Thomas, M.D., D.Sc. ix

Contributors xiii

SESSION I.
GASTROINTESTINAL MOTOR ACTIVITIES

The Contractile Process in Smooth Muscle
Marion J. Siegman 1

Electrical Activity of Gastrointestinal Muscle
Alexander Bortoff 17

The Hormonal Control of Gastrointestinal Motor Function
Sidney Cohen 31

The Regulation of Gastric Emptying
J. N. Hunt 47

The Entero-Enteric Reflexes
M. H. F. Friedman 57

The Intestinal Intrinsic Mucosal Reflex: A Possible Mechanism of Propulsive Motility
Marjorie V. Baldwin and J. E. Thomas 75

Choledochoduodenal Junction
Martin F. Tansy and Francis M. Kendall 93

SESSION II.
GASTROINTESTINAL SECRETORY ACTIVITIES 121

Basic Mechanism of HC1 Production
Warren S. Rehm 123

Regulation of Gastric Secretion
Basil I. Hirschowitz 145

Histamine H_2-Receptor Antagonists and Gastric Secretion
M. E. Parsons and J. W. Black 167

Hormonal Control of Secretion
Leonard R. Johnson 179

Factors Influencing Mesenteric Blood Flow
David G. Reynolds, John C. Kerr and Kenneth G. Swan 195

The Role of the Brain in the Control of Gastric Secretion
Frank P. Brooks 207

Pharmacologic Control of Gastric Secretion
David A. Brodie and Y. H. Lee 221

SESSION III.
SECRETORY AND ABSORPTIVE ACTIVITIES OF INTESTINE AND BILIARY TRACT 245

Ion Transport in Large and Small Intestine
Henry J. Binder 247

Amino Acid Homeostasis in the Small Gut
E. S. Nasset 259

Mechanism of the Intestinal Absorption of Sugars and Amino Acids
Robert K. Crane 273

Fat Absorption
Peter R. Holt and Susanne Bennett Clark 285

Enterohepatic Circulation of Bile Acids
Gershon W. Hepner 301

Absorptive Functions of Gallbladder
Richard C. Rose 329

Drug Interactions in the Gastrointestinal Tract
Ruth R. Levine and Carol T. Walsh 349

SESSION IV.
PATHOLOGIC PHYSIOLOGY 375

Dysfunction of the Esophagogastric Junction
Donald O. Castell 377

Gastrointestinal Motor Dysfunctions
Alastair M. Connell 389

Dysfunction of Gastric Secretion
S. P. Bralow 405

Endogenous Inhibitors of Gastric Secretion
George B. Jerzy Glass 423

Intestinal Malabsorption
O. Dhodanand Kowlessar 447

Index to Charts and Tables 459

Subject Index 463

PREFACE

The objective of this Symposium is to bring together scientists known for their research studies on the functions of the stomach and intestine, so that they may summarize for us the present state of knowledge and suggest directions for further investigations. These subjects occupied the interests of the late Professor J. Earl Thomas and this Symposium is in honor of the man who made so many important advances in these areas.

The Symposium Committee, comprising S. Philip Bralow, M.D., Frank P. Brooks, M.D., M. H. F. Friedman, Ph. D., and Alexander Scriabin, M.D., express their sincere thanks to the many essayists and to all the participants in the audience. They are especially grateful to the several section chairpersons for the time and effort spent in conducting the sessions. We wish also to express our gratitude to Ms. Sallie O'Donnell, Ms. Francine Vassallo, Ms. Alexandra Janson and Mr. Peter Panasjuk for the many hours they spent on preparation and arrangements for the Symposium.

We wish to acknowledge with appreciation the aid of the Thomas Physiology Fund of Thomas Jefferson University and the Philadelphia Physiological Society for their sponsorship of the Symposium.

To Ms. Setsu Nakai go my sincerest thanks for her work in preparing the manuscripts for publication.

M. H. F. F.

J. EARL THOMAS, B.S., M.S., M.D., D. Sc.
January 31, 1891—February 2, 1972

Jacob Earl Thomas was born on January 31, 1891, in Steilacoom, Washington, only a little more than a year after that territory was admitted to the Union. His parents, John and Nettie (Wyckoff) Thomas, had migrated from Indiana and Kentucky to homestead in the Great Northwest. Earl attended the Free Methodist Church School (founded the year he was born, and now known as Seattle Pacific College) and the University of Washington. Later he attended St. Louis University from which he graduated with the degrees of B.S., M.D., in 1918 and M.S. in 1924.

In his boyhood Earl spent his summer months as an apprentice in the mechanical trades. To his early acquaintance with the machine shop may be traced his genius for designing and making numerous pieces of laboratory equipment that came to be widely used in teaching and research. Several seasons spent in his youth working in the old Chautaugua circuit afforded him the opportunity of hearing orations and lectures by outstanding speakers of the day and this probably laid the groundwork for the clarity of his own lectures.

Dr. Thomas was Associate Professor of Physiology at West Virginia University in 1920 and 1921. He then returned to St. Louis University as an Associate Professor where he remained until 1927 when he came to Jefferson as Professor of Physiology and Head of the Department. He remained at Jefferson until his retirement in 1956 as Emeritus Professor of Physiology. He could not, however, stay away from experimental research and accepted an appointment of Professor of Physiology and Chairman of the Department at the College of Medical Evangelists in California (now Loma Linda University). In 1964 he relinquished the Chairmanship but continued to teach and participate in research until his terminal illness.

Earl's good humor, kindliness, clear thinking, and inspirational lectures and conferences are cherished memories. The high esteem in which he was held by students and colleagues at Jefferson were demonstrated in his selection by the Class of 1948 as the subject of an oil portrait, and by his election to the Chairmanship of the

Executive Faculty of the College. Appreciative Jefferson alumni established the Thomas Physiology Fund and the Thomas Physiology Library: similar appreciation was demonstrated at Loma Linda University by naming the new student laboratories as the Thomas Physiology Laboratories.

During World War II Dr. Thomas was an advisor to the Quartermaster Corps and carried out studies on appetite, digestibility, and nutritional quality of rations for combat troops. He was a member of numerous national and international academic and professional societies in many of which he held high office. For his rich and mellow learning, for his humanitarianism, and for his great service to medical research and education, he was awarded the Honorary Degree of Doctor of Science by Jefferson in 1960. For his meritorious contributions to gastrointestinal physiology he was awarded posthumously in May 1972 the prestigious Friedenwald Medal by the American Gastroenterological Association.

Dr. Thomas' skill in experimental surgery and his ingenuity in instrumentation placed him high among physiologists. The Thomas drop recorder, the Thomas wrench, the Thomas gastric pouch, the Thomas pancreatic fistula, the Thomas intestinal cannula are only a few of his many contributions which have added immeasurably to the advance of physiology. To him we owe much of our present understanding of the regulation of gastric emptying, the filling and evacuation of the gallbladder, the autoregulation of gastric secretion, the complexities of the entero-enteric reflexes, and the mechanisms of pancreatic secretion. His more than two hundred scientific papers on the physiology of the digestive system, his encyclopedic reviews in reference books, including the Handbook of Physiology and the Encyclopedia Britannica, and his definitive monograph on "The External Secretion of the Pancreas" marked him as an outstanding experimental gastroenterologists.

Though he acknowledged the influence of several medical school teachers, Earl was essentially self-taught. His innate curiosity drove him to seek answers to questions; if he found no answers in the published literature he embarked on projects to obtain them. This questing showed itself early, while he was still an undergraduate student. His major investigations were in the field of gastrointestinal physiology but he also did outstanding work in toxicology and the autonomic nervous system, some while still an undergraduate student.

In 1917 Doctor Thomas married Ursula May Johnson and to them were born two children, J. Earl Thomas, Jr. and Marjorie Ellen (Mrs. John Frederick Larkin). After the death of his wife in 1957, Doctor Thomas was married to Grace Neal Webster.

The artist Frederick Roscher, who painted Doctor Thomas' portrait, had also portrayed Queen Wilhelmina, Pope Benedict XV, Pope Pius XI, Mrs. Eleanor Roosevelt, and others. His comments about Doctor Thomas summed up what all his friends and colleagues felt about him. He wrote, "Doctor Thomas has a remarkable face, in which you feel warmth, friendship, and integrity...the curiosity of one who is dedicated to establishing truth through research."

The Philadelphia Physiological Society and the Physiology Department of Thomas Jefferson University think it most fitting to honor the memory of this distinguished scientist thru a symposium in an area of physiology to which he contributed so much, "The Functions of the Stomach and Intestine".

M. H. F. F.

CONTRIBUTORS

Marjorie V. Baldwin, M.D.
Dept. of Physiology
Loma Linda University
Loma Linda, Calif.

Henry J. Binder, M.D.
Dept. of Internal Medicine
Yale University
New Haven, Conn.

J. W. Black, M.D.
Dept. of Pharmacology
University College
London, England

Alexander Bortoff, Ph. D.
Dept. of Physiology
State University of New York
Syracuse, N.Y.

S. Philip Bralow, M.D.
Dept. of Medicine
Thomas Jefferson University
Philadelphia, Pa.

David A. Brodie, Ph. D.
Research Division
Abbott Laboratories
North Chicago, Ill.

Frank P. Brooks, M.D., D. Sc.
Dept. of Physiology
University of Pennsylvania
Philadelphia, Pa.

Donald O. Castell, M.D.
Gastroenterology Section
Naval Regional Medical Center
Philadelphia, Pa.

Susanne Bennett Clark, M.D.
Dept. of Medicine
Columbia University
New York, N.Y.

Sidney Cohen, M.D.
Dept. of Medicine
University of Pennsylvania
Philadelphia, Pa.

Alastair M. Connell, M.D.
Division of Digestive Diseases
University of Cincinnati
Cincinnati, Ohio

Robert K. Crane, Ph. D.
Dept. of Physiology
Rutgers Medical School
Piscataway, N.J.

M. H. F. Friedman, Ph. D.
Dept. of Physiology
Thomas Jefferson University
Philadelphia, Pa.

George B. Jerzy Glass, M.D.
Gastroenterology Research Laboratory
New York Medical College
New York, N.Y.

Gershon W. Hepner, M.D.
Dept. of Medicine
The Milton S. Hershey Medical Center
Hershey, Pa.

Basil I. Hirschowitz, M.D.
Dept. of Medicine
University of Alabama
Birmingham, Alabama

Peter R. Holt, M.D.
Dept. of Medicine
Columbia University
New York, N.Y.

J. N. Hunt, M.D.
Dept. of Physiology
Guy's Hospital
London, England

Leonard R. Johnson, Ph. D.
Program in Physiology
University of Texas
Houston, Texas

Francis M. Kendall, Ph. D.
Health Sciences Center
Temple University
Philadelphia, Pa.

John C. Kerr, M. Tech.
Division of Surgery
Walter Reed Army Institute of Research
Washington, D.C.

O. Dhodanand Kowlessar, M.D.
Dept. of Medicine
Thomas Jefferson University
Philadelphia, Pa.

Y. H. Lee, M.D., Ph. D.
Research Division
Abbott Laboratories
North Chicago, Ill.

Ruth R. Levine, Ph. D.
Dept. of Pharmacology and Experimental Therapeutics
Boston University
Boston, Mass.

E. S. Nasset, Ph. D.
Children's Hospital Medical Center of Northern California
Oakland, Calif.

M. E. Parsons, M.D.
The Research Institute
Smith Kline & French Laboratories
Welwyn Garden City
Hertfordshire, England

Warren S. Rehm, M.D., Ph. D.
Dept. of Physiology and Biophysics
University of Alabama
Birmingham, Alabama

David G. Reynolds, M.D.
Division of Surgery
Walter Reed Army Institute of Research
Washington, D.C.

Richard C. Rose, Ph. D.
Dept. of Physiology
The Milton S. Hershey Medical Center
Hershey, Pa.

Sue S. Sanders, Ph. D.
Dept. of Physiology and Biophysics
University of Alabama
Birmingham, Alabama

Marion J. Siegman, Ph. D.
Dept. of Physiology
Thomas Jefferson University
Philadelphia, Pa.

Kenneth G. Swan, M.D.
Dept. of Surgery
New Jersey College of Medicine and Dentistry
Newark, N.J.

Martin F. Tansy, Ph. D.
Dept. of Physiology and Biophysics
Health Sciences Center
Temple University
Philadelphia, Pa.

†J. Earl Thomas, M.D., D. Sc.
Dept. of Physiology
Loma Linda University
Loma Linda, Calif.

Carol T. Walsh, Ph. D.
Dept. of Pharmacology and Experimental Therapeutics
Boston University
Boston, Mass.

† Deceased

SESSION I.

GASTROINTESTINAL MOTOR ACTIVITIES

THE CONTRACTILE PROCESS IN SMOOTH MUSCLE

Marion J. Siegman

INTRODUCTION

My assignment in this Symposium is to review some of the fundamental physiological properties of smooth muscle. Because of the restrictions of time and the broad scope of the topic, I shall limit my remarks to the subject of the Contractile Process, with emphasis on morphology and dynamics. I want to acknowledge, at the outset, the collaboration of Dr. Allen Gordon in the studies from my own laboratory which will be discussed.

THE CONTRACTION PROCESS IN SKELETAL MUSCLE

Contractile Elements and Stages of Contraction

Our present concepts of muscle contraction in general have been derived largely from investigations of striated muscle. These will be reviewed briefly for the purpose of gaining some perspective on the problems facing investigations of smooth muscle.

Figure 1 shows the basic architecture of an amphibian skeletal muscle fiber in diagramatic form. The muscle fiber is surrounded by a membrane, the sarcolemma, which is continuous with a tubular structure, the transverse tubular (T) system. The T system extends from the surface membrane into the interior of the cell, and the fluid within its lumen is identical with the extracellular fluid (Porter and Palade, 1957; Endo, 1964; Huxley, 1964). The T-system comes in close apposition to an intracellular longitudinal tubular system, or

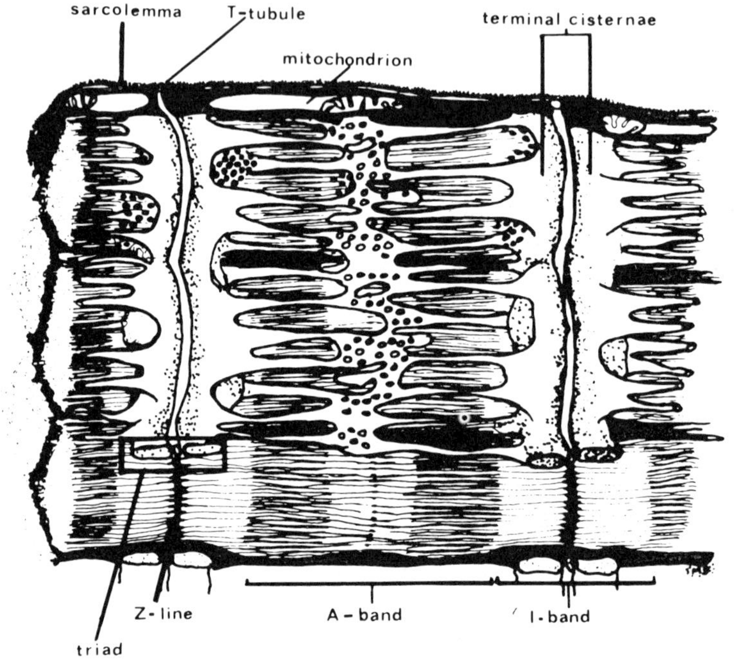

Fig. 1. Diagramatic three-dimensional reconstruction of a frog sartorius fiber, with the longitudinal axis running horizontally. Each myofibril is surrounded by a system of internal membranes which constitute the sarcoplasmic reticulum (SR); the terminal cisternae of this system are indicated. The T-tubular system is continuous with the sarcolemma. (From Peachey, 1965 and Fawcett et al., 1969).

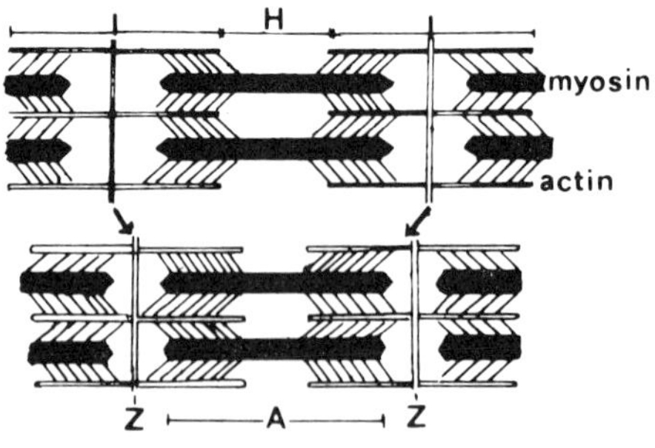

Fig. 2. Diagramatic representation of a sarcomere from a striated muscle. Globular heads of myosin molecules form cross-bridges between the thick (myosin) filaments and thin (actin) filaments. During short-ending (lower figure) the filament length remains constant but the H band narrows.

sarcoplasmic reticulum (SR), which surrounds the myofibrils. The area at which the membranes of both systems approach one another is the triad.

Contraction can be considered as three stages of complex processes which occur in rapid succession: (1) excitation, (2) contraction of the myofibrils and (3) relaxation. Functionally, the sarcolemma and T system are the sites of propagation of the action potential. The longitudinal tubular system is the site of calcium storage (in areas called terminal cisternae) and have the special property of actively accumulating calcium. When an electrical signal reaches the triad, it causes the release of calcium from the cisternae; calcium then moves rapidly down its concentration gradient into the myofibrillar space. The calcium ions react with the contractile proteins to cause muscle contraction, and it is the reuptake of calcium by the sarcoplasmic reticulum that causes relaxation. In resting muscle, calcium is bound and concentrated in the cisternae, keeping the myofibrillar calcium concentration at a low level (less than 10^{-7}M). During excitation, Ca^{++} is released from the cisternae so that the myofibrillar calcium concentration increases about 100-fold, inducing contraction. Following excitation, the calcium concentration is lowered through its sequestration by the SR, and the muscle returns to the relaxed condition. Thus calcium is a controlling factor for the contractile machinery.

Contraction Process

The striated appearance of skeletal muscle under the light microscope is due to the different refractive indices of the interdigitating contractile protein filaments, actin and myosin. With the advent of sophisticated technology in electron microscopy and x-ray diffraction, a more detailed picture of the ultrastructure of muscle has emerged (Hanson and Huxley, 1953, 1955). The thick filaments, which are composed of myosin, have a series of projections along their length except at the middle. These projections, which are globular "heads" of myosin molecules, form cross-bridges which come into contact with the neighboring thin actin filaments (Huxley, 1969), figure 2. The thin filaments consist of three proteins: actin, and, in lesser quantities, tropomyosin and troponin. Tropomyosin and troponin are crucial for the regulation of contraction by calcium; in the absence of calcium, these proteins prevent the interaction of actin and myosin. During excitation, when intracellular free calcium is plentiful, this inhibitory action is lost as calcium becomes bound to troponin; cross-bridges can form and contraction proceeds.

Tension Development

According to the sliding filament theory of contraction (Hanson and Huxley, 1953, 1955; Huxley, 1971), it is through a cyclic "rowing" motion that the cross bridges cause the ends of the actin filaments to draw closer towards one another, thereby causing shortening of the sarcomere. The energy for the cyclic attachment and detachment of cross bridges, hence contraction, comes from the hydrolysis of adenosine triphosphate (ATP). In the absence of calcium the ATPase activity is low. However, in the presence of calcium ATPase activity increases and there is interaction of the filaments with vigorous hydrolysis of ATP (Weber et al., 1964). The maximum speed at which muscles shorten (V_{max}) has been shown to be directly related to their myofibrillar ATPase activity (Barany, 1967). In addition, the relationship between tension development and myofibrillar calcium concentration has been investigated (Natori, 1954). The curve describing calcium concentration and tension is similar to that for myofibrillar ATPase (Hellam and Podolsky, 1969). Therefore, calcium regulates shortening through the hydrolysis of ATP and cross-bridge cycling, and tension development through the number of sites of interaction (cross-bridging) between actin and myosin. The relationship between tention development and ATPase activity is still not understood and requires further study.

The greater the overlap of the myofilaments, the greater the possible number of sites of interaction of the filaments (Huxley and Hanson, 1954). It has been known for some time that tension development depends on the initial length of a muscle, and that there is an optimum length for tension development, usually normal resting length (L_o) in situ (Ramsey and Street, 1940). The ultrastructural basis of this relationship was investigated by Gordon and co-workers (1966a, b) who measured sarcomere length (hence myofilament overlap) of single fibers in relation to tension development. Their work showed that there is an "ideal" degree of overlap of the actin and myosin filaments at which maximum force could be generated because at lengths greater or less than L_o, tension diminshed. The increases in length decreased the degree of filament overlap, resulting in fewer sites of interaction and thus less tension. At shorter lengths, an overlap of actins from opposite Z lines occurred, which presumably reduced the efficiency of cross-bridge formation, and thereby tension was reduced. These experiments are essential to and in agreement with the sliding filament model of contraction.

THE CONTRACTILE PROCESS IN SMOOTH MUSCLE

Comparison with Striated Muscle

We may query, does our concept of contraction as just described apply to smooth muscle as well? First, there are some vital questions to be answered. (1) Are the contractile proteins, actin and myosin, organized in vertebrate smooth muscle in two sets of filaments that contract through a sliding filament mechanism? (2) Is there a sarcoplasmic reticulum or some other structure that can serve as a calcium store, to release calcium during excitation and re-accumulate it to allow relaxation? (3) Are there portions of the SR associated with the surface membrane comparable to the triad which serves as the site of excitation-contraction coupling? (4) How are contraction and relaxation regulated by calcium in smooth muscle? We shall attempt to answer these important questions in light of current evidence.

The ultrastructure of smooth muscle has been studied extensively in recent years, using modern electron microscope and x-ray diffraction techniques. The progress, although remarkable, has not lacked controversy. For some time, the occurrence of myosin in a filamentous form was doubted (Lowy and Small, 1970), but recent investigations show clearly that a thick filament, about 155 Å in diameter does, indeed, exist (Devine and Somlyo, 1971; Rice et al., 1971; Somlyo et al., 1971). Furthermore, projections from these filaments resembling cross-bridges have been noted (Somlyo et al., 1973). Thin filaments (50–80 Å diameter) identified as actin, occur in association with the thick filaments. The actin filaments enter structures called dense bodies, which may be functional counterparts of the Z line of striated muscles. In addition, a non-contractile thin filament (100 Å diameter) has been found which is usually associated with the dense bodies (Cooke and Chase, 1971; Cooke and Fay, 1972). Although the function of these filaments is not well understood, it has been suggested that they may be analogous to a cytoskeleton (Somlyo et al., 1971; Cooke and Fay, 1972), forming the structural basis of passive tension in resting smooth muscle (Cooke and Fay, 1972).

The transverse tubular system of striated muscle has not been observed in smooth muscle. Rather, there exist surface vesicles or "caveolae", which are in communication with the extracellular space (Devine et al., 1972a, 1973; Gabella, 1971, 1973). A sarcoplasmic reticulum, a truly intracellular tubular system, has been shown in various smooth muscles (Devine et al., 1972, 1973; Somlyo et al., 1971b). Often the sarcoplasmic reticulum forms fenestrations around the caveolae, and more peripheral elements approach the surface membrane over considerable distances. Because of the occurrence of opaque connections in the gap separating the SR and surface membrane, it has been suggested that these may be sites of electrical-mechanical coupling in smooth muscle (Somlyo, 1972). That is, the SR in close apposition to the surface membrane may be the site of stored calcium that can be released by the action potential, initiating a twitch.

Although the volume of the SR of smooth muscle is considerably smaller and less developed than skeletal muscle, it can bind enough calcium to fully activate the contractile machinery. Furthermore, there is convincing evidence that microsomal fractions with ATPase activity can accumulate calcium (Carsten, 1969) and that the SR can accumulate divalent cations, such as strontium, which can substitute for calcium in contraction (Somlyo and Somlyo, 1971). The inference is that the SR of smooth muscle can serve as a calcium sink. It is interesting that the cations were also localized in mitochondria, but the role of these structures in the contractile process remains to be established.

MECHANICAL PROPERTIES OF SMOOTH MUSCLE

Length-Tension and Force-Velocity Relationships

We have, I think, satisfactorily answered many of the questions raised earlier: the morphology of smooth muscle can support the contractile process and a sliding filament model as we know it in cardiac and striated muscle. Let us now consider the dynamic aspects of smooth muscle contraction, in order to determine whether it conforms functionally to a sliding filament model. The studies to be described were done in my laboratory, on the isolated taenia coli of the rabbit. In order to eliminate spontaneous activity, we cooled the tissues and bathing media to 22°C, and were able to obtain reliable, reproducible responses that could be treated quantitatively.

A prerequisite to acceptance of the sliding filament model is that tension development bear a certain relationship to contractile filament overlap. Put another way, a length-tension relationship similar to that of skeletal muscle would have to operate. The length-tension relationship for taenia coli is shown in figure 3. We can see that passive tension rises monotonically with length. Active tension shows an optimum length for tension development. From this curve we can also estimate that the muscle should be able to contract to about 25% of its resting length, a figure which is in good agreement with estimates based on light microscopy measurements of contracting dissociated cells (Gordon and Siegman, 1971a).

The relationship that defines the two fundamental properties of muscle, the ability to shorten and to bear a load, would be expected to be similar to that observed in striated muscles. The force-velocity relationship would be described by a hyperbolic curve (Hill, 1938). In figure 4 we see the force-velocity curves obtained for smooth muscles at their optimum length, L_o, and at a length some 40% shorter. To begin with, we note that the curve is similar to that of striated muscles. The result of decreasing the initial muscle length is a shift of the curve toward the origin, with proportional decreases in the intercepts P_o and V_{max}. The dynamic constants _a_ and _b_ defined by Hill, however, are independent of length. It is interesting that these relationships conform well to those of skeletal muscle. When compared to skeletal muscle, the Hill constants obtained for smooth muscle suggest that the molecular mechanisms for contraction may be the same, but that smooth muscles operate by expending energy at a much lower rate (Gordon and Siegman, 1971a).

Role of Calcium

The calcium requirement for smooth muscle contraction is well known from the work of Edman and Schild (1961), Schatzmann (1964) and others. However, all studies involving the requirement for calcium, until recently, were done on potassium-depolarized, glycerinated, or spontaneously contracting preparations. In my laboratory, we were interested in determining how alterations in the

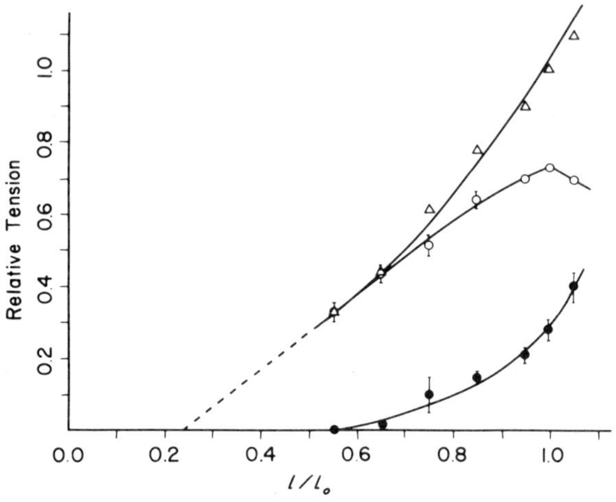

Fig. 3. Length-tension relation. Abscissa: muscle length normalized to optimum length. Ordinate: muscle tension normalized to total tension at length l_0. Passive tension, closed circles; total tension during tetanic stimulation, triangles. Active tension, open circles, is obtained by subtracting passive tension from total tension at each muscle length. SEM are shown in brackets except when smaller than symbol. (From Gordon and Siegman, 1971a).

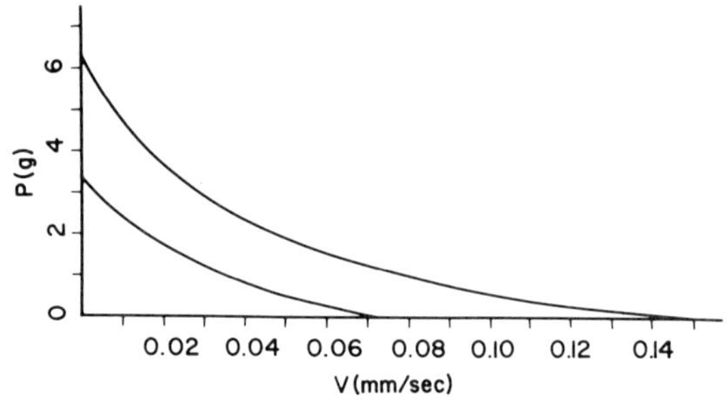

Fig. 4. Force-velocity relations at 2 muscle lengths. Curve at right was determined at l_0 and curve at left at a shorter length. (From Gordon and Siegman, 1971a).

mechanisms governing calcium delivery and removal operate to affect contraction during a single twitch. In all cases, muscles were given single supramaximal DC shocks, and isometric twitch responses were monitored.

To begin with, we examined the effects of alterations of the extracellular calcium concentration on tension development. As the calcium concentration of the bathing medium was increased in the range from 0.5 to 8.0 mM, dramatic changes in twitch tension occurred (figure 5). Both twitch tension and rate of tension development (shown by the slope of the rising phase of tension development) increased as the calcium concentration increased. It is interesting that in the range of calcium concentrations tested tetanus tension remained constant.

From the fact that twitch responses increased as calcium concentration increased it is inferred that some change in the active state of the contractile machinery had occurred. To test this hypothesis, we determined the time course of the active state, using the classical quick-stretch method of Hill (1949), and this is shown in figure 6 (Gordon and Siegman, 1971b). The time course of the active state can be considered the mechanical counterpart of the calcium concentration and interaction with the contractile apparatus. Following a stimulus, the active state rises rapidly, reaching its maximum intensity in about 1 second. It then decays exponentially, presumably as calcium is removed by the SR. Figure 6 also shows the rise in tetanus tension, which reaches a maximum that exceeds the peak of the active state curve. This finding is contrary to the classical view of Hill and others that mechanical saturation is achieved during a twitch. According to the classical view, the maximum intensity of the active state is equal to tetanus tension; it follows that any agent that potentiates contraction acts by prolonging the active state. This erroneous view delayed understanding of twitch potentiation, or staircase phenomena, some twenty years.

When we examined the effects of calcium on the active state, we noted that the primary effect of increasing calcium concentrations was to increase the intensity of the active state, with little change in its duration [figure 7; (Siegman and Gordon, 1972)]. By electrically differentiating the tension signals, we also noted that (1) the maximum rate of tension development (maximum dP/dt, or $\dot{P}$) was directly proportional to maximum tension, and that (2) tension, dP/dt, and the maximum intensity of the active state all varied in the same way as a function of the calcium concentration [figure 8; (Siegman and Gordon, 1972)].

These studies showed that twitch tension can be potentiated by increasing calcium delivery, and when this occurs, proportional changes will be seen in the active state intensity, twitch tension, and in the maximum rate of tension development (figure 9). This is the type of response we see in rate-dependent potentiation, such as

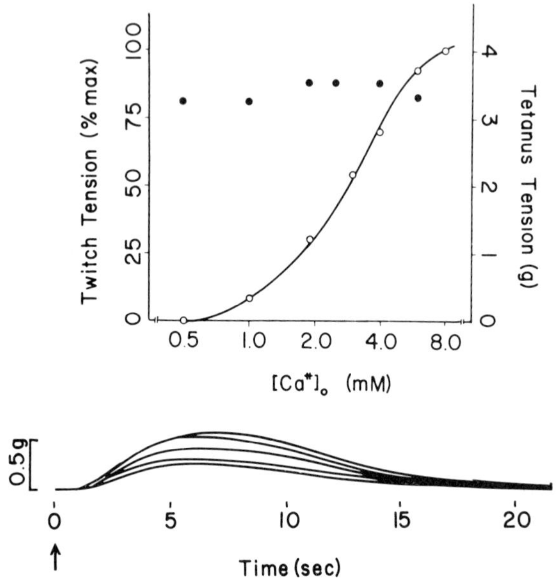

Fig. 5. The effect of increasing $[Ca^{++}]_O$ on twitch (open circles) and tetanus (solid circles) tension. Lower panel shows traces of isometric twitch responses in increasing Ca^{++} media, with smallest response in low Ca^{++}. Note that as $[Ca^{++}]_O$ increases, the rate of tension development and peak tension increase.

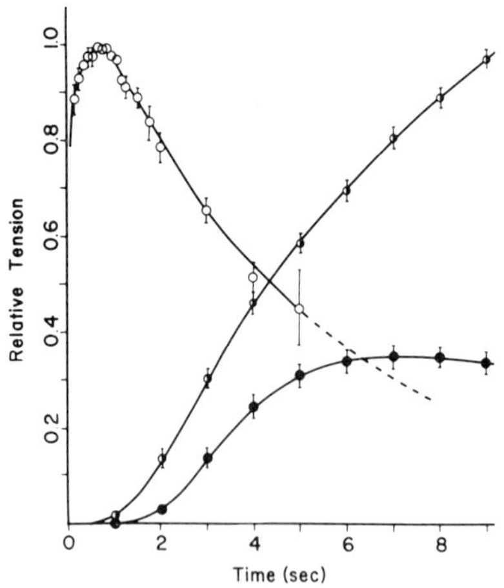

Fig. 6. Time course of active state. Normalized mean values of active-state intensity at each increment of time are shown by open circles. Filled circles are isometric twitch response. Rise in tetanus tension is represented by half-filled circles. Abscissa: time from application of stimulus. SEM are shown by brackets except when smaller than symbols. (From Gordon and Siegman, 1971b).

Fig. 7. Effect of $[Ca^{++}]_o$ on active state and twitch tension. Upper curves show early time course of active state. Lower curves are corresponding twitch responses. Results are from a typical experiment using a single muscle. (From Siegman and Gordon, 1972).

Fig. 8. Effect of $[Ca^{++}]_o$ on twitch tension (P), maximum rate of tension development (dP/dt), and maximum intensity of active state (MIAS). Each point is mean value, $n \gtrsim 12$. At a given $[Ca^{++}]_o$ no, significant differences ($P \gg 0.05$) between P, dP/dt, and MIAS were noted. (From Siegman and Gordon, 1972).

Fig. 9. Analog computer simulation of model showing effects of varying maximum intensity of active state on twitch response. Upper curves are active-state time courses and lower curves are corresponding computer-generated twitch responses. Ordinate: arbitrary units. Abscissa: 1 sec/div. Rate constant of decay of active state was 0.195 sec^{-1}. Calibration mark = 1 sec. (From Gordon and Siegman, 1971b).

Fig. 10. Computer simulation showing effects of changing rate constant for decay of active state. Rate constants of upper curves, from bottom to top, are 0.250, 0.195, and 0.150 sec^{-1}, respectively. Bottom curves are corresponding computer-generated twitch responses. Scale is same as figure 9. Calibration mark = 1 sec. (From Siegman and Gordon, 1971b).

---

treppe, or staircase.

A second mechanism for potentiation involves a prolongation of contractile machinery activity, and this can be accomplished by interfering with calcium removal by the SR. In our experiments, we treated the tissues with 1 mM caffeine, which increased myofibrillar calcium by (1) causing calcium release from, and inhibition of its re-uptake by ,the SR (Bianchi, 1961; Herz and Weber, 1965; Weber, 1968; Weber and Herz, 1968), (2) by increasing membrane permeability to calcium (Bianchi, 1961), and (3) by causing calcium release from membrane binding sites (Ito and Kuriyama, 1971). The mechanical consequences are shown in figure 10. In this case, the intensity of the active state was constant, but its rate of decay was slowed, and the extent to which it was slowed increased as the calcium concentration increased. The corresponding twitch responses were progressively potentiated, but these effects were not accompained by a change in P. We could induce a plateau in the active state, keeping the intensity and the rate of decay constant. Here, too, twitch tension increased, but these changes were not accompanied by changes in P (figure 11). Chemical agents, such as caffeine, act by a combination of the schemes just shown, and these can be selectively demonstrated by proper concomitant manipulation of the calcium supply. Essentially, agents which increase calcium delivery elicit changes seen early in the contractile cycle, so that the rate of tension development and maximum tension are increased. Agents which impede calcium removal affect a later part of the contractile cycle, so that tension increases as a result of a prologation of activity (Siegman and Gordon, 1972).

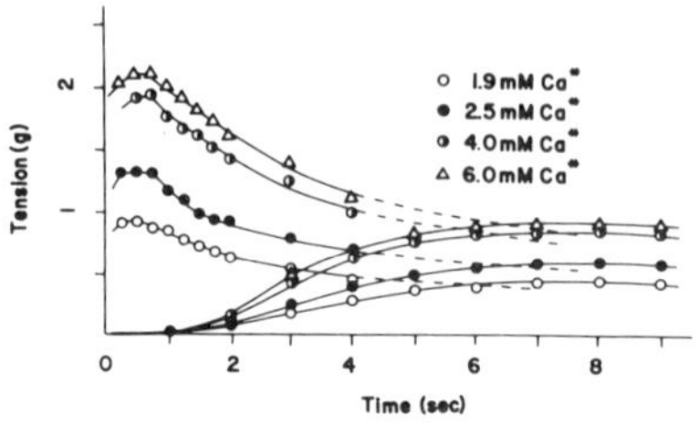

Figure 7

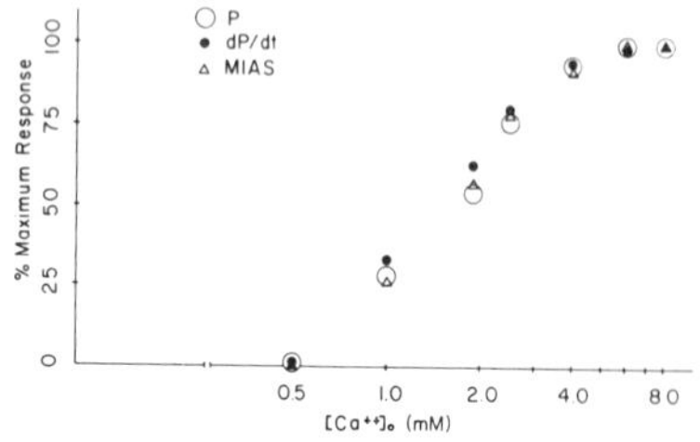

Figure 8

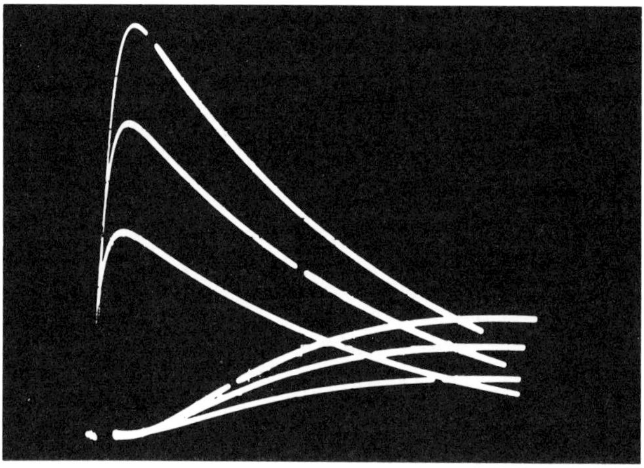

Figure 9

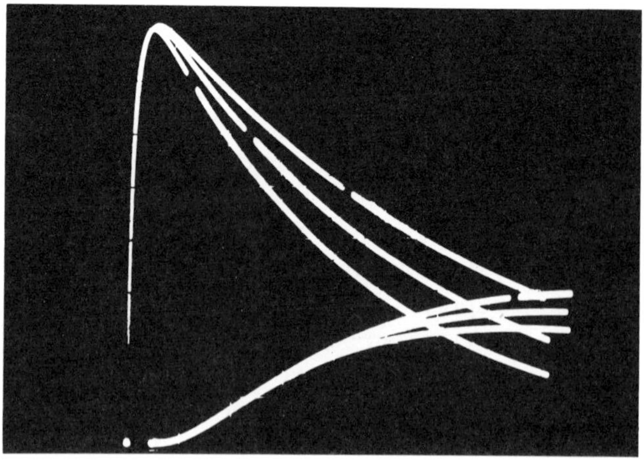

Figure 10

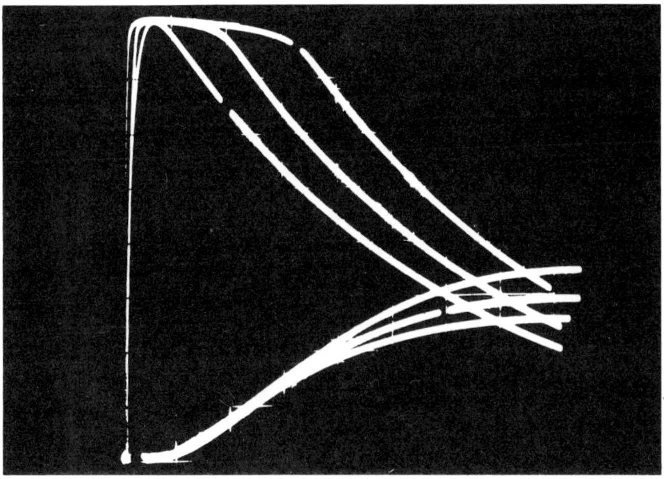

Fig. 11. Computer simulation showing effects of introducing a plateau phase of active state. Rate constant for decay of active state in all 3 cases in 0.195 sec^{-1}. Scale is same as figure 9. Calibration mark = 1 sec. (From Gordon and Siegman, 1971b).

CONCLUSION

A few basic principles have been shown from these experiments which contribute to our understanding of smooth muscle contraction. We have shown that mechanical activation is variable during a twitch, and can be regulated by either the rate of calcium delivery or the rate of calcium removal, or both. This type of regulation operates in the direction of potentiation as well as reduction of tension development. We have also shown that a sliding filament model is compatible with observations on the mechanical behavior of smooth muscle. The correlation of structure and function in smooth muscle is in its infancy. Hopefully, collaborative efforts which are already in progress will further our understanding of these fascinating tissues.

REFERENCES

Barany, M., 1967. ATPase activity of myosin correlated with speed of muscle shortening. J. Gen. Physiol., 50: 197.

Bianchi, C. P., 1961. The effect of caffeine on radio-calcium movement in frog sartorius. J. Gen. Physiol., 44: 845.

Carsten, M. E., 1969. Role of calcium binding by SR in the contraction and relaxation of uterine smooth muscle. J. Gen. Physiol., 53: 414.

Cooke, P. H. and Chase, R. H., 1971. Potassium chloride-insoluble myofilaments in vertebrate smooth muscle cells. Exptl. Cell Res., 66: 417.

Cooke, P. H. and Fay, F., 1972. Correlation between fiber length, ultrastructure, and the length-tension relationship of mammalian smooth muscle. J. Cell. Biol., 52: 105.

Devine, C. E. and Somlyo, A. P., 1971. Thick filaments in vascular smooth muscle. J. Cell. Biol., 49: 636

Devine, C. E., Somlyo A. V. and Somlyo, A. P., 1972. Sarcoplasmic reticulum and excitation-contraction coupling in mammalian smooth muscles. J. Cell Biol., 52: 690

Devine, C. E., Somlyo, A. V. and Somlyo, A. P., 1973. Sarcoplasmic reticulum and mitochondria as cation accumulating sites in smooth muscle. Phil. Trans. R. Soc. London. B. 265: 17.

Edman, K. A. P. and Schild, H. O., 1962. The need for calcium in the contractile responses induced by acetylcholine and potassium in the rat uterus. J. Physiol., 161: 424.

Endo, M., 1964. Entry of a dye into the sarcotubular system of muscle. Nature, 202: 1115.

Fawcett, D. W. and McNutt, N. S., 1969. The ultrastructure of the myocardium. I. Ventricular papillary muscle. J. Cell. Biol., 42: 1

Gabella, G., 1971. Caveolae intracellulares and sarcoplasmic reticulum in smooth muscle. J. Cell Sci., 8: 601.

Gabella, G., 1973. Fine structure of smooth muscle. Phil. Trans. R. Soc. London B. 265: 7.

Gordon, A. M., Huxley, A. F. and Julian, F. J., 1966a. Tension development in highly stretched vertebrate muscle fibers. J. Physiol. (London) 184: 143.

Gordon, A. M., Huxley, A. F. and Julian, F. J., 1966b. The variation in isometric tension with sarcomere length in vertebrate muscle fibers. J. Physiol. (London), 184: 170.
Gordon, A. R. and Siegman, M. J., 1971a. Mechanical properties of smooth muscle. I. Length-tension and force-velocity relations. Am. J. Physiol., 221: 1243.
Gordon, A. R. and Siegman, M. J., 1971b. Mechanical properties of smooth muscle. II. Active state. Am. J. Physiol., 221: 125.
Hanson, J. and Huxley, H. E., 1953. The structural basis of the cross-striations in muscle. Nature, 172: 530.
Hanson, J. and Huxley, H. E., 1955. The structural basis of contraction in striated muscle. Symp. Soc. Exptl. Biol., 9: 228.
Hellam, D. C. and Podolsky, R. J., 1969. Force measurements in skinned muscle fibers. J. Physiol., 200: 807.
Herz, R. and Weber, A., 1965. Caffeine inhibition of Ca uptake by muscle reticulum. Federation Proc., 24: 208.
Hill, A. V., 1938. The heat of shortening and the dynamic constants of muscle. Proc. Roy. Soc. London, B. 126: 136.
Hill, A. V., 1949. The abrupt transition from rest to activity in muscle. Proc. Roy. Soc. London, B. 136: 399.
Huxley, H. E., 1964. Evidence for the continuity between the central elements of the "triad" and extracellular space in frog sartorius muscle. Nature, 202: 1067.
Huxley, H. E., 1971. The structural basis of muscular contraction. Proc. Roy. Soc. London, B. 178: 131.
Huxley, H. E. and Hanson, J., 1954. Changes in the cross-striation of muscle during contraction and stretch and their structural interpretation. Nature, 173: 973.
Ito, Y. and Kuriyama, H., 1971. Caffeine and excitation-contraction coupling in the guinea-pig taenia coli. J. Gen. Physiol., 57: 448.
Lowy, J. and Small, J. V., 1970. The organization of myosin and actin in vertebrate smooth muscle. Nature, 227: 46.
Natori, R., 1954. The property and contraction process of isolated myofibrils. Jikeikai Med. J. 1: 119.
Peachey, L. D., 1965. The sarcoplasmic reticulum and transverse tubules of the frog's sartorius. J. Cell Biol., 25: 209.

Porter, K. R. and Palade, G. E., 1957. Studies on the endoplasmic reticulum. III. Its form and distribution in striated muscle cells. J. Biophys. Biochem. Cytol., 3: 269.

Ramsey, R. W. and Street, S. F., 1940. The isometric length-tension diagram of isolated skeletal muscle fibers of the frog. J. Cell. Comp. Physiol., 15: 11.

Rice, R. V., McManus, G. M., Devine, C. E. and Somlyo, A. P. 1971. A regular organization of thick filaments in mammalian smooth muscle. Nature New Biology, 231: 242.

Siegman, M. J. and Gordon, A. R., 1972. Potentiation of contraction: effects of calcium and caffeine on active state. Am. J. Physiol. 222: 1587.

Schatzmann, H. J., 1964. Excitation, contraction and calcium in smooth muscle. In: The Pharmacology of Smooth Muscle. edited by E. Bulbrings. London; Pergamon Press.

Somlyo, A. P., 1972. Excitation-contraction coupling in vertebrate smooth muscle: correlation of ultrastructure with function. The Physiologist, 15: 338.

Somlyo, A. P., Devine C. D. and Somlyo, A. V., 1971a. Thick filaments in unstretched mammalian smooth muscle. Nature New Biology, 233: 218.

Somlyo, A. P., Devine, C. E., Somlyo, A. V., and North, 1971b. Sarcoplasmic reticulum and the temperature-dependent contraction of smooth muscle in calcium-free solution. J. Cell Biol., 51: 722.

Somlyo, A. P., Devine, C. E., Somlyo, A. V., and Rice, R. V., 1973. Filament organization in vertebrate smooth muscle. Phil. Trans. R. Soc. London, B. 265: 223.

Somlyo, A. V. and Somlyo, A. P., 1971. Strontium accumulation by SR and mitochondria in vascular smooth muscle. Science, 174: 955.

Weber, A., 1968. Mechanism of the action of caffeine on SR. J. Gen. Physiol., 52: 760.

Weber, A. and Herz, R., 1968. The relationship between caffeine contracture of intact muscle and effect of caffeine on reticulum. J. Gen. Physiol., 52: 750.

Weber, A., Herz, R., and Reiss, I., 1964. The regulation of myofibrillar activity by calcium. Proc. Roy. Soc. London, B. 160: 489.

ELECTRICAL ACTIVITY OF GASTROINTESTINAL MUSCLE

Alexander Bortoff

INTRODUCTION

Although J. Earl Thomas was never, to my knowledge, actively engaged in electrophysiological studies of gastrointestinal muscle, many of his observations and ideas regarding gastrointestinal function have stimulated work in this area. In his review of intestinal peristalsis in 1955 Thomas pointed out that the two most characteristic mechanical properties of the intestine are: (1) its inherent rhythmicity, and (2) its polarity, which related to the tendency for contractions to propagate in the aboral direction. These mechanical properties of the intestine are reflected in its electrical activity, and indeed are the end result of the patterns of electrical activity generated by the muscle layers of the intestine and modulated by neural and humoral influences.

ELECTRICAL ACTIVITY

The basic pattern of electrical activity recorded from the small intestine of most species of mammal, consists of spontaneous slow waves (sometimes called the "basic electrical rhythm" or BER), and spike potentials. The temporal relationship between slow waves and spike potentials is illustrated in figure 1A, which is a tracing of electrical activity recorded from a segment of cat jejunum, with a pressure electrode. This type of recording, which can also be obtained with suction electrodes or intracellular microelectrodes,

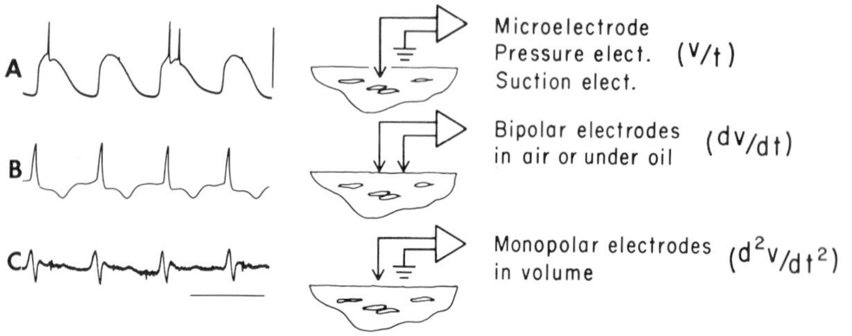

Fig. 1. Effect of type and orientation of recording electrodes on configuration of slow waves recorded from cat jejunum. A: time course of membrane potential; B: direction and magnitude of longitudinal current; C: direction and magnitude of membrane current. Horizontal bar, 5 sec.

reflects the time course of changes in membrane potential occurring in longitudinal muscle and probably circular muscle, although it is technically more difficult to record from the latter in intact segments of intestine. Four slow waves are shown in figure 1A, each consisting of a rapid depolarization of approximately 10 mv, a plateau and a gradual repolarization which is terminated by depolarization of the next slow wave, i.e., there is no isopotential period between successive slow waves. Spike potentials occur during the plateau of the first and third slow waves in this tracing. As a rule, spike potentials occur only during the slow wave plateau. Hence, it appears that the slow waves function to periodically increase and decrease the probability of spike discharge.

Figures 1B and 1C illustrate how the configuration of the recorded slow wave is affected by the type and orientation of the recording electrodes. When recorded with bipolar wick electrodes, the configuration of the slow wave approximates the first time derivative of the monophasic potential (fig. 1B), and when recorded with monopolar electrodes in volume the slow wave approximates its second derivative (fig. 1C). Since these are the expected configurations for changes in membrane potential which propagate uniformly past the recording electrode, they constitute evidence for propagation of slow waves. With the electrodes arranged as in figure 1C the recorded potentials reflect the direction and time course of membrane current occurring during the slow wave. The initial depolarization is associated with outward current flow which becomes inward as the membrane continues to depolarize. The pattern of membrane current indicated first, that slow wave propagation occurs by way of local circuit currents, with proximal membrane near or at its peak of slow wave depolarization providing outward flowing current for the membrane ahead of it, and second, that slow wave depolarization is initiated by cathodal current which triggers a potential-dependent change in the properties of the membrane, making it more conducive to net inward current flow which results in further depolarization. Propogation by local circuit currents is also indicated by the findings that slow waves can be driven by cathodal or anode-break current (Specht and Bortoff, 1972), and that the velocity of propagation is inversely related to the refractoriness of the tissue (Specht, 1972) and to its internal resistance (Haiman, unpublished).

The nature of the change in membrane properties which results in increased net inward current flow is presently the subject of much speculation. It could result either from an increase in inward current, such as would occur if the membrane conductance to sodium or calcium were increased, or to a reduction of outward current, such as would occur if the conductance to potassium were decreased. The sensitivity of slow waves to ouabain and to sodium-free solutions (Liu, Prosser and Job, 1969, El-Sharkaway and Daniel, 1973) and an apparent increase in sodium influx during depolarization is associated with an increase in inward sodium current, while repolarization has been attributed to an electrogenic sodium pump (Job, 1969, El-Sharkaway and Daniel, 1973). However, recent double sucrose gap experiments on cat longitudinal muscle (Weems, Connor and Prosser, 1973) have failed to detect the decrease in membrane resistance which must accompany an increase of inward sodium current during slow wave depolarization. Thus, although the sodium ion seems to be established as the major current carrier during generation of the slow wave, the precise mechanisms responsible for its influx and efflux remain to be determined. Most evidence, both physiological and pharmacological, indicates that spike potential depolarization is effected primarily by an increase in calcium influx (Bulbring and Tomita, 1970; Liu, Prosser and Job, 1969; Golenhofen and Lammel, 1972).

RELATIONSHIP BETWEEN ELECTRICAL AND MECHANICAL ACTIVITY

Because electrical recordings are usually restricted to a much smaller area of intestinal muscle than mechanical recordings, absolute correlations cannot be made between electrical and mechanical activity of the intestine. However, it appears as though intestinal contractions are normally triggered by spike potentials. As shown in the top tracings of figure 2, circular muscle contractions, detected as increases in intraluminal pressure, are well correlated with the occurrence of spike potentials during the slow wave plateau. In the absence of spike potentials, no contraction is evident even though slow waves continue to be generated. Since the occurrence of spike potentials is usually limited to the plateau region of the slow wave, it follows that contractions are temporally related to slow waves even though they are not triggered by them.

A similar relationship seems to exist between slow waves, spikes and contractions in the cat antrum (fig. 2, middle) although the slow wave frequency is lower than that of the intestine, and its configuration is somewhat more complex. In the dog antrum spike potentials are recorded much less frequently, although the temporal relationship between slow waves and contractions is similar to that found in the antrum and small intestine of the cat (fig. 2, bottom). From records such as those of figure 2 it is evident that the rhythmical nature of gastrointestinal contractions is due to the slow wave periodically increasing and decreasing the excitability of the muscle membrane. In most cases if the excitability is sufficiently increased, spike potentials are generated and a contraction ensues.

Since slow waves are propagated, and since they can give rise to spike potentials which trigger contractions, it seems reasonable to ask whether propagated slow waves are related to peristalsis. Our studies indicate not only that they are related, but that the propagated slow wave constitutes the myogenic basis for peristalsis. In the experiment represented by figure 3, a 5 cm segment of cat jejunum was placed in a bath of oxygenated Tyrode solution at 37° C. Its lumen was perfused with Tyrode solution through its oral end at the rate of

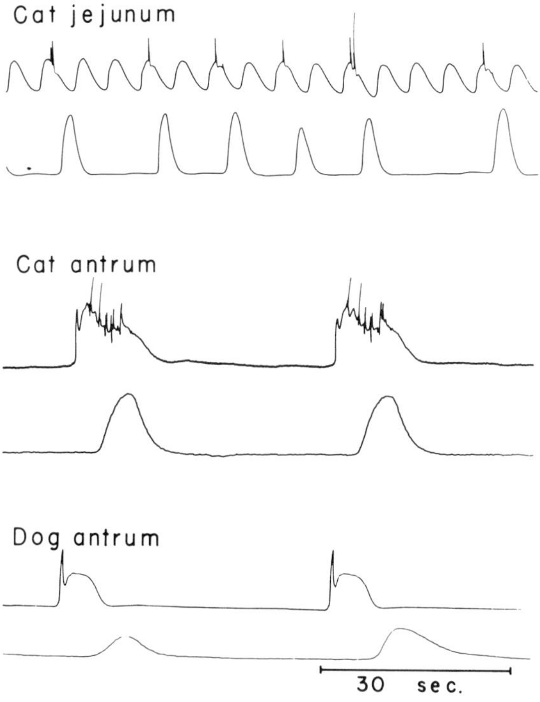

Fig. 2. Electrical (top) and mechanical (bottom) activity simultaneously recorded from cat jejunum, cat antrum and dog antrum.

7 ml/min. The outflow at the aboral end passed through a fixed resistance consisting of a tapered glass tube. The lumen of the tube was attached to a pressure transducer by means of which pressure in the tube, which was proportional to rate of outflow, could be monitored. Three suction electrodes were placed on the segment in order to record monophasic potentials at the oral end, the middle and the aboral end of the segment. Following a period of equilibration slow waves began to propagate from electrode 1, at the oral end, to electrode 3, at the aboral end, at a velocity of approximately 2.0 cm/sec. Hexamethonium chloride was then added to the bath and perfusing fluid at a concentration of 10^{-5}M, sufficient to block synaptic transmission in the myenteric plexuses. Atropine sulphate was then added to the bath at a concentration of 10^{-4}M, sufficient to stimulate both muscle layers directly (Bortoff and Müller, un-

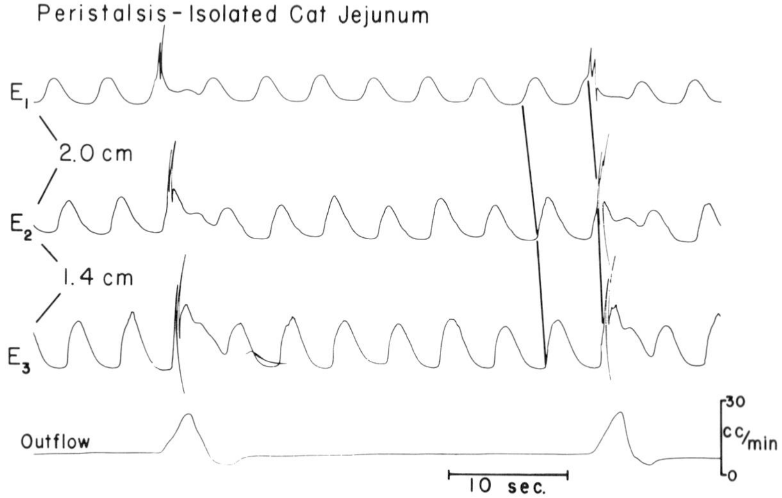

Fig. 3. Monophasic electrical activity recorded from three loci, E_1, E_2, E_3, along a 5 cm segment of cat jejunum as two peristaltic waves traverse the length of the segment. Each peristaltic wave was preceded at each point by burst of spike potentials, and resulted in increased rate of outflow from aboral end of preparation. Preparation bathed in Tyrode solution containing 10^{-5}M hexamethodium to block reflex activity of myenteric plexus and 10^{-4}M atropine to stimulate the preparation. Solid lines at right indicate propagation of slow waves and spike potentials between electrodes E_1 to E_3.

published). The records of figure 3 were obtained 20 min later. The first two slow waves propagated from electrode 1 to electrode 3, but since they were not associated with spike potentials, no contraction was evident and the outflow rate remained constant at 7 ml/min. The third slow wave gave rise to spike potentials which propagated along with the slow wave past electrode 3. The resulting contraction was also propagated as a peristaltic wave, and transiently increased the rate of outflow more than threefold. The next seven slow waves were devoid of spikes, hence no contractions occurred. The rate of outflow transiently fell to zero immediately after the first peristaltic wave, gradually increasing again to equal the rate of inflow. The following slow wave was again associated with spike potentials, again triggering a peristaltic wave.

Similar experiments have been done on intact intestines of anesthetized animals. An example of records obtained from such a preparation is shown in figure 4. In this preparation electrical activity was monitored with suction electrodes placed 2 cm apart along the jejunum. Circular muscle contractions were measured with strain gauge transducers along the circumferential plane of each suction electrode so that M_1 corresponds to E_1, M_2 to E_2, etc. (cf Bortoff and Sacco, 1973). Hexamethonium was administered intravenously at a dosage of 2 mg/Kg and atropine was later given at a concentration sufficient to induce spiking and contractile activity. In other experiments Urecholine was administered with similar results. In the tracings of figure 4, propagated slow waves, spike potentials and peristaltic waves are evident. As indicated by the solid line, the peristaltic wave and the slow wave propagate at essentially the same velocity of about 2 cm/sec.

If the slow waves or the spike potentials fail to propagate from one electrode to the next the resulting mechanical activity is more localized, resembling segmental rather than peristaltic contractions. An example of limited propagation of slow waves is shown in figure 5. The records were taken from a region of cat ileum where the slow waves were undergoing waxing and waning. The slow wave frequency at E_1 was slightly higher than at E_2 and E_3, which in turn were slightly higher than that at E_4. Slow waves appeared to propagate only from E_2 to E_3. As a result the mechanical activity recorded from this region was segmental rather than peristaltic.

These studies indicate that peristalsis can occur in the absence of any reflex activity providing propagating slow waves are present and the level of excitability is sufficient for spike potentials to be generated and propagated in the muscle. Hence, they indicate that peristalsis is basically a myogenic phenomenon which may be modulated by neural and hormonal influences.

This concept of peristalsis is essentially similar to that suggested almost twenty years ago by J. Earl Thomas (1955), and also by Milton, Smith and Armstrong (1955). Thomas proposed the presence of pacemakers in the intestine which he described as "areas of superior excitability and rhythmicity capable of initiating impulses at regular intervals which would be conducted along the intestine." He went so far as to imply that the impulses might be electrical slow waves which increase the excitability of the area over which they pass without causing contraction. "In this way", he

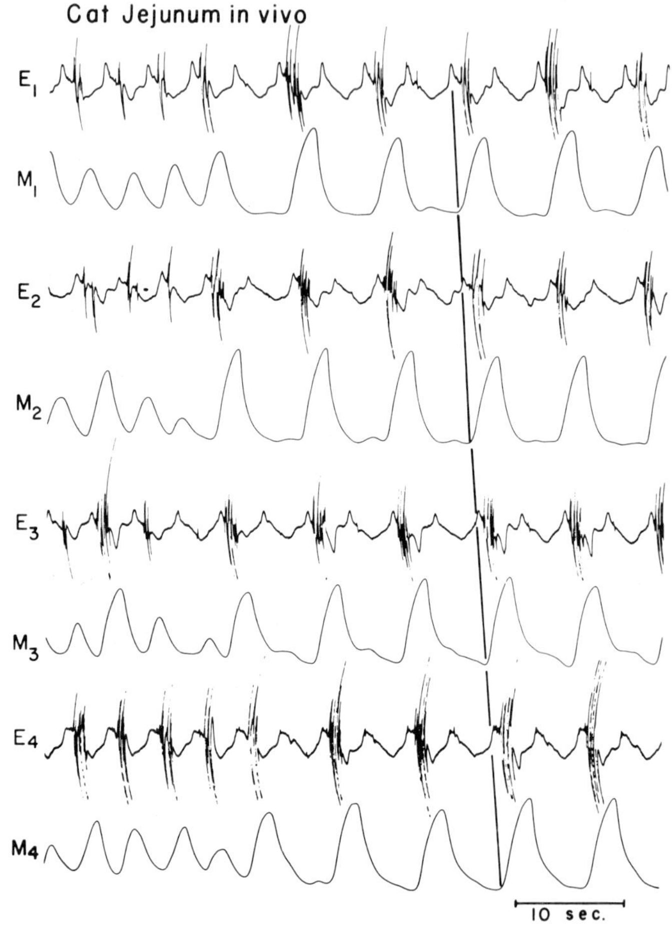

Fig. 4. Electrical (E_1 to E_4) and corresponding mechanical (M_1 to M_4) activity recorded from 4 loci 2 cm apart along the jejunum of an anesthetized cat. Solid line drawn from beginning of contraction at M_1 to beginning of contraction at M_4, i. e., the peristalitic wave. Same line intersects slow waves and spike potential bursts at corresponding points, indicating that contractile wave propagates at same velocity as slow waves. Preparation contains 2 mg hexamethonium chloride per kilogram. Intestinal activity stimulated with atropine sulphate administered intravenously.

suggested, "they would merely increase the effectiveness of local stimuli and actual contraction would be the result of summation of local and conducted impulses." Thomas, however, conceived of the impulses, or slow waves, "as being generated and conducted in the myenteric plexus and not in the muscle."

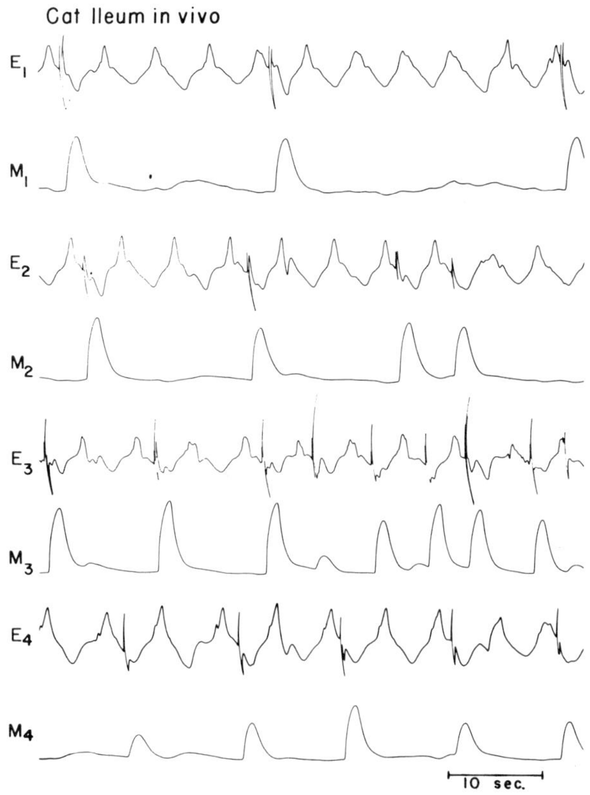

Fig. 5. Spontaneous electrical (E_1 to E_4) and corresponding mechanical (M_1 to M_4) activity recorded from 4 loci 2 cm apart along the distal ileum of an anesthetized cat. Slow waves do not propagate from E_1 to E_4 because electrodes are situated on three different frequency plateaus. In the absence of slow wave propagation contractile activity is localized, i. e., segmental.

THE SLOW WAVE FREQUENCYGRADIENT

To Doctor Thomas, one of the more intriguing problems of gastrointestinal physiology involved the polarity of the intestine, which he related to the well-known intestinal frequency gradient. In a paper published with Robert Hasselbrack (1961), he showed that the frequency of intestinal contractions decreases in step-wise fashion from duodenum to ileum. Several years later, when attemptying to reconcile the fact of slow wave propagation with the aboral decrease in slow wave frequency, Nick Diamant and I found, not unexpectedly, that the frequency of slow waves also exhibits a step-wise decrease along the intestine (Diamant and Bortoff, 1969a, b). The length of each resulting frequency plateau was found to be variable, especially beyond the mid-jejunum, and each was separated from the next by a region of waxing and waning. Within each plateau the intrinsic frequency of consecutive small segments of intestine was found to decrease aborally in a linear fashion. Thus, it appears that within a plateau slow waves are driven by a pacemaker, situated at the oral end of the plateau and necessarily having the highest intrinsic frequency within that plateau. Subsequent computer simulations of the slow wave frequency gradient indicate that the frequency of a pacemaker oscillator can be increased by the slow wave oscillators in the adjacent more proximal plateau (Diamant, Rose, and Davison, 1970; Sarna, Daniel, and Kingma, 1971), thus giving credence to the concept of a dominant pacemaker in the first part of the duodenum (Smith and Armstrong, 1956). Such studies have helped to establish the concept that the slow wave frequency gradient determines the direction of peristaltic activity in the intestine.

GASTRO-DUODENAL JUNCTION

Based on an early observation by Thomas and Crider (1935) we attempted some years ago to determine whether antral slow waves would influence the electrical and mechanical activity of the proximal duodenum (Bortoff and Davis, 1968). Thomas and Crider observed that during antral peristalsis the duodenum is relatively quiescent. Immediately after the antral wave passes over the pylorus, one or two duodenal contractions occur, even when the stomach is empty. By recording the electrical activity on either side of the gastroduodenal junction we found that antral slow waves spread electrotonically across the gastroduodenal junction and into the proximal duodenum where they periodically augment the depolarizations produced by duodenal slow waves themselves. This added amount of depolarization further increases the probability of spiking during those duodenal slow waves associated with antral slow waves. When the background level of excitability is raised, such as during vagal stimulation (fig. 6) or gastric emptying, the probability of spiking is even further increased, causing proximal duodenal spike activity to be temporally related to the arrival of the antral slow

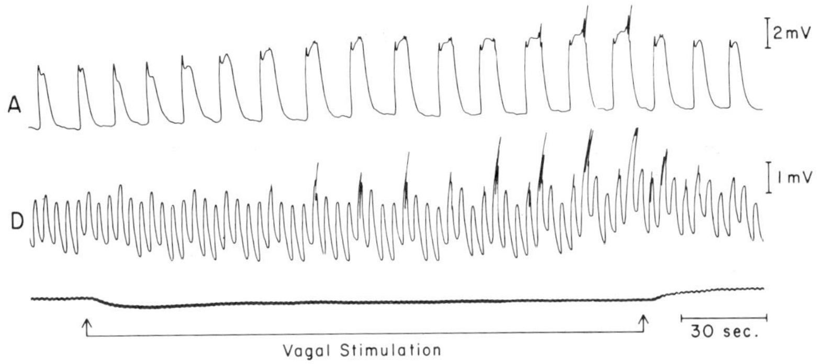

Fig. 6. Effect of vagal stimulation on monophasic potentials recorded simultaneously from both sides of the cat gastroduodenal junction in situ. The antral electrode (A) was 4 mm oral to the junction, (D) was 2 mm aboral. Bottom tracing is blood pressure. Note periodic augmentation of duodenal slow waves corresponding to antral slow waves, further augmentation and synchrozined spiking on either side of the junction during vagal stimulation (Bortoff and Davis, 1968).

wave at the gastroduodenal junction. Antral and duodenal contraction would likewise be temporally related to one another exactly as described by Thomas and Crider.

REFERENCES

Bortoff,A., and Davis,R.S., 1968.
Myogenic transmission of antral slow waves across the gastroduodenal junction in situ.
Am. J. Physiol. 215:889.

Bortoff,A., and Sacco,J., 1973.
Myogenic control of intestinal peristalsis.
(In Press).

Bulbring,E., and Tomita,T., 1970.
Effects of Ca removal on the smooth muscle of the guinea pig taenia coli.
J. Physiol. (London), 210:217.

Diamant,N.E., and Bortoff,A., 1969a.
Nature of the intestinal slow-wave frequency gradient.
Am. J. Physiol. 216:301.

Diamant,N.E., and Bortoff,A., 1969b.
Effects of transection on the intestinal slow-wave frequency gradient.
Am. J. Physiol. 216:734.

Diamant,N.E., Rose,P.K., and Davison,E.J., 1970.
Computer simulation of intestinal slow-wave frequency gradient.
Am. J. Physiol. 219:1684.

El-Sharkaway,T.Y., and Daniel,E.E., 1973.
The ionic basis of intestinal control potentials (slow waves).
Rendiconti Gastroent. 5:

Golenhoffen,K., and Lammel,E., 1972.
Selective suppression of some components of spontaneous activity in various types of smooth muscle by Iproveratril (Verapamil).
Pfugers Arch., 331:233.

Hasselbrack,R., and Thomas,J.E., 1961.
Control of intestinal rhythmic contractions by a duodenal pacemaker.
Am. J. Physiol. 201:955.

Job,D.D., 1969.
Ionic basis of intestinal electrical activity.
Am. J. Physiol. 217:1534.

Liu,J., Porsser,C.L., and Job,D.D., 1969.
Ionic dependence of slow waves and spikes in intestinal muscle.
Am. J. Physiol. 217:1542.

Milton,G.W., and Smith,A.W.M., 1956.

The pacemaking area of the duodenum.
J. Physiol. (London), 132:100.
Milton,G.W., Smith,A.W.M., and Armstrong,H.I.O., 1955.
The origin of the rhythmic electropotential changes in the duodenum.
Q. J. Exp. Physiol. 40:79.
Sarna,S., Daniel,E.E., and Kingma,Y.J., 1971.
Simulation of slow-wave electrical activity of small intestine.
Am. J. Physiol. 221:166.
Specht,P., 1972.
Excitation and propagation of the slow electrical wave in the cat intestine.
Ph.D. Thesis, State University of New York Upstate Medical Center, Syracuse, New York.
Specht,P., and Bortoff,A., 1972.
Propagation and electrical entrainment of intestinal slow waves.
Am. J. Dig. Dis. 17:311.
Thomas,J.E., 1955.
The gradient theory versus the reflex theory of intestinal peristalsis.
Am. J. Gastroenterol, 23:13.
Thomas,J.E., and Cridder,J.O., 1935.
Rhythmic changes in duodenal motility associated with gastric peristalsis.
Am. J. Physiol., 111:124.
Weems,W.A., Connor,J.A., and Prosser,C.L., 1973.
Ionic mechanisma of slow waves in cat intestinal muscle.
Fed. Proc.

THE HORMONAL CONTROL OF GASTROINTESTINAL MOTOR FUNCTION

Sidney Cohen

INTRODUCTION

During the past several years, there have been a number of studies describing the effects of the gastrointestinal hormones on gastrointestinal motor function. It is not the purpose of this discussion to detail each hormonal action described to date. Rather, I would like to discuss several model systems and show the possible mechanisms by which the hormones may act and interact to regulate gastrointestinal motility. The specific areas to be considered are: (1) characteristics of hormonal action on gastrointestinal smooth muscle, in vitro; and (2) the physiological role of hormones in the regulation of motor function, in vivo.

IN VITRO STUDIES

A number of studies have been published in which the effect of a hormone on muscle from a specific area of the gastrointestinal tract has been tested. These studies have suggested that muscle from specific anatomic regions may respond differently to a given hormone. Studies performed in our laboratory on the esophageal circular muscle of the opossum (Didelphis virginiana) suggested certain principles that should be followed in evaluating the hormonal responses of muscle, in vitro (Christensen and Lund, 1969; Lipshutz and Cohen, 1971; Lipshutz and Cohen, 1972). First, in comparing the hormonal responses of muscles from different portions of the gastrointestinal tract, appropriate adjustments must be made for differences in the length-tension properties of the muscle. Secondly, full dose response curves should be performed to truly compare the responses of different muscles. Both principles will be discussed in detail.

Length-Tension Properties of Smooth Muscle

In figure 1 are shown the length-tension determinations for muscles from three areas of the gastrointestinal tract, the lower esophageal sphincter (LES), the stomach and the pyloric sphincter (Lipshutz and Cohen, 1972). The passive tension was achieved by gradually increasing the muscle length by a screw micrometer. Passive tension curves were quite similar. Active tension curves obtained at each change in muscle length were quite different. The active tension curves were obtained in response to 10^{-4} M acetylcholine. Each muscle achieved its peak active tension (Po) at different passive tensions. The length at which the Po was achieved was termed the length of optimal tension development (Lo). In further studies, each muscle was evaluated at its respective Lo. This normalized for differences in length-tension properties of the muscle. When the active tensions were corrected for muscle weight, each muscle achieved a similar Po.

The Dose Response Curve: Differences in Hormonal Effects on Muscles from Specific Areas of the Gastrointestinal Tract

The second important aspect of studying the different muscles, *in vitro*, was the performance of full dose response curves for each hormone. Because of the response of the muscle to the hormones, single doses might have missed the entire range of response.

In figure 2 is shown the effect of gastrin I on the circular muscle of the LES, gastric antrum and the pyloric sphincter (Lipshutz and Cohen, 1972). The response, expressed as a percent of the maximum response achieved on the LES muscle, was plotted against the log dose of gastrin I (residues 2–17). The LES muscle responded at a lower threshold dose and achieved a greater tension at a lower dose than muscle from the gastric antrum. The pyloric sphincter muscle did not respond at any dose of gastrin I. These dose response curves performed on isolated circular muscle at Lo illustrated that each

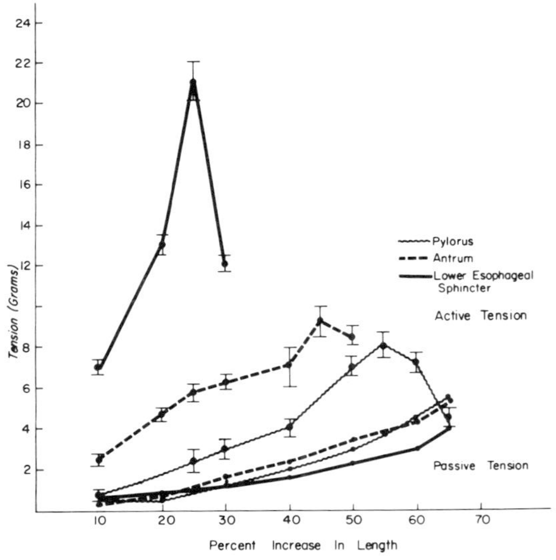

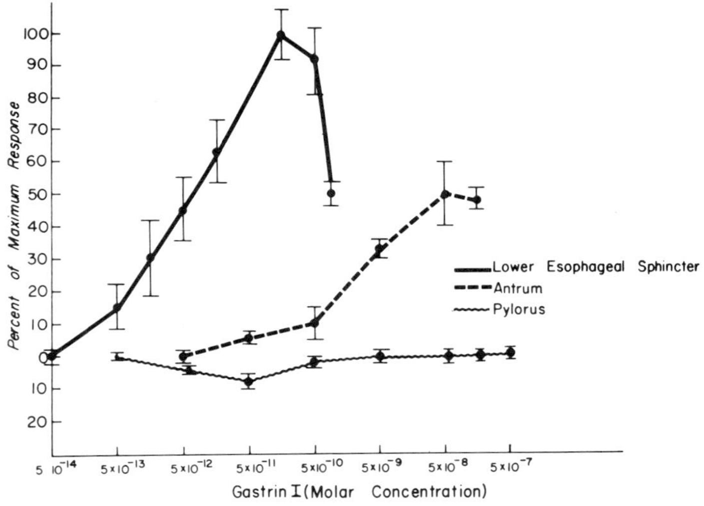

Fig. 1. (Left) Length-tension curves for lower esophageal sphincter, stomach, and pylorus. Tension in grams corrected for muscle weight is plotted as a function of percent increase in muscle length. Passive tension is shown on lower set of curves, and active tension produced by chemical stimulation with 10^{-4} M acetylcholine is shown in upper set of curves. Each point represents mean ± SE for 20 separate experiments. SEM values for passive tension measurements are ± 0.1 to ± 0.5 g. Length of maximum active tension development, Lo, is different for muscles from different anatomic regions. (Reprinted from the Am J Physiol 222: 775–781, 1972).

Fig. 2. (Right) Dose-response curves, at Lo, for increasing molar concentration of gastrin I and active tension. Active tension is expressed as a percent of maximum response of lower esophageal sphincter (LES) muscle. Each point represents mean ± SE for 20 separate experiments. LES muscle responds at a lower threshold dose and attains a greater maximum active tension. Pyloric muscle is inhibited by gastrin, but this response is not statistically significant ($P > .05$). (Reprinted from the Am J Physiol 222: 775–781, 1972).

portion of the gastrointestinal tract responded specifically to each gastrointestinal hormone, in vitro. In addition, these curves illustrated that simple comparison of a single dose of a hormone on a muscle strip may give an erroneous impression. The characteristic dose response curve for a hormone showed a prominent phase of diminished responsiveness at doses greater than that which gave the maximum response. This diminished response at higher doses has been called autoinhibition and may reflect hormone combining with a low affinity inhibitory receptor. Thus, the entire dose response range may be missed if only a single high dose of gastrin was tested on a muscle. The gastrointestinal smooth muscle responded at much lower molar concentrations of the polypeptide hormones than generally noted with the neural transmitters acetycholine or norepinephrine (Lipshutz and Cohen, 1971).

In figure 3 is shown the effect of secretin on the muscle from the three areas discussed previously (Lipshutz and Cohen, 1972). Secretin was the other structural prototype for the gastrointestinal hormone receptor as suggested by Grossman (Grossman, 1970). Secretin had a reciprocal effect as compared to gastrin. The pyloric muscle contracted at a low molar concentration of secretin but the antral and LES muscles showed a minimal response at higher concentrations. Again, it seemed that each portion of the gastrointestinal tract responded specifically to this hormone in vitro. As will be discussed, these specific hormone dose response curves obtained on circular muscle correlated closely with intact sphincter function, in vivo.

Interaction of the Gastrointestinal Hormones

The gastrointestinal hormones can be shown to interact with each other on circular muscle, in vitro. In figure 4 is shown the interaction of secretin and gastrin on LES circular muscle (Lipshutz and Cohen, 1972). Secretin, alone, had a minimal effect on the LES muscle. However, in the presence of secretin, the entire dose response relationship to gastrin I was shifted to the right. That is, it now took a larger dose of gastrin to achieve the same response, but in the presence of secretin the maximum response to gastrin could still be achieved. Thus, secretin did not have a significant independent effect on the muscle when given alone but when given in combination with another hormone, gastrin, it behaved as a potent

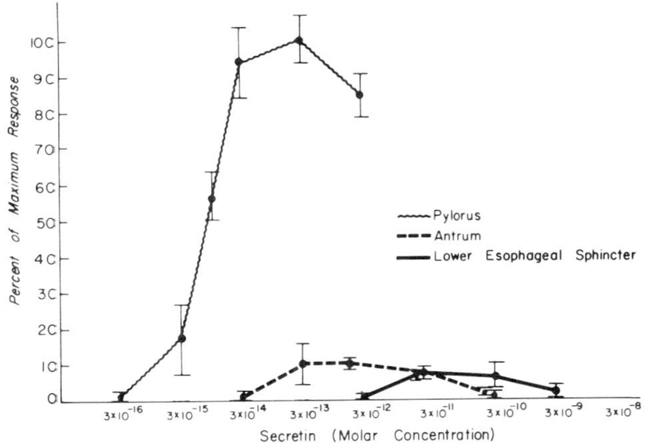

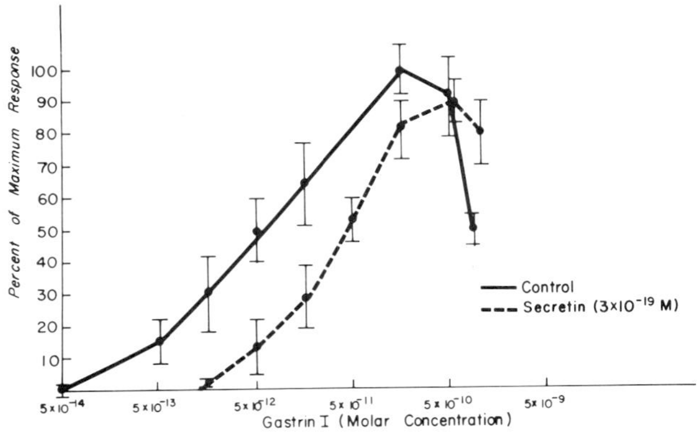

Fig. 3. (Left) Dose-response curves, at Lo, for increasing molar concentration of secretin, and active tension. Active tension is expressed as a percent of maximum response of pyloric muscle. Each point represents mean ± SE for 20 separate experiments. Pyloric muscle responds at a lower threshold dose and attains a greater maximum active tension. (Reprinted from the Am J Physiol 222: 775–781, 1972).

Fig. 4. (Right) Dose-response curves, at Lo, for increasing molar concentration of gastrin alone, and in the presence of 3×10^{-19} M secretin on LES muscle. Active tension is expressed as a percent of maximum response to gastrin I, when given alone. Each point represents mean ± SE for 20 separate experiments. In the presence of secretin, threshold dose of gastrin I is increased, linear phases of dose-response curves are parallel, and same maximum response is still attained at a higher gastrin I concentration. (Reprinted from the Am J Physiol 222: 775–781, 1972).

antagonist. This antagonism suggested that secretin combined with its receptor on the LES muscle but is combination with the receptor was only manifest in the presence of another hormone. The competitive kinetics of this antagonism were similar to those observed on the LES in man (Cohen and Lipshutz, 1971).

In figure 5 is shown the interaction of secretin and cholecystokinin on the pyloric circular muscle (Fisher et al., 1973). Each hormone contracted the pyloric muscle when given alone. The combination of hormones gave an active tension that was slightly greater than the peak tension in response to cholecystokinin, alone. However, this additive effect at lower concentrations did not fulfill the criteria for true potentiation since the peak response to the hormone combination did not exceed the peak response to cholecystokinin. To date, no evidence for true potentiation of a hormone effect on sphincter function, in vitro or in vivo, has been shown. Secretin and cholecystokinin do potentiate each other for gall bladder contraction and for pancreatic secretory function.

The interaction of gastrointestinal hormones on circular smooth muscle, in vitro, can be demonstrated for each hormone combination on muscle from different areas. Under those conditions where tested, the in vitro interactions correlated closely with findings, in vivo. Both secretin and cholecystokinin antagonized the action of gastrin I on LES muscle in vitro, and on sphincter function in man and the opossum, in vivo. Secretin and cholecystokinin contracted pyloric muscle in vitro and increased pyloric sphincter pressure in man, in vivo. In both situations, the combination showed neither potentiation nor antagonism. Gastrin was an antagonist to secretin and cholecystokinin on the pylorus in vitro and in vivo.

Selectivity of Hormone Interaction

As shown in figure 6, the interaction of hormones on muscle strips, in vitro, was highly selective (Lipshutz and Cohen, 1972). A hormone did not nonselectively diminish the effect of all agonists on a muscle. Secretin reduced the response of LES muscle to gastrin to approximately 5% of its control value. However, secretin at concentrations of 3×10^{-17} M and 3×10^{-15} M (not shown) had no significant effect on the LES response to histamine, dimethylpiperazinium (DMPP), norepinephrine and acetylcholine. It was of special interest that the response to DMPP, a ganglionic stimulant,

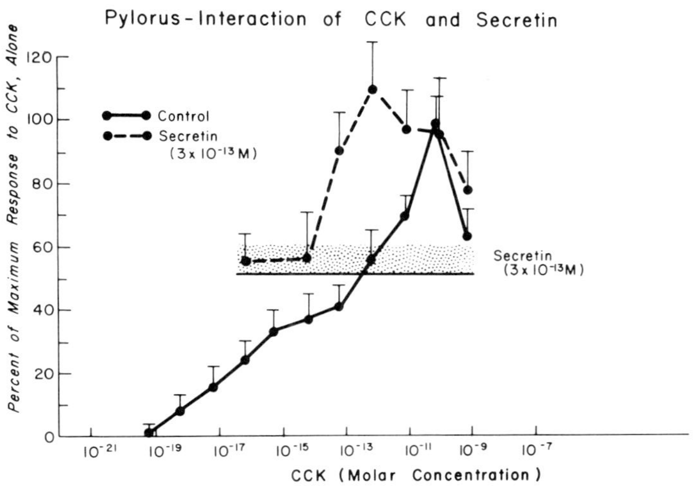

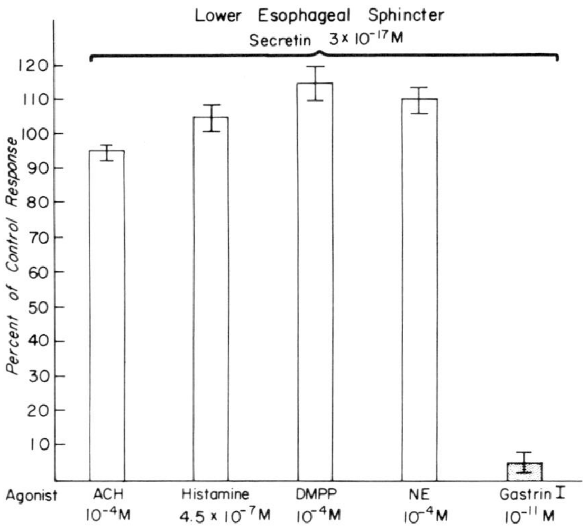

Fig. 5. (Left) Dose-response curves, at Lo, for cholecystokinin (CCK) alone, and in the presence of 3 X 10^{-13} M secretin, on pyloric muscle. Active tension is expressed as a percent of maximal response to cholecystokinin alone. Each point represents mean + SE for 12 separate experiments. The horizontal line represents the maximal tension to secretin alone. In the presence of secretin, the maximal response to cholecystokinin occurred at a lower concentration but the maximal response was not altered ($P > 0.05$). (Reprinted from J Clin Invest 52: 1289–1296, 1973).

Fig. 6. (Right) Percent of maximum gastrin I and other agonist control responses in presence of 3 X 10^{-17} M secretin on LES muscle. Molar concentration of secretin was chosen as that concentration that provided near-maximum inhibition of a maximum gastrin I response. Molar concentration of agonist, shown on bottom, is that concentration which produces a maximum response on LES muscle. Each bar represents ± SE for 10 separate experiments. Secretin significantly inhibits a maximum gastrin I response ($P < .001$), but does not affect response to other agonists ($P > .05$). (Reprinted from the Am J Physiol 222: 775–781, 1972).

was not altered. DMPP acted at a site proximal to the action of gastrin on the postganglionic cholinergic nerve (Lipshutz et al., 1971). This observation indicated that secretin antagonized the effect of gastrin at the postganglionic site without altering neural function through other stimuli. This finding of the highly selective interaction of these hormones suggested that the specific receptors for gastrin and secretin were closely related, an observation supporting the hormone receptor hypothesis of Grossman (Grossman, 1970).

Inotropic Effect of Gastrin

Generally, hormone effects on smooth muscle were considered to be either stimulatory or inhibitory. These effects have been discussed based on the observations made on muscle contracting under isometric conditions. However, recent studies suggested that the hormone effects on smooth muscle may be more complex. In figure 7 is shown the effect of gastrin I on the force velocity characteristics of LES circular muscle (Cohen and Green, 1973). A force velocity curve provides an index of muscle contractility or the inotropic state of the muscle. It shows how rapidly a muscle contracts while moving a load. In the presence of gastrin, the LES muscle contracted more rapidly and moved a greater load. Thus, gastrin not only initiated contraction of this muscle, as shown previously, but gastrin also changed the basic inotropic state of the muscle when a contraction was elicited to an electrical stimulus. It was of interest that glucagon had an inotropic effect on cardiac muscle. It is also possible that other hormones may have an inotropic action on other gastrointestinal smooth muscles. The implications of this observation were that hormones may have a major role in modulating gastrointestinal luminal propulsive force and strength of sphincter closure. These inotropic effects may occur while other factors are acting to initiate contraction.

The physiological significance of inotropic effects of hormones on both the heart and gastrointestinal tract must await further studies, in vivo.

IN VIVO STUDIES

The Role of Gastrin in the Genesis of Basal LES Pressure

To best determine the role of a hormone in the physiological

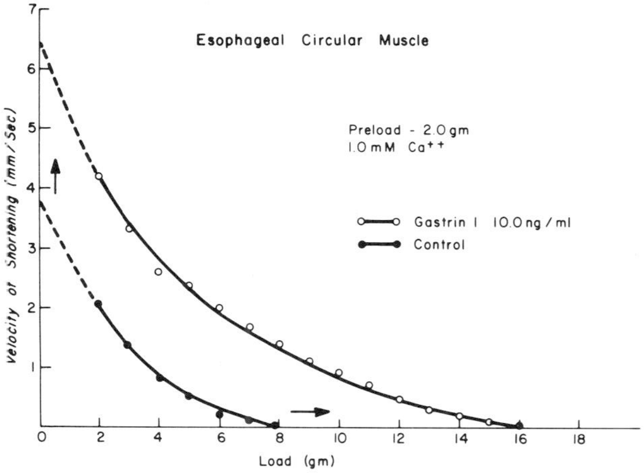

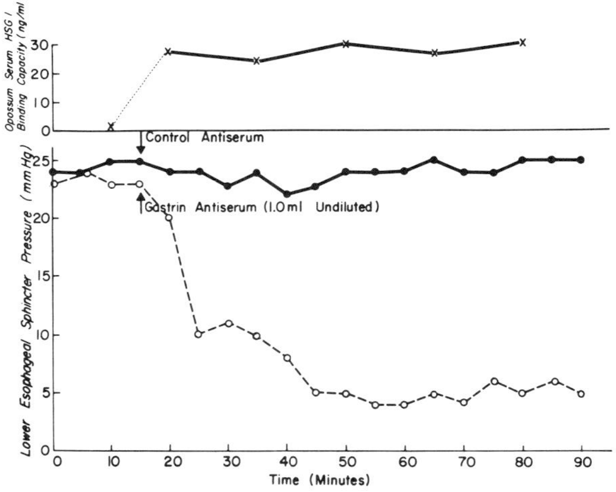

Fig. 7. (Left) Effect of gastrin I on LES circular muscle force-velocity relation. The muscle was studied at its Lo (1.5 g preload) at calcium concentration of 1.0 mM. Gastrin I shifted the entire force-velocity curve of LES muscle. The V max and Po were markedly increased. (Reprinted from J Clin Invest 52: 2029–2040, 1973).

Fig. 8. (Right) The effect of 1.0 ml of control serum and 1.0 ml of gastrin antiserum on the resting lower esophageal sphincter pressure of a single animal. Binding capacity of opossum serum for HSG 1 after the intravenous injection of gastrin antiserum, shown at the top, remained unchanged while LES pressure was reduced. (Reprinted from J Clin Invest 51: 522–529, 1973).

control of a motor organ, one could observe the function of that organ once the hormone effect has been removed. This may be accomplished by ablating the source of the hormone or by neutralizing the biological effect of the hormone. In studies performed in the opossum, in vivo, circulating gastrin was rendered biologically inactive by the intravenous administration of rabbit serum with a high titre of antibodies to gastrin (Lipshutz et al., 1973). The antiserum was first shown to abolish the effect of gastrin on the LES muscle strips, in vitro. Additionally, studies were also performed using a control rabbit antiserum. In figure 8 is shown the LES response in a single animal to the control antiserum and to the antigastrin antiserum. The antigastrin antiserum reduced the LES pressure by over 70%. While the LES pressure remained at its reduced level, the opossum could be shown to have a high level of passively transferred circulating antigastrin activity. The control antiserum had no effect on LES pressure. These studies indicated that gastrin played a major role in determining the genesis of basal LES pressure. We have shown recently that the additional 20–30% of basal LES pressure not accounted for by gastrin was determined by alpha adrenergic stimulation (DiMarino and Cohen, in press). Reduction in LES pressure in man similar to that achieved in the opossum with antiserum could be obtained by acidification of the gastric antrum. These observations indicated that the gastrin effect in vivo could be correlated directly with the marked sensitivity of the LES circular muscle, in vitro.

It would seem that the observations in vitro might be used as an index of a hormone's importance in the control of the motor function, in vivo. This suggestion has not been tested fully. However, it has been shown that if a specific hormone contracts the circular muscle of a given area at a low threshold dose and produces a prominent increase in muscle tension, one can show that in vivo, the hormone contracts that area and may play a major role in its control. The role of a hormone in maintaining basal tone or pressure has only been demonstrated at the LES.

The Action of Hormones on Gastrointestinal Sphincters

To date, each internal gastrointestinal sphincter has been shown to respond to hormonal stimulation. Although the LES, pyloric, choledochal and ileocecal sphincters respond to exogenous and endogenous hormonal stimulation, the role of the hormones in maintaining basal tone has only been documented for the LES. A clue to the role of hormones in maintaining basal sphincter tone may be derived from the observations, in vitro (see figure 6). The inability of a hormone, in vitro and in vivo, to produce inhibition of a nonhormonal agonist would suggest that each gastrointestinal sphincter showing an inhibitory response to a hormone was indeed under the basal control of another hormone. Since the basal tone of the choledochal and ileocecal sphincters were inhibited by gastrin, it would suggest that the basal pressure of these sphincters was dependent upon either secretin or cholecystokinin. This hypothesis has not been tested.

The Action of Hormones on Luminal Gastrointestinal Myoelectrical and Motor Activity

Gastrointestinal hormones may increase the motor function of either the stomach, small intestine or colon. Due to limitations in methodology, it is not certain whether this increase in motor activity is directly correlated with an increase in propulsive movement. In figure 9 is shown the effect of secretin on the motor activity and myoelectrical activity of the human duodenum (DiMarino et al., in press). Secretin increased the number of spike bursts and thus the amplitude of duodenal contractions. The hormone had no effect on frequency of slow waves or their propagation velocity. The effect of hormones on luminal activity generally follows this pattern. Slow wave frequency and thus the rhythmicity of contractions are not affected. The incidence of spike bursts and the force of contractions are increased. The contractile force may be increased by both an activation of the muscle and by the hormones' inotropic effect. The specificity of hormone action and interaction, in general, holds true for luminal activity as discussed previously for smooth muscle being studied, in vitro. Hormonal actions on gastrointestinal myoelectrical activity in vivo have not been completely explored to date.

Physiological Role of Hormones in the Control of Gastrointestinal Motility

It is not certain whether the many actions of hormones on gastrointestinal motility are of physiological significance. An effect to the

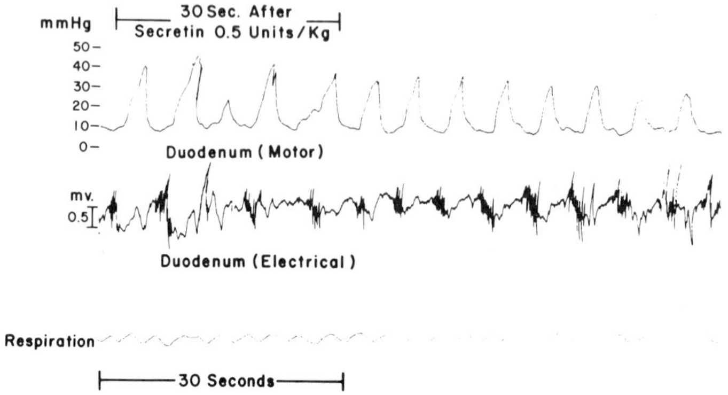

Fig. 9. Myoelectric and pressure record obtained in a normal subject following the intravenous injection of secretin (0.5 units/kg). After the injection of secretin each slow wave showed a burst of action potentials. Increases in duodenal luminal pressure followed each burst of action potentials. Respirations are shown below. (Reprinted from New Engl J. Med.—in press).

exogenous administration of a hormone certainly cannot be directly correlated with a physiological role. Similarly, the motor response of an organ to the endogenous release of a hormone to unphysiological stimuli cannot be readily interpreted as being physiological. The problem is further complicated because the function of specific regions of the gastrointestinal tract are not clearly defined. For example, how does one interpret the physiological response of the ileocecal sphincter if its function is not known? A major challenge will be to determine the physiological significance of the diverse hormonal activities being described. It is quite possible that the importance of hormones in the regulation of gastrointestinal motility may eventually be ascertained from experiments of nature, i.e., diseases. It is possible that specific diseases of altered hormone responsiveness of portions of the gastrointestinal tract will point to the importance of a particular hormone in controlling the function of that specific area. Certain examples of diseases of the LES and pylorus have been reported (Lipshutz et al., 1973; Fisher and Cohen, 1973).

CONCLUSIONS

Based on the studies presented on muscle strips, in vitro, and in animals and man, in vivo, several conclusions can be put forth.

1. Each gastrointestinal hormone has a specific effect on each portion of the gastrointestinal tract, and these hormonal effects are intrinsic to the smooth muscle itself.

2. The specific interaction of hormones on smooth muscle, in vitro, suggests that hormone induced inhibition, in vivo, occurs only in the presence of the stimulatory action of another hormone.

3. Gastrointestinal hormones can alter the inotropic state of gastrointestinal smooth muscle and thus may alter the force of closure of a sphincter or the propulsive force of a luminal structure.

4. Gastrointestinal hormones increase the incidence of spike bursts in the small intestine as well as other luminal structures but do not seem to have a marked effect on slow wave frequency or propagation velocity.

5. Each gastrointestinal sphincter and luminal structure tested responds to the hormones, but the physiological significance of the hormonal control of motor function has not been clarified in all cases.

The future evaluation of gastrointestinal motor function and its hormonal regulation should be a productive area of investigation in coming years. The most difficult problem to resolve will be the determination of the physiological significance of the observations concerning hormonal effects on gastrointestinal sphincters.

REFERENCES

Christensen,J., and Lund,G.F., 1969.
Esophageal responses to distension and electrical stimulation.
J. Clin. Invest. 48:408.

Cohen,S., and Green,F., 1973.
The mechanics of esophageal muscle contraction.
J. Clin. Invest. 52:2029.

Cohen,S., and Lipshutz,W.H., 1971.
Hormonal regulation of human lower esophageal sphincter competence: interaction of gastrin and secretin.
J. Clin. Invest. 50:449.

DiMarino,A.J., Carlson,G., Myers,A., Schumacher,H.R., and Cohen,S.
Duodenal myoelectric activity in schleroderma: abnormal responses to mechanical and hormonal stimuli.
N. Eng. J. Med. (In Press).

DiMarino,A.J., and Cohen,S., 1974.
The adrenergic control of lower esophageal sphincter function.
J. Clin. Invest. (In Press).

Fisher,R., and Cohen,S., 1973.
Pyloric sphincter dysfunction in patients with gastric ulcer.
N. Eng. J. Med. 288:273.

Fisher,R.S., Lipshutz,W., and Cohen,S., 1973.
The hormonal regulation of pyloric sphincter function.
J. Clin. Invest. 52:1289.

Grossman,M.I., 1970.
Hypothesis: gastrin, cholecystokinin and secretin act as one receptor.
Lancet 1:1088.

Lipshutz,W.H., and Cohen,S., 1971.
Physiological determinants of lower esophageal sphincter function.
Gastroenterology 61:16.

Lipshutz,W.H., and Cohen,S., 1972.
Interaction of gastrin I and secretin on gastro-intestinal circular muscle.
Am. J. Physiol. 222:775.

Lipshutz,W.H., Gaskins,R., Lukash,W. and Sode,J.,1973.
Lower esophageal sphincter incompetence.
N. Eng. J. Med. 289:182.

Lipshutz,W., Hughes,W., and Cohen,S., 1973.
The genesis of lower esophageal sphincter pressure: its identification through the use of gastrin anti-serum.
J. Clin. Invest. 51:522.

Lipshutz,W., Tuch,A., and Cohen,S., 1971.
A comparison of the site of action of gastrin I on lower esophageal sphincter and antral circular smooth muscle.
Gastroenterology 61:454.

THE REGULATION OF GASTRIC EMPTYING

J. N. Hunt

INTRODUCTION

It has been known for a long time that glucose added to test meals slows gastric emptying (Carnot and Chassevant, 1905). Glucose acts on duodenal osmoreceptors, since glucose and potassium chloride in test meals slow gastric emptying equally when they exert equal osmotic pressures (Barker et al., 1974). Glucose, boiled starch, and most disaccharides have an almost equal action per gram in slowing gastric emptying (Hunt, 1960; Elias et al., 1968). This has been explained by suposing that duodenal osmoreceptors see all carbohydrates as monosaccharides because the receptors lie distal to the hydrolysis of starch by pancreatic amylase, and deep to the disaccharidases of the brush border of the cells of the mucosa of the small intestine. In patients with deficiency of pancreatic amylase starch solutions leave the stomach more rapidly than the corresponding solutions of glucose (Mallison, 1968).

IS THE ENERGY CONTENT OF FOOD A DETERMINANT OF GASTRIC EMPTYING?

Since starch and sugars have almost equal energy per gram, the control system ensures that the molecular weight of the carbohydrate does not influence the rate at which energy is transferred to the duodenum. This conclusion prompted the question, is the rate of gastroduodenal transfer of the energy of food independent of the source of energy, whether it be carbohydrate, fat or protein?

As well as duodenal osmoreceptors there are also duodenal receptors responding to fat or rather to anions of fatty acids (Quigley and Meschan, 1941). Consistent with this, it is found that fats are relatively ineffective in slowing gastric emptying in patients with deficiency of pancreatic lipase, showing that the receptors do not respond to undigested triglycerides (Knox and Mallinson, 1971). If the slowing of gastric emptying, say by 9g carbohydrate (9 x 4 kcal/g = 36 kcal) were equal to that produced by 4g triglyceride (4 x 9 kcal/g = 36 kcal), then variation in the ratio of fat to carbohydrate in the gastric content would leave the rate of transfer of energy from stomach to duodenum unchanged.

Contrary to the effect of fat and carbohydrate, pure protein, as distinct from lean meat which always contains fat, has not been demonstrated to slow gastric emptying. However, the control system might offset changes in the protein content of food in two ways.

1. The ratio of fat to protein in many diets, 1.3 to 1.0, has a standard deviation of only 15%. If this ratio is accepted as constant, and the fat receptor were suitably tuned, a transfer of energy independent of composition of the gastric contents would be achieved.

2. The secretion of acid in response to food is largely determined by the buffer formed in the stomach. In the duodenum there is a system which slows gastric emptying in response to acid by titrating it to pH 6.5 (Hunt and Knox, 1972). In essence this system measures the amount of acid secreted by the stomach, determined by the amount of protein in the food, and slows gastric emptying accordingly (Saint-Hilaire et al., 1960). It was noted that, in principle, a system might transfer isocaloric amount of contents to the duodenum, independent of the proportions of carbohydrate and fat in the food. This was tested using results from six papers summarised in table 1.

RATE OF GASTRIC EMPTYING AND THE HALF-LIFE OF MEAL

Calculation

It has become customary to describe the emptying of meals in terms of the time required for the volume of meal in the stomach to fall by half. Figure 1 shows how the volume of meal emptied in 30 min may be computed from the volume at time zero and the half-

GASTRIC EMPTYING IN HEALTHY PEOPLE

Author	Volume of meal (ml)	kcal/ml	Content	Half life (min)
Harvey et al. 1970	350	2.3	egg breakfast	56 (5)
Brömster 1968	300	1.4	milk glucose	37 (13)
Griffiths et al. 1968	550	1.0	egg breakfast milk	66 (19)
Hunt et al. 1951	750	0.84	sucrose	82 (10)
Berg 1969	750	0.4	glucose	50 (14)
Hunt 1951	750	0.15	sucrose	22 (21)

Table 1. Gastric emptying in healthy people. Numbers in parenthesis are numbers of persons. 1 kcal = 4.2 MJ.

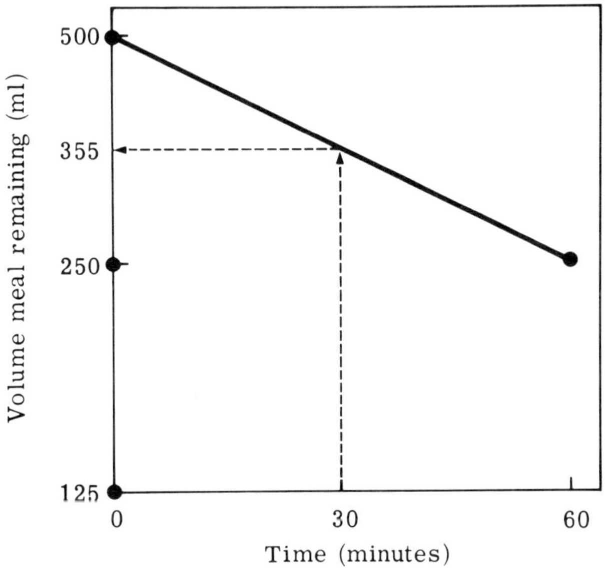

Fig. 1. Method of calculating volume of meal emptied in 30 min.

life. Since the emptying process is exponential, a plot of log volume of meal remaining in the stomach against time gives a straight line. Two points on this line are log of initial volume at zero time, and $\log \frac{(\text{initial volume})}{2}$ at the half-time. By interpolation or extrapolation, the log volume remaining at 30 min may be found. The antilog gives the volume remaining. The volume emptied into the duodenum in the period 0–30 min can be found by subtracting the volume remaining at 30 min from the volume at zero time. This method was used in the present study.

Details of Experimental Studies

Table 1 sets out some features of the work providing the data for this enquiry. There are five points to be made about these six papers by five groups of authors:—

1. The volumes of test meal given varied between 750 and 300 ml.
2. The percentage of total energy as fat was 62%, 40% and 51% for the first three papers, respectively, and zero for the remainder.
3. The kcal/ml in the given meal varied from 2.3 to 0.15.
4. The half-lives of the emptying process varied from 82 to 22 min.
5. The dates of the papers span 20 years.

Relation between Energy Transferred to Duodenum in 30 Min and Kcal/ml of Meal

The products of the volume of meal emptied in 30 min and the kcal/ml meal were plotted for six sets of results set out in table 1. The regression was: kcal transferred in 30 min = 66 + 79 (kcal/ml meal). This is brought out in figure 2.

Since the meals range in composition from pure carbohydrate to one having 60% of its energy in the form of fat, and all the points fall close to the line, it is clear that kcal/ml determines the rate of energy transferred, independent of the ratio of fat to carbohydrate in given meal. However, there is a weakness in this conclusion because kcal/ml which is the abscissa in figure 2, also appears on the ordinate, which is a product of volume emptied and kcal/ml. This form of plotting exaggerates any correlation which may exist. This difficulty was overcome by taking several points on the fitted line (not the six experimental points) and dividing the value on the ordinate by the

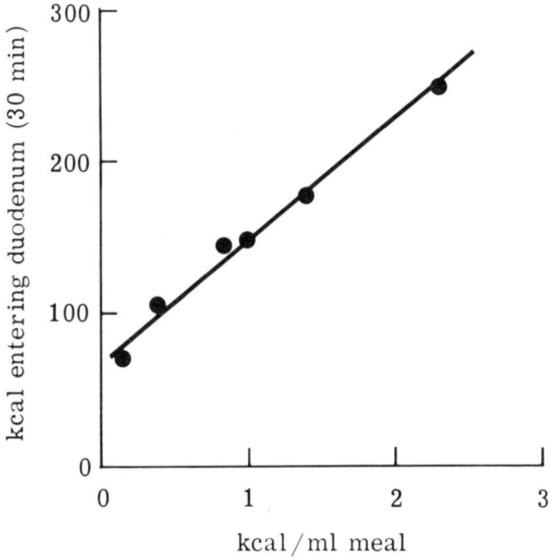

Fig. 2. Relation between kcal/(MJ) ml meal and kcal entering duodenum in 30 min.

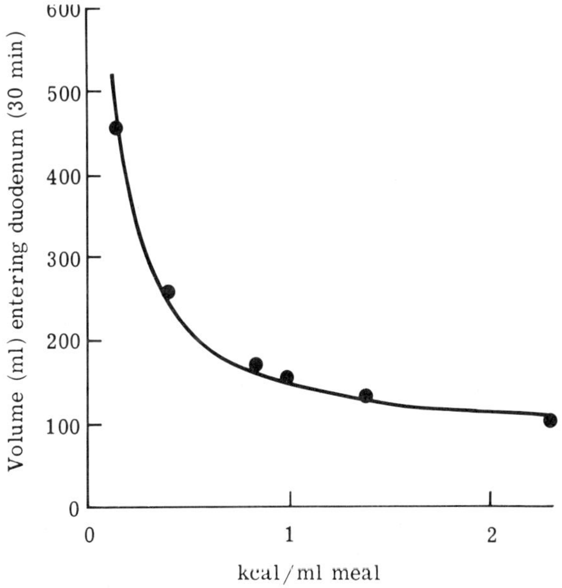

Fig. 3. Relation between kcal/(MJ) ml meal and volume of meal entering duodenum in 30 min.

corresponding value on the abscissa. The volume emptied in 30 min was obtained from the formula $\frac{\text{volume emptied (ml) x kcal/ml}}{\text{kcal/ml meal}}$.
The values for volumes emptied, computed from the fitted line of figure 2, are the basis for the fitted line of figure 3. The points on figure 3 are the experimental values of volume emptied in 30 min computed from the six papers of table 2 as shown in figure 2. The close fit of the points to the line in figure 3 shows that kcal/ml in the given meal does dominate the volume emptied in 30 min in spite of the variation in composition of the six meals.

It might appear from figure 3 that the system of regulation is indifferent to the volume of the meal given. However, this is not so. The ordinate, volume emptied in 30 min was computed as shown in figure 1 from volume of meal ingested and the half-life of the emptying process.

There is a further method of making the curvilinear relation of figure 2 into a rectilinear relation between volume emptied and kcals/ml. This can be done by plotting volume emptied in 30 min against $\frac{1}{\text{kcal/ml meal}}$. Student's t values for this regression are 23 with a fair degree of freedom. The corresponding t values for the relation for volume emptied in 15 min and 60 min are 15 and 9 respectively, and p much less than 0.001. However, there are unresolved anomalies in the analysis so far undertaken and therefore the conclusions drawn below are essentially tentative.

The first tentative conclusion is that duodenal receptors control gastric emptying as though they were responding to kcal/ml meal ingested although, of course, they presumably do this by responding to related properties of the food. The second tentative conclusion is that the regulated transfer of amounts of kcals shown in figure 2 is achieved with precision in spite of a two-fold range in the volume of meal given. Thus the system is computing a function of volume and concentration, that is amount. Such systems as I am aware of, determine amount by responding to concentration in fixed volume. In the gastroduodenal control system there is apparently something more complex than is usually found. Referring back to table 1, it can be seen that the groups of subjects were in some instances small, and the techniques used were various. Yet the true variance of the output of the control system, as judged from figure 3, is astonishingly small and the constraints applied by the gastroduodenal control system are severe.

REFERENCES

Barker,G.R., Cochrane,G.McL., Corbett,G.A., Hunt,J.N., and Roberts,S.K., 1973.
Actions of glucose and potassium chloride on osmoreceptors slowing gastric emptying.
(In Press).

Berger,T., 1969.
The gastric emptying mechanism.
Acta. Chir. Scand. (Suppl.), p. 414.

Bromster,D., 1968.
Measurement of gastric emptying rate using I-HSA. A methogological study in man.
Scand. J. Gastroent., 3:651.

Carnot,P., and Chassevant,A., 1905.
Sur le passage pylorique des solutions de glucose.
C.r.Seanc. Soc. Biol., 58:1069.

Elias,E.G., Gibson,J., Greenwood,L.F., Hunt,J.N., and Tripp,J.H., 1968.
The slowing of gastric emptying by monosaccharides and disaccharides in test meals.
J. Physiol., 194:317.

Griffiths,G.H., Owen,G.M., Campbell,P.H., and Shields, R., 1968.
Gastric emptying in health and gastroduodenal disease.

Harvey,R.F., Mackie,D.B., Brown,N.J.G., and Keeling, D.H., 1970.
Measurement of gastric emptying time with a gamma camera.
Lancet, 1:16.

Hunt,J.N., and Spurrell,W.R., 1951.
The pattern of emptying of the human stomach.
J. Physiol., 113:157.

Hunt,J.N., MacDonald,T., and Spurrell,W.R., 1951.
The gastric response to meals of high osmotic pressure.
J. Physiol., 115:185.

Hunt,J.N., 1960.
The site of receptors slowing gastric emptying in response to starch in test meals.
J. Physiol., 154:270.

Hunt,J.N., and Knox.M.T., 1972.
The slowing of gastric emptying by four strong acids and three weak acids.
J. Physiol., 222:187.

Knox,M.T., and Mallinson,C.N., 1971.
Gastric emptying of fat in patients with pancreatitis.
Tendiconti, 3:115.

Mallinson,C.N., 1968.
Effect of pancreatic insufficiency and intestinal lactase deficiency on the gastric emptying of starch and lactose.
Gut, 9:737.

Quigley,J.P., and Meschan,I., 1941.
Inhibition of the pyloric sphincter region by the digestion products of fat.
Am. J. Physiol., 134:803.

THE ENTERO-ENTERIC REFLEXES

M. H. F. Friedman

INTRODUCTION

The early investigations in digestive physiology were directed more often at elucidating the processes of secretion and absorption than movement of ingested food. Formation of acid by the stomach, the nature of peptic digestion, the role of the pancreas, the role of the intestinal lymphatics, received attention since they were understandably phenomena of popular concern. The early studies on gastrointestinal motor activities likewise dealt with readily observed activities, for example the process of vomiting studied by Magendie and the transit time through the gastrointestinal tract (described by Stevens in 1777). Some observations on gastric motor activities were recorded by Helm (1801) and Beaumont (1833) in man and by Bassov (1842) and Blondlot (1843) in the unanesthetized dog, but these were made incidental to their studies on gastric secretion. A number of studies dealing specifically with motor activities followed Ludwig's description in 1861 of both stationary and moving contractions of the small intestine. However, when describing his own pioneer work on gastric movements as seen by Roentgen ray, Cannon (1898) summed up the earlier observations reported in the literature as "full of conflicting statements and uncertain results".

Important advances made in the 1890's soon established some order. Mall (1896) showed that normal peristaltic movements in the small intestine always progressed in an aboral direction. Meltzer

(1897, 1899) described the transit of food through the esophagus and cardia. Cannon (1898) showed the usefulness of the newly discovered X-ray in studying gastric motility and most important, Bayliss and Starling (1899) formulated their "law of the intestine" to provide an explanation for peristalsis.

THE MYENTERIC REFLEX

Law of the Intestine

In their studies of the movements and innervation of the small intestine, Bayliss and Starling (1899, 1901) ennunciated what they called the "law of the intestine". Concisely stated, this holds that the response of the small intestine to local stimuli consists of contraction of the muscle immediately above and relaxation immediately below the point of stimulation. They attributed this response to a reflex which involved the myenteric plexus but was independent of the extrinsic innervation of the intestine. Cannon (1912) designated this as the "myenteric reflex". The biphasic wave of relaxation-contraction would pass over the muscle in an aboral direction for short distances from the point of stimulation (figure 1). It was later postulated also that the phase of relaxation under certain conditions could be initiated before, and advance aborally more rapidly than, the phase of contraction (Thomas and Friedman, 1950, unpublished). Some later workers (Alvarez, 1948, Posey and Bargen, 1951) failed to note the forward relaxation phase, probably through inappropriate application of the stimulus (see Baldwin and Thomas, 1975) but the myenteric reflex as originally described has been repeatedly confirmed (Thomas and Baldwin, 1968) and is now widely accepted.

It should be emphasized that the "law of the intestine" refers to a localized response of the bowel to stimulation. The total area involved in the myenteric reflex was stated by Bayliss and Starling (1901) to extend only from about 5 cms above to 4 cms below the point of stimulation.

In addition to the myenteric reflex, stimulation of the gastroenteric tract by mechanical or chemical means may elicit other reflex responses which may be conveniently categorized on the basis of the effectors involved. The entero-enteric reflexes comprise associated effects of inhibition and excitation in regions of the digestive tract which are remote from the area of moderate stimulation. The entero-visceral reflexes comprise effects on the cardiovascular, respiratory and renal systems. The entero-somatic reflex comprise effects on muscles of the limbs and abdomen. This presentation will be limited mostly to a general discussion of the entero-enteric reflexes and only briefly touch on entero-visceral reflexes.

THE ENTERO-ENTERIC REFLEX

Second Law of the Intestine

Stimulation of the gastrointestinal tract in a discrete area can be shown to modify the smooth muscle activities of segments of the bowel which are at some distance from that local of stimulation where the myenteric reflex in being evoked. Except when the stimulus is of excessive strength, the response is one of inhibition of gastrointestinal segments located some distance above the point of stimulation with concurrent increase in activity of bowel segments some distance distal to this point. Unlike the myenteric reflex, the entero-enteric reflex is dependent on the extrinsic innervation. Under optimum conditions of stimulus strength, digestive state, etc., the reflexes are evoked so consistantly that Thomas and Friedman (1961) were led to designate the phenomena as comprising a "second law of the intestine". The entero-enteric reflex is illustrated in figure 2.

It must be stressed that the entero-enteric reflex which is characterized in the following discussion is elicited only with moderate intensities of stimuli. However, stimuli which are strong enough to evoke pain or are of sub-pain threshhold result almost always in inhibition throughout most of the digestive tract (Pearcy and Van Liere, 1926). When due to excessive intraluminal pressure, such a reflex was designated by Hermann and Morin (1934) as the "intestino-intestinal inhibitory reflex". This reflex has been extensively reviewed by Youmans (1949, 1968) and will not be discussed further.

Distension as the Stimulus

The only impulse which reaches the sensorium from the normal intestine is that induced by tension. Distension as a stimulus to produce muscle tension allows for a better degree of grading stimulus strength than do other means. Production of excessive tension and pain, resulting in mass intestino-intestinal inhibition, can be avoided readily by controlling distension. For these reasons Youmans (1949) and others used distension as the appropriate stimulus for deter-

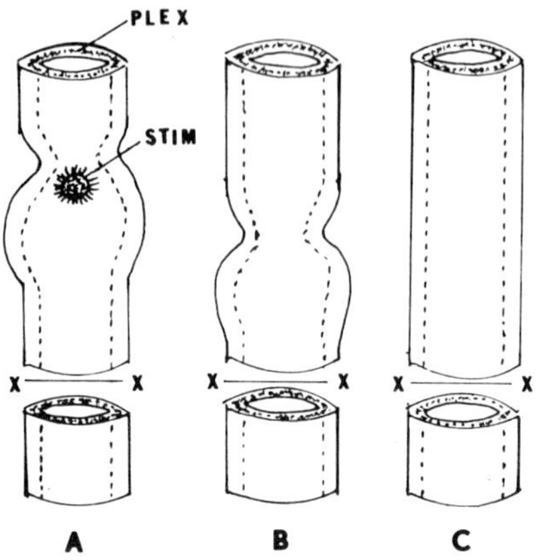

Fig. 1. The myenteric reflex, illustrating the "Law of the Intestine" (Bayliss and Starling, 1898). A. An intraluminal stimulus, applied to the intestine deprived of extrinsic innervation, results in contraction immediately above and relaxation immediately below the point of stimulation. B. The coupled relaxation-contraction moves as a wave in an aboral (down) direction. C. The myenteric reflex is dependent on the integrity of the myenteric plexus since the contraction wave does not cross the intestine sectioned at X–X. PLEX–myenteric plexus. STIM–stimulus.

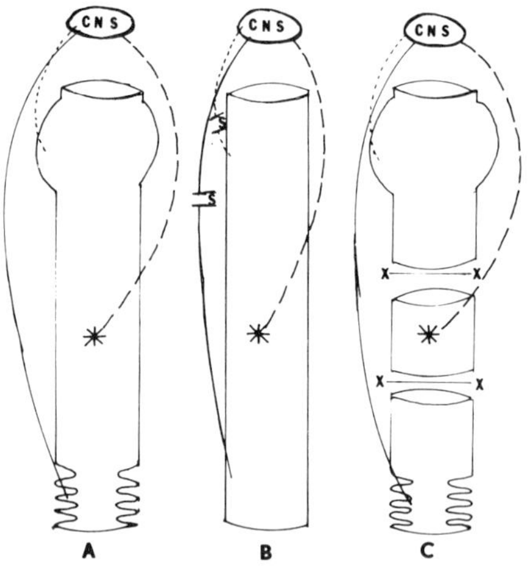

Fig. 2. The entero-enteric reflex, illustrating the "Second Law of the Intestine". (Thomas and Friedman, 1961). A. An intraluminal stimulus (starburst), in addition to resulting in the local myenteric reflex, reflexly inhibits the motility some distance above (proximal to) the stimulation and augments the motility some distance below (distal to) the stimulation. B. The inhibitory and excitatory components of the entero-enteric reflex are abolished by section (S) of the vagal innervation. C. The reflex responses are independent of the integrity of the myenteric plexus, since they persist after transection of the gut at X–X either above or below the stimulation point. (Modified from Friedman, 1964).

mining afferent pathways.

Our studies were carried out on unanesthetized dogs equipped with chronic fistulas of the stomach and intestine. These were supplemented by special acute experiments on dogs under chloralose-urethane, dial, or thiobarbital-pentobarbital anesthesia. Distension of the stomach and intestine to various pressures was produced by inflation of balloons of different sizes.

The entero-enteric motor reflex was found to be elicited more readily when the distension stimulus was applied to some areas of the digestive tract than to others. The body of the stomach, the duodenum in the region of the pancreatic duct papilla, the mid-jejunum and the colon showed lower threshholds than other areas tested.

Moderate distension (10—20mm Hg balloon pressure) applied rapidly to the duodenum was more effective in producing gastric inhibition than when applied slowly. Rapid distension of the colon produced more prolonged inhibition of the ileum than of the stomach or duodenum. Increasing the area of duodenum subjected to rapid distension by using a larger balloon required a lower pressure to inhibit the stomach or increase colonic activity. Essentially similar conclusions were drawn by Peterson and Youmans (1945) and Youmans (1949).

When a moderate distension stimulus was applied to the upper ileum, inhibition of the proximal segment (duodenum) resulted in 64 per cent of the responses and activation of the distal segment (terminal ileum) in 60 per cent of the responses. In 45 per cent of the distension trials the two responses, proximal inhibition and distal activation, occurred simultaneously. In table 1 are shown the correlations between the two responses.

The Entero-Enteric Reflex

Increased motor activity when elicited in a distal bowel segment by jejunal distension consisted of peristaltic contraction waves as well as non-propagated contractions. The peristaltic contractions originated about 20 cms distal to the point of stimulation and traversed distances of 10 to 25 cms before dimunition. On the other hand, inhibition of the cephalid segment (duodenum or stomach) occurred about 10 to 20 cms above the area stimulated and consisted of arrest in activity and fall in tonus which did not spread along the bowel. It is interesting to note that antiperistaltic movements were

Table 1

Response of Bowel Segment		Responses	
Proximal	Distal	Frequency	Percent
—	—	9	7
—	0	16	12
—	+	59	45
+	—	8	6
+	0	2	2
+	+	9	7
0	—	3	2
0	0	14	11
0	+	10	8
		n = 130	

Combined data from 5 dogs. The distension stimulus was applied by an intraluminal balloon in the upper ileum. Proximal recordings were taken from the duodenum and distal recordings from the terminal ileum. (Recordings from the stomach and colon are not shown). Increase in motor activity indicated by +, inhibition by —, no apparent effect by 0.

rarely noted in the chronic experiment but were found frequently in the experiment under light anesthesis.

An important determinant of the response was the digestive state of the animal at the time of the experiment. Inflation of either stomach or intestine increased the contractions of the colon in proportion to the degree of colonic filling. Little activity was induced when the colon was empty, as shortly after defecation. The optimum time of inhibition of the stomach and duodenum produced by inflation of the terminal ileum was 30 to 90 minutes after eating. Welch and Plant (1926) found in the dog and man that feeding increased colon activity when the bowel was full but not when the bowel was empty. In their study of the gastrocolic reflex in the dog,

Tansy et al. (1972) concluded that the primary determinant of the response is the degree of colonic distension rather than the type or intensity of the applied gastric or duodenal stimulus.

Receptors

At this time we do not know whether both the inhibition of the proximal segment and the excitation of the distal segment resulted from activation of the same receptors. Since normally the intestinal stimulus is food we believe that, unlike balloon distension, food also involves chemoreceptors and osmoreceptors in addition to mechanoreceptors. The topographic distribution of these receptors, their depth in the mucosa and their stimulation threshholds are all unknown.

We must also consider the possibility that not all the effects of intraluminal distension by balloon were necessarily evoked by excitation of mechanoreceptors in the mucosa. The existence of stretch receptors in gastric (Paintal, 1954) and intestinal muscle (Hukuhara et al., 1957) has been postulated. In studies on entero-visceral reflexes performed by Freundlich (1967) in our laboratory, evidence was obtained that increase in tension of the muscle fibers alone may be effective. Simple mechanical stretch applied by a device directly to the muscle of the stomach produced definite cardiovascular and respiratory effects. In another study in our laboratory, Holmes (1968) working with Doemling found this also to be true for stretch applied to the jejunum and colon. We do not know whether such muscle stretch would induce both entero-enteric and intestino-intestinal inhibitory reflexes in the unanesthetized animal.

"Gastrocolic" Reflex

Relatively few studies have embraced the entire entero-enteric motor reflex as here described. However, the two components, inhibition some distance above and excitation some distance below the point of stimulation, have each been studied separately as individual reflexes. An example of the distal effects is the gastrocolic excitatory reflex while the enterogastric inhibitory reflex is an example of the proximal effects. These are imprecise designations for reflexes with wider ranging effects: each is used here to designate a class of responses of which it is a prototype.

It has long been known that motor activities of the ileum, cecum, and colon are increased after eating (Cannon, 1902; Mac Ewan, 1904; Hurst, 1907; Hertz, 1913; Welch and Plant, 1926; Douglas and Mann, 1940; Misiewicz et al., 1966; Tansy et al., 1972b). A composite picture of the many studies is one of increased segmentation and peristalsis in the ileum sweeping its contents into the cecum and colon: in the colon also are seen increased segmental activity and mass movements. These may culminate in a separate defecation reflex, especially in the infant or puppy that has not yet been subjected to conditioned inhibition of defecation by toilet training.

The events described as the gastrocolic reflex have been attributed to distension of the stomach and duodenum. This is supported by finding in the dog (but according to Welch and Plant, 1926, not in man) that introduction of food directly into the stomach or the duodenum via a fistula provokes motor responses in the ileum and colon. Similar effects have been noted in isolated loops of the small intestine (Puestow, 1932). The responses are abolished after vagus nerve section but are still obtainable following section of the bowel between the point of stimulation and the affected distal segments (figure 2).

However, the simple process of eating has been shown to produce similar motor responses. Welch and Plant (1926) in controlled studies on colon motility in man, found that feeding by mouth, but not by fistula, always increased bowel activity. Connell et al. (1964) reported that unappetizing foods gave a small colonic response. Preshaw and Knauf (1966) found that sham feeding in the dog increased motor activity of the innervated isolated duodenal loop.

From studies in Pavlov's laboratory, it is clear that the feeding reflex is a conditioned reflex. The present consensus is that the distension "gastrocolic" reflex and the feeding reflex are activated concurrently and that one reinforces the other.

Fig. 3. Comparative effects of mild and excessive distension of balloon in jejunum on gastric hunger contractions and motility of terminal ileum in unanesthetized dog. Preinflation movements of stomach and ileum constituted the respective base-lines. On left, jejunal balloon inflated to 9 mm Hg pressure: result was reflex inhibition of gastric motility with augmentation of motility of terminal ileum. On right, jejunal balloon inflated to 50 mm Hg pressure: result was profound inhibition of all movements in stomach and terminal ileum.

Fig. 4. Representative entero-enteric reflexes. In each case the starburst is the site of an intraluminal stimulus. The solid line directed aborally from a stimulation point indicates the respective area of increased reflex motility. The broken line directed cephalad indicates the respective area of reflex inhibition. The afferent and efferent extrinsic nerve pathways of the reflex arcs are not shown.

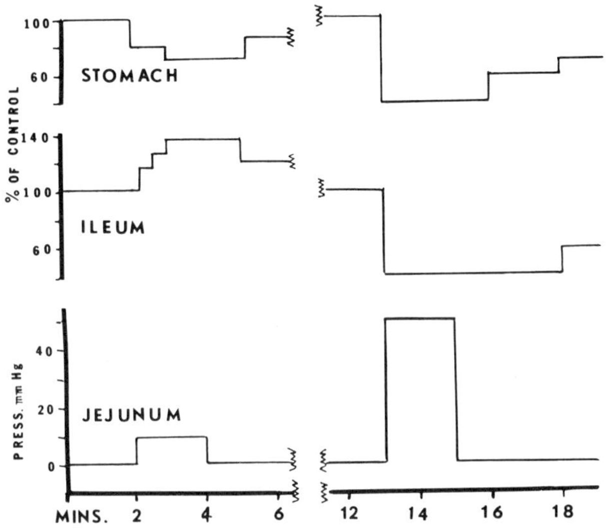

Figure 3

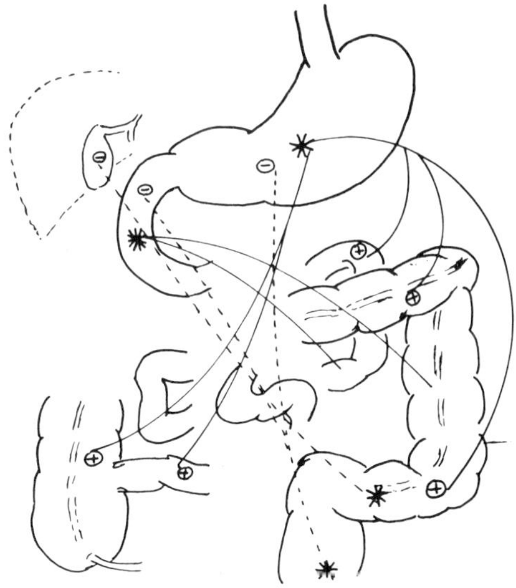

Figure 4

"Enterogastric" Inhibitory Reflex

In his pioneer study on the stomach, von Mering (1893) noted that gastric evacuation was delayed by introduction of water and food substances into duodenum. The delay was shown by Thomas and Mogan (1931) to be due to inhibition of gastric motility and tonus and not to closure of the pylorus as proposed earlier by Cannon. Two mechanisms, a vagal reflex and the liberation of a hormone, may be responsible.

Water, protein digestion products and distension act from the duodenum as stimuli for an enterogastric inhibitory reflex. Fats (Lim, 1933) and concentrated solution of carbohydrate (Quigley and Phelps, 1934) act through liberation of an inhibitory hormone from the duodenal mucosa, but probably also through the enterogastric reflex.

The inhibitory hormone for gastric motility has been designated enterogastrone, but recent studies indicate that more than one gastro-intestinal hormone may be involved. Acid in the duodenum inhibits gastric movements by both the enterogastric reflex and the liberation of the hormone secretin. The inhibition of gastric motility which is due to the enterogastric reflex occurs after a relatively brief latent period and is of short duration. On the other hand, the latent period for inhibition produced by the intestinal hormone(s) is much longer but the inhibitory effect is sustained.

As shown by figure 3, stimulation of the jejunum by moderate (less than 10 mm Hg pressure) distension of an intralumenal balloon will cause inhibition of hunger contractions of the stomach and motility of the ileum (Thomas and Friedman, 1950, unpublished). Distension of the ascending colon will produce similar effects (Pearcy and Van Liere, 1926). The inhibitory effects are due to a vagal-vagal reflex and apparently do not involve intestinal hormones. Inhibition is not dependent on transmission through intrinsic nervous connections since transection of the bowel between the distension area and the effector site has little effect (figure 2). Sympathectomy has little effect: however, the sympathetics mediate the inhibition which occurs when the distension is strong enough to produce discomfort or pain.

Loew and Patterson (1938) and others (see Youmans, 1949) showed in the unanesthetized dog that inhibition of gastric hunger contractions and movements of the small intestine also occurred on mechanical stimulation of the anorectal region. According to Youmans (1949) this is an adrenergic sympathetic reflex. Many observers, ourselves included, have seen that during the act of defecation there will be arrest of gastric hunger contractions and intestinal motility. Presumably the gastric and duodenal inhibition during defecation is due to anorectal stimulation by the feces but central inhibition has not been ruled out.

It should be noted that inhibitory effects of distension as described above are not limited to the stomach and intestine. Patterson (1940, personal communication) observed that mechanical stimulation of the lower bowel and anorectal region resulted in impaired gall bladder evacuation. This is in agreement with clinical experience that defective gall bladder motor function sometimes is relieved by removal of irritants or impacted stool from the sigmoid colon.

Utility of Entero-Enteric Reflex

"Receptive relaxation" is a phenomenon of accomodation to incoming digestive content seen in those segments of the digestive tract immediately distal to the sphincters. The efficiency of this process would be reduced if the relaxed segments were already filled. The increased motility induced by the "gastrocolic reflex" may be regarded as serving to clear the bowel well in advance of the digestive content and thereby also to increase the accomodative capacity of the bowel segments immediately distal to the pyloric and ileocecal sphincters.

Occurring concurrently with the distal activation, the inhibition in motor activities produced in proximal segments by the digestive content may serve to prevent overloading. If I may permitted, I would like to suggest that the two components of the entero-enteric reflex are analogous to the operation of traffic control. When traffic flow is heavy and there is danger of congestion at any point on the route, the traffic control officer (or an electronic device) signals ahead to the next check point to implement speeding up of movement. At the same time, a signal is passed back to the preceding check point to slow up traffic flow. Figure 2 may be viewed in this light. Several entero-enteric reflexes are illustrated in figure 4.

The entero-enteric reflexes are independent of the myenteric nerve plexus but are dependent on the extrinsic innervation. The relative roles of the vagi and splanchnic nerves in the reflex arc are still unknown. In accord with the facts is the concept that the reflex due to the normal chemical and mechanical stimuli of food is mediated from the stomach and upper small intestine over the vagus nerves (Thomas and Friedman, 1951). Reflexes from stimuli in the large bowel and ano-rectal region are mediated over the splanchnic nerves (Youmans, 1949).

We again express the view that the vagus is part of the normal regulatory mechanism of digestive functions. On the other hand, the sympathetic is part of the sympatheco-adrenal emergency system and, as such, is concerned primarily with regulatory processes during stress. This is illustrated by the finding that mild ("normal") intestinal distension elicits the entero-enteric reflex, but only if the vagi are intact. However, distension which produces discomfort or pain results in the intestino-intestinal inhibitory reflex throughout the bowel (excepting the sphincters) but not after splanchrectomy.

REFERENCES

Alvarez, Walter, C., 1948.
An introduction to gastroenterology.
4th Edit.
New York, Paul B. Hoeber.

Baldwin, M. V. and Thomas, J. E., 1975.
The intestinal intrinsic mucosal reflex: a possible mechanism of propulsive motility.
In Functions of Stomach and Intestine., Edit. by M. H. F. Friedman, Baltimore, University Park Press.

Bassov, R., 1842.
Fistules gastriques artificielles sur des chiens.
Soc. imperiale des naturalistes des Moscou, 16: 39.

Bayliss, W. M., and Starling, E. H., 1899.
The movements and innervation of the small intestine.
J. Physiol. (London), 24: 99.

Bayliss, W. M., and Starling, E. H., 1901.
The movements and innervation of the small intestine.
J. Physiol. (London), 26: 125.

Beaumont, Wm., 1833.
Experiments and observations on the gastric juice and the physiology of digestion.
Plattsburgh, 1833, reprinted Boston, 1926.

Blondlot, N., 1843.
Traite analytique de la digestion considerée particulierement dans l' homme et dans les animaux vertebres.
Nancy. (Extensive English exerpts in Friedman, 1943).

Cannon, W. B., 1898.
Movements of the stomach studied by means of the roentgen ray.
Am. J. Physiol., 1: 359.

Cannon, W. B., 1902.
The movements of the intestine studied by means of the roentgen ray.
Am. J. Physiol., 6: 251.

Cannon, W. B., 1912.
Peristalsis, segmentation, and the myenteric reflex.
Am. J. Physiol., 30: 114.

Connell, A. M., Gaafer, M., Hassanein, M. A., and Khayal, N., 1964.
Motility of the pelvic colon. III Motility responses in patients with symptoms following amoebic dysentery.
Gut, 5: 443.

Douglas, D. M., and Mann, F. C., 1940.
The gastro-ileac reflex: further experimental observations.
Am. J. Digest. Diseases. 7: 53.

Freundlich, J. J., 1967.
Cardiovascular and respiratory effects of stomach distension and wall stretch in anesthetized dogs.
Doctoral Dissertation, Jefferson Medical College, Philadelphia.

Friedman, M. H. F., 1943.
Early experimental fistulas of the stomach.
Am. J. Digest. Dis., 10 : 447.

Friedman, M. H. F., 1964.
Animal techniques for evaluating laxatives Chap. 67 in "Pharmacologic Techniques in Drug Evaluation". Edit. by J. H. Nodine and P. S. Siegler.
Chicago, Year Book Medical Publishers, Inc.

Helm, Jacob, 1803.
Zwei Kranken-Geschichten (1) Ein Weib mit einem Loche in dem Magen. (2) Eine durch die Brust in den Magen...Stichwunde.
Vienna, Cameseinaische Buchhandlung.
(Extensive English exerpts by Kisch, 1954).

Hermann, H., and Morin, G., 1934.
Mise en évidence d'un réflexe inhibiteur intestino-intestinal.
Comp. Rend. Soc. de Biol., 115: 529.

Hertz, A. F., 1913.
The ileo-cecal sphincter.
J. Physiol (London), 47: 54.

Holmes, M. D., 1968.
Cardiovascular and respiratory responses to intestinal stimulation.
Doctoral Dissertation, Jefferson Medical College, Philadelphia.
Hukuhara, T., Yamagami, M., and Nakayama, S., 1957.
The intestinal intrinsic reflexes.
J. Physiol. Japan, 8: 9.
Hurst, A. F., 1907.
Passage of food along the human alimentary tract.
Guy's Hosp. Report, 61: 389.
Kisch, B., 1954.
Jacob Helm's observations and experiments on human digestion.
J. History Med., 9: 311.
Lim, R. K. S., 1933.
Observations on the mechanism of inhibition of gastric function by fat.
Quart. J. Exper. Physiol., 23: 263.
Loew, E. R. and Patterson, T. L., 1938.
Reflex influence of the lower portion of the large gut on the tonus and movements of the empty stomach in dogs.
Quart. J. Exper. Physiol., 28 : 305.
Ludwig, C., 1861.
Lehrbuch der Physiologie des Menschen. Vol. 2.
Wintersche, Leipzig, 1861.
Mac Ewan, W., 1904.
The function of the caecum and appendix.
Lancet 2: 995.
Mall, F. P., 1896.
A study of the intestinal contractions.
Johns Hopkins Hosp. Report, 1: 37.
Meltzer, S. J., 1897.
A further experimental contribution to the knowledge of the mechanism of deglutition.
J. Exp. Med., 2: 453.
Meltzer, S. J., 1899.
On the causes of the orderly progress of the peristaltic movements in the esophagus.
Am. J. Physiol., 2: 266.

Mering, J. von, 1893.
Über die Funktion des Magens.
Verh. Kongr, inn. Med., 12: 471.
Misiewicz, J. J., Connell, A. M., and Pontes, F., 1966.
A comparison of the effects of meals on the proximal and distal colon in patients with and without diarrhea.
Gut, 7: 468.
Paintal, A. S., 1954.
A study of gastric stretch receptors.
J. Physiol. (London), 126: 255.
Pearcy, J. F., and Van Liere, E. J., 1926.
Studies on the visceral nervous system.
XVII. Reflexes from the colon: (1) Reflexes to the stomach.
Am. J. Physiol., 78: 64.
Peterson, C. G., and Youmans, W. B., 1945.
The intestino-intestinal inhibitory reflex: threshold variations, sensitization and summation.
Am. J. Physiol., 143: 407.
Posey, E. L., Jr., and Bargen, J. A., 1951.
Observations of normal and abnormal human intestinal motor function.
Am. J. Med. Sci., 221: 110.
Preshaw, R. M., and Knauf, R. S., 1966.
The effect of sham feeding on the secretion and motility of canine duodenal pouches.
Gastroenterol., 51: 193.
Puestow, C. B., 1932.
The activity of isolated intestinal segments.
Arch. Surg., 24: 565.
Quigley, J. P., and Phelps, K. R., 1934.
The mechanism of gastric motor inhibition from ingested carbohydrates.
Am. J. Physiol., 109: 133.
Stevens, Edward, 1777.
Dissertatio De Alimentorum Concoctiore.
Inaugral Dissertation, Edinburgh, 1777.
English transcription in "Edward Stevens, Gastric Physiologist, Physician and American Statesman".

Edit. by Stacey B. Day; Cultural and
Educational Productions Inc., Montreal.

Tansy, M. F., Kendall, F. M., and Murphy,J.J. 1972a.
The reflex nature of the gastrocolic propulsive response in the dog.
Surg. Gynecol. Obstet., 135: 404.

Tansy, M. F., Kendall, F. M., and Murphy,J.J. 1972b.
Pharmacologic analysis of the gastroileal and gastrocolic reflexes in the dog.
Surg. Gynecol. Obstet., 135: 763.

Thomas, J. E., and Baldwin, M. V., 1968.
Pathways and mechanisms of regulation of gastric motility.
In Handbook of Physiology, Sect. 6., Vol. 4.
Washington, American Physiological Society.

Thomas, J. E., and Friedman, M. H. F., 1951.
Physiology of the upper gastrointestinal tract as it relates to peptic ulcer.
Chapt. 3 in Peptic Ulcer. Edit. by D. S. Sandweiss.
Philadelphia, W. B. Saunders.

Thomas, J. E., and Friedman, M. H. F., 1961.
The normal physiology of the digestive system.
In Handbuch der allgemeinen Pathologie, Vol. 5., Edit. by F. Buchner.
Heidelberg, Springer.

Welch, P. B., and Plant, D. H., 1926.
The muscular activity of the colon, with specific reference to its response to feeding.
Am. J. Med. Sci., 172: 261.

Youmans, W. B., 1949.
Nervous and humoral regulation of intestinal motility. 148p.
New York, Interscience Publishers, Inc.

Youmans, W. B., 1968.
Innervation of the gastrointestinal tract.
In Handbook of Physiology, Sect. 6, Vol. 4.
Washington, American Physiological Society.

THE INTESTINAL INTRINSIC MUCOSAL REFLEX; A POSSIBLE MECHANISM OF PROPULSIVE MOTILITY

Marjorie V. Baldwin and J. E. Thomas

INTRODUCTION

Propulsive motility in the small intestine has long been a subject of controversy. Except for the rarely observed rush peristalsis described by Meltzer and Auer (1907) there has been no definitive explication available of either the movements responsible for the aboral progress of the intestinal contents or the underlying mechanisms that control them. Bayliss and Starling's "law of the intestine" (Bayliss and Starling, 1899), which Cannon attributed to a "myenteric reflex" (Cannon, 1912), seemed at one time to provide a satisfactory explanation, but has subsequently been questioned by numerous observers (Alvarez, 1948; Alvarez and Zimmermann, 1927; Alvarez and Hosoi, 1930; Henderson, 1928; White et al., 1934; Forster and Hertzman, 1938; Ganter, 1923; Posey and Bargen, 1951). It appears, however, to be readily demonstrated in the cat small intestine (Lenz et al., 1971), in the large intestine in experimental animals (Auer and Krueger, 1947; Crema and Frigo, 1969), and has also been observed, although rarely, in human subjects (Torsoli et al., 1969; Ritchie et al., 1969). The gradient theory of Alvarez, although based on sound observations (Alvarez, 1914; Alvarez and Starkweather, 1918), gives no indication of the specific motor phenomena involved in propulsion.

The principle difficulty in accepting Bayliss and Starling's "law" (contraction above and relaxation below a stimulated point) has been the failure of most observers to elicit relaxation "below" a point of stimulation and failure to observe relaxation in advance of "spontaneous" peristaltic contractions.

One of us (Thomas, 1951; Thomas, 1955; Thomas, 1961), while attempting to demonstrate the "law of the intestine" to students, observed contractions above and relaxation below a point of stimulation of the intestinal mucosa by various chemical substances in fistula dogs. Hukuhara and his associates (1958) independently observed the same phenomena on chemical or mechanical stimulation of the exposed intestinal mucosa in anesthetized animals. They reported also that chemical or mechanical stimulation of the serosa or muscular coat caused relaxation of the muscle both above and below the point of stimulation. Thus they distinguished two intrinsic intestinal reflexes, a "mucosal reflex" conforming to Bayliss and Starling's law and a "muscular" reflex of a different nature. They proved by appropriate experiments that both reflexes were dependent on the integrity of the intrinsic nerve plexus and independent of the extrinsic innervation. They suggested that failure of some investigators to elicit responses in accordance with the law of the intestine might be due to failure to distinguish between the two reflexes. The electrical equivalent of Hukuhara's mucosal reflex was observed by Nakayama and Nanba (1961) who reported increased amplitude and frequency of spike potentials in the muscle above and decrease below the site of mucosal stimulation. These observations, along with our own previous findings, suggested to us that a restudy of the mucosal reflex might provide a basis for a rational analysis of propulsive motility. This report deals with those of our experiments that bear on the occurrence and physiological significance of this reflex. Preliminary reports of some of these studies have been published elsewhere (Baldwin and Thomas, 1969a, 1969b, 1970; Thomas and Baldwin, 1969).

METHODS

Seven adult mongrel dogs with tubulated gastric and duodenal fistulae of a type previously described (Thomas, 1941; Thomas, 1951) were used for this study. Four were neurally intact, three had received bilateral supradiaphragmatic vagotomy and, in two of these, the major splanchnic serves had been severed bilaterally. They were trained to stand quietly in a Pavlov type hammock during the recording sessions which lasted two to four hours. Intraluminal pressures

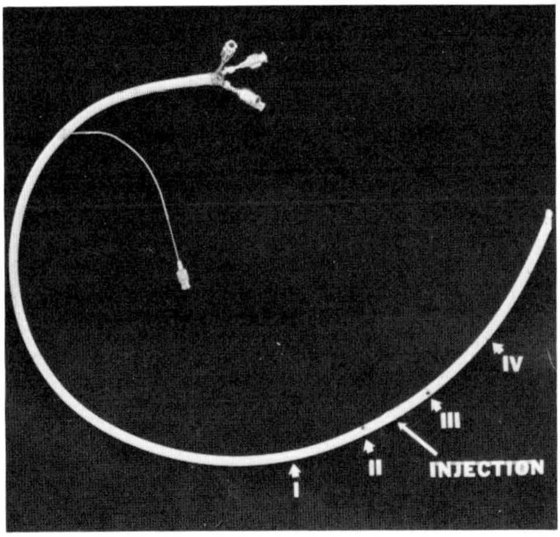

Fig. 1. Four lumen rubber tube assembly used in measurement of intraluminal pressures. Side openings at sites I, II, III, and IV are 5 cm apart. The small polyethylene injection tube which enters one lumen near the upper end of the tube delivers solutions at "I". Level of recording is determined by depth to which tube is placed in the intestine.

were recorded using four-lumen tubing with side openings in each of the four channels. As illustrated in figure 1, the openings were numbered from I to IV from above downward. Water solutions of mucosal stimuli were injected through a small polyethylene tube threaded through one lumen and brought out between side openings II and III.

For recording, the tube was placed with the side openings located in the duodenojejunal or midjejunal area. Opening number I was either 15 or 60 cm from the duodenal fistula. To insure patency of the narrow tubal lumens, constant infusion of normal saline solution through each of the four channels at a rate of 0.1 ml/min was maintained by a Harvard infusion pump. Intraluminal pressures were measured by Statham transducers and recorded by a Grass polygraph. They were also integrated by a 4 channel electronic integrator with a time constant of 4.5 seconds, and the integrated pressures were recorded simultaneously on a second Grass polygraph.

Solutions used as stimuli included 0.075 N HCl, 2% Ivory soap, 2% potassium oleate, 2% sodium desoxycholate, and dog bile drained from the duodenal fistula. Locke-Ringer solution was used as a control. Solutions were injected in volumes of 0.2, 0.5 or 1.0 ml. The smaller volumes were used most frequently since increasing the volume did not improve the results.

Not all solutions were precisely neutral and isotonic (table 3), so the possible role of hydrogen ion and osmolar concentrations was investigated by use of solutions of non-stimulating substances of varying acidity and osmolality.

In one series of experiments, as a means of determining whether the reflex could be elicited through extrinsic nervous pathways, a length of intestine between the area of stimulation and the recording balloon was chilled until contraction frequency below the area of cooling decreased from about 18 per minute to 12–15 per minute. For this purpose cold brine (effluent temperature 4–10°C) was circulated through a latex balloon in the intestine by a modification of the method described by Hasselbrack and Thomas (1961).

For comparison of balloon and intraluminal pressures, a similar tube was provided with four balloons in tandem; recording and integration of balloon pressures were done as in the intraluminal pressure method. The overall responses indicated by balloon pressures and intraluminal pressures did not differ substantially. This report is based primarily on intraluminal pressure recordings.

RESULTS

The frequently described alternation of periods of activity with periods of inactivity were manifest. During activity the minimal intraluminal pressure was usually slightly above atmospheric and the pressure fluctuated at a frequency corresponding to the known frequency of segmenting contractions. During periods of inactivity the pressure was low, sometimes appearing to be below atmospheric, and either exhibited minor changes at irregular intervals or remained constant. The effects of mucosal stimuli were manifest in characteristic form only during periods of activity. During inactive periods the response was either absent or so equivocal as to be useless for purposes of analysis.

Changes in muscular activity affecting intraluminal pressures were indicated by changes in amplitude, duration and regularity of pressure fluctuations, and by minimal pressure levels (tone). Comparisons of these parameters as observed during, and for suitable

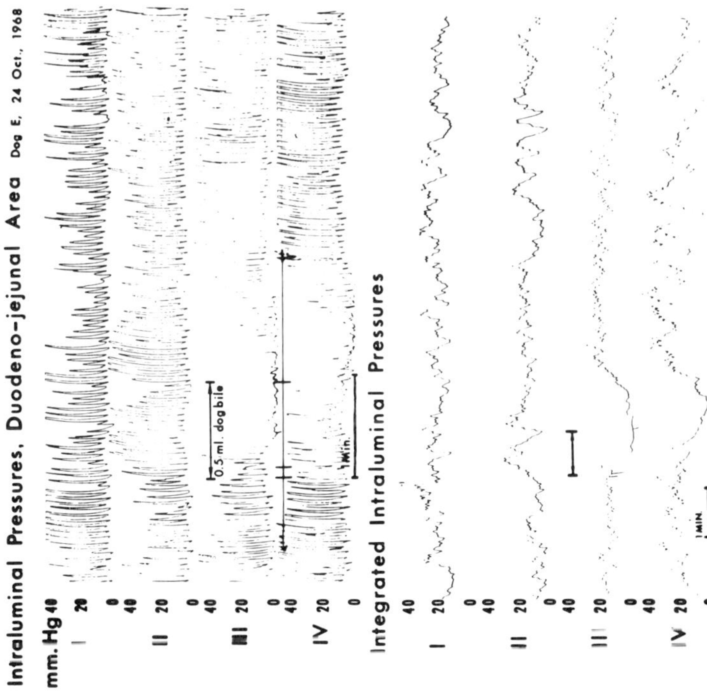

Figure 2

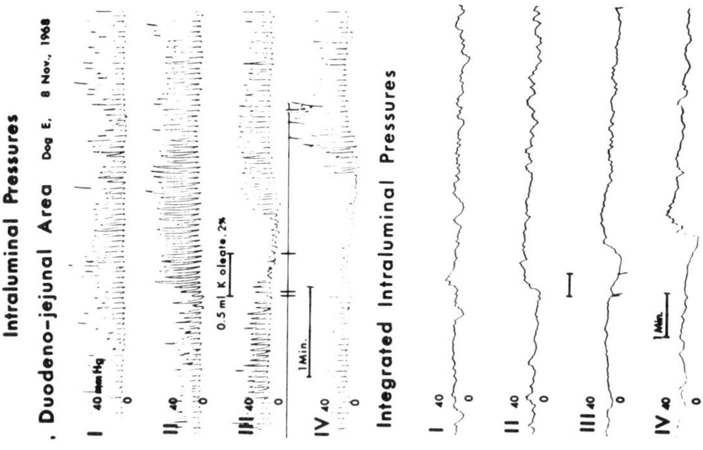

Figure 3

periods before and after, application of a stimulus were made. The integrated pressure records provided a means of estimating the mean pressures resulting from interaction of these variables.

Typical changes in intraluminal pressures following effective stimulation of the mucosa with bile and potassium oleate are illustrated in figures 2 and 3 respectively. Mean intraluminal pressures below the site of stimulation immediately decreased; the decrease was transmitted at least as far as the caudalmost recording site. Mean pressure above the stimulated area usually increased; this increase was transmitted at least as far as the highest site. Variations in mean pressure were associated with appropriate changes in rhythmic elevations in pressure. These were diminished or abolished below the site of stimulation, while above it they were increased in one or more of the following parameters: amplitude, regularity, or duration. The minimal pressure level ("tone level") usually showed corresponding changes. Pressure changes similar in pattern to the initial response were occasionally repeated in cyclic fashion.

The entire complex, both proximal pressure increase and distal pressure decrease, appeared to be propagated caudally. Often the inhibitory phase immediately distal to site of mucosal stimulation (channel III), seemed to be interrupted by the arrival of the excitatory phase from upper levels. In these instances inhibition at channel IV was more prolonged than that at III, consistent with the later arrival of the propagated excitatory phase.

The numbers and percentages of occasions on which one or more recording sites exhibited this typical response to each of the several stimuli are listed in table 1. On statistical analysis no significant differences were noted between these parameters as recorded from duodenojejunal and midjejunal areas, as indicated in table 2. No significant difference in degree of frequency of characteristic response was seen between neurally intact dogs and those with vagotomy and splanchnicotomy. Except in 3 instances, involving 1

Fig. 2. Records of intraluminal pressure changes at 4 levels, indicative of a typical mucosal reflex. Stimulus was 0.5 ml autogenous bile injected between levels II and III. Upper panel: direct pressure recording from the four sites. Lower panel: integrated record approximating mean pressures. Beginning and end of injection marked by signal; initial double signal indicates filling of dead space. Signal is shown in lower panel by downstrokes in record of channel III. Note difference in paper speed between upper and lower panels.

Fig. 3. Similar to figure 2, showing response to 0.5 ml 2% potassium oleate.

dog, there was no significant difference between any of the dogs as studied individually. The appearance of the pressure decrease distal to stimulation was more consistently present than the increase proximally. Locke-Ringer solution had no effect.

Responses to solutions of various osmolar concentrations ranging from distilled water to 5% NaCl are summarized in table 3. Also summarized in table 3 are results from solutions with hydrogen ion concentrations ranging from pH 3 (glutamic acid) to pH 10 (carbonate-bicarbonate buffer). Figure 4 shows the response in the same dog, sequentially, to carbonate-bicarbonate buffer at pH 9.1 compared with that to Ivory soap adjusted to pH 9.1 by carbonation.

The failure of these solutions of varying osmolalities and hydrogen ion concentrations to elicit the mucosal reflex except at the extremes listed (table 3), indicates that these were not, per se, adequate stimuli within the ranges and in the amounts used. They were therefore not responsible for the results obtained with the test solutions. Since we were testing these only as a control against our test substances, the same minute quantities were used. The possible effects of larger quantities cannot be inferred from these experiments.

In the experiments in which local conduction was blocked by cold, stimuli were applied above the chilled region before, during and after the establishment of a presumed cold block. Typical inhibition, as indicated by decrease in balloon pressure below the region of the block, was consistently present before the application of cold but failed regularly when block was present. It reappeared when the chilled area was rewarmed. A typical sequence is illustrated in figure 5. It may be pointed out here that proof of complete conduction block is not essential to the objective of these experiments. The fact that interference with local conduction, whether complete or not, can prevent the reflex effectively eliminates long reflex arcs as conduction pathways.

Of additional interest was the occasional spontaneous appearance during control periods of a sequence of pressure changes appearing first at site I and moving progressively to sites II, III, and IV (fig. 6), similar to what could have been expected had a mucosal stimulus been applied somewhere proximal to site I.

Due to limitation in the number of channels, respiration was not usually recorded. In a few experiments records of respiratory movement were substituted for pressure records in channel I. No relation between respiratory movements and the records of intraluminal

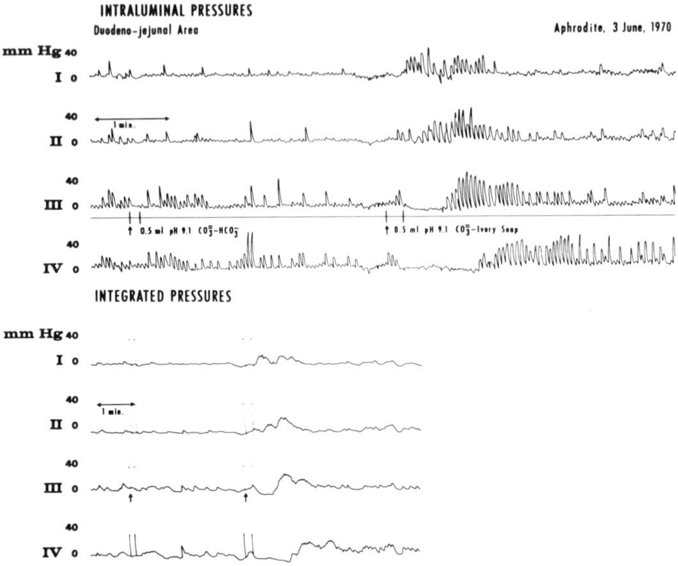

Fig. 4. Comparison of response to 0.5 ml carbonate-bicarbonate buffer with that to the same quantity of 2% Ivory soap solution both at pH 9.1. See figure 2 for explanation of traces.

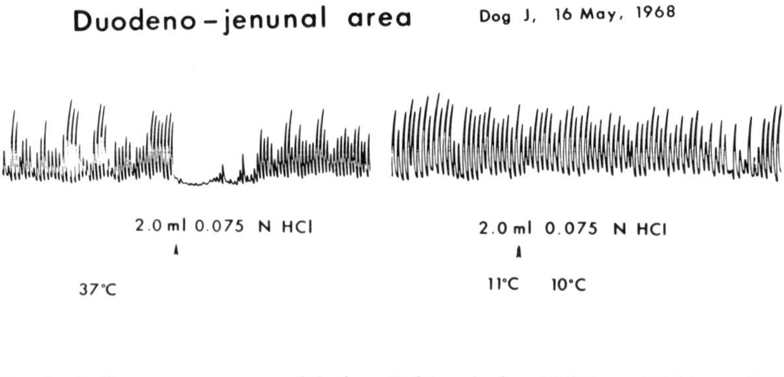

Fig. 5. Balloon pressure record before (left) and after (right) establishing cold block between the point of injection and the recording balloon. Stimulus: 2.0 ml 0.075 N HCl. Time of injection indicated by arrows.

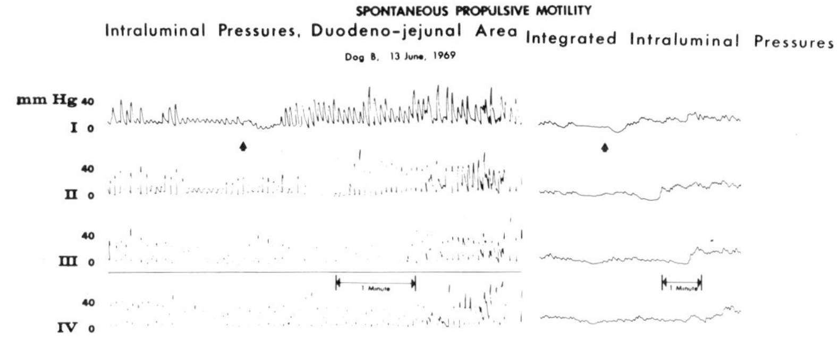

Fig. 6. Record of pressure changes of a type that occurred occasionally without experimental intervention. Left and right panels correspond to upper and lower panels respectively of figure 2. Arrows mark synchronous points on the 2 panels.

pressure changes was observed.

DISCUSSION

Our pressure records are not suitable for precise determination of absolute intraluminal pressures. They are subject to two uncontrolled errors. The first is hydrostatic error, resulting from the fact that the openings in the tube leading to the various channels were probably not all at the same horizontal level in the animal; the actual level was known only approximately. Our baselines were referred to the level of the fistula. The second is the effect of intraabdominal pressure; this was not controlled and may have affected different channels differently. However, our interpretations are based on brief local variations in pressure, and these were accurately recorded.

Our method of pressure measurement would probably not record motor responses in a relaxed intestine. For differences in pressure that result from muscular movement to be recorded, the tone of the muscle must be such that closed spaces can be created around the tubular openings. This is not likely to be the case in a quiescent gut. Doubtless some information is lost but since our results with balloon pressure recording, which are a direct result of changes in muscle activity, do not differ materially with these from intraluminal pressure, we think the loss is not significant.

Our observations were limited to those portions of the small intestine between the level of the fistula (pancreatic papilla) and a distance of 60 cm from the papilla. Our results therefore do not necessarily represent the response of lower levels of the small intestine.

The intrinsic mucosal reflex, as described by Hukuhara (1958), comprises not only responses to chemical stimulation but also qualitatively identical responses to mechanical stimulation (e. g. stroking) of the mucosa. We have investigated only responses to chemical stimuli but are aware that mechanical stimulation may be equally important. The question arises whether the intrinsic mucosal reflex response to mechanical stimulation may not be one aspect of the peristaltic reflex described by Trendelenburg (1917). The latter has been shown to be triggered by radial stretching of receptors in the vicinity of the mucosa (Ginzel, 1959; Kosterlitz and Robinson, 1959), which could also result from stroking the mucosa. A typical inhibitory phase preceding the contraction phase of the peristaltic reflex has not usually been reported but the experimental conditions may not have been suitable for its demonstration. The limitations of the excised material in which the reflex has been demonstrated must also be taken into account.

Much of the experimental work on small intestinal motility has been done on acutely operated, anesthetized animals in which the intestine is usually in a relaxed state. For reasons cited above an inhibitory phase of "peristalsis" is not likely to be manifest in such circumstances. This fact may explain the numerous denials in the literature of such a phase. Also, as Hukuhara et al. (1958) have pointed out if the stimulus is applied elsewhere than to the mucosa (e. g. the muscularis or serosa) responses of a different character are obtained.

Our observations and our interpretation of the literature have led us to the conclusion that propulsion of contents in the small intestine is usually accomplished principally by reflex modulation of local motor activity. The most noticeable effect is on the rhythmic contractions, and the result is a transient gradient of mean pressure in the affected areas.

The rhythmic contractions are triggered by the interaction of caudally conducted pacemaker potential waves arising in the duodenum, and the effects of other stimuli acting locally. The depolarizing effect of the pacemaker potential is below the threshold for causing muscular contraction, hence the rhythmic contractions are largely dependent on accessory stimuli. Such stimuli may act mechanically on the muscle or through the local nerve plexuses. Our interest is in the latter.

The intrinsic neural plexuses contain cells of afferent and efferent function (Kuntz, 1922–3; Schofield, 1960), and the latter comprise excitatory (depolarizing) and inhibitory (hyperpolarizing) neurons (Burnstock et al., 1966; Bennett et al., 1966; Day and Warren, 1968). Local stimuli that activate excitatory cells increase tension in the muscle and cause rhythmic contractions to appear in an otherwise quiescent intestine or increase the vigor of contractions in an active intestine. Activation of inhibitory cells has an opposite effect.

Our experiments indicate that some of the afferent cell processes are associated with receptors in the mucosa which are responsive to the chemical composition of the intestinal contents. They imply that these cells also have synaptic connections with excitatory motor neurons that activate the muscle orad to the point of stimulation,and with inhibitory neurons that influence the muscle for some distance below that point. The resulting local gradient of mean intraluminal pressure may be expected to move the contents from the higher to the lower pressure area. In our experience the whole process, once initiated, tends to move downstream for a variable distance, probably because there is a built-in aboral conducting mechanism in the plexus but also doubtless because the effective stimulus is carried downstream with the gut contents. The response becomes weaker as it travels (decremental conduction) hence the reflex is not likely to initiate rush peristalsis.

We do not believe that the intrinsic mucosal reflex is the sole mechanism of aboral transit. The postulated overall intraluminal pressure gradient (Alvarez, 1948) no doubt makes a substantial contribution. Likewise, the occasional contraction waves that seem to ride the crest of the pacemaker potential wave (Code, 1968) probably move the contents rapidly over a long distance. We have occasionally seen such waves in a very active intestine. Szurszewski (1969) observed in the small intestine of chronic conscious fasting dogs a caudad-moving electrical complex which started in the duodenum and continued the entire length of the small bowel. This he interpreted as producing a caudally migrating band of rhythmic segmentation which serves a propulsive function. In such records of "spontaneous" electrical activity, as in ours of motor activity, one would like certainty as to whether these action potentials are causing intestinal contractions, or are the result of chemical substances or distension in the intestine stimulating mucosal or muscle receptors. Whichever came first, we agree that it no doubt represents forward propulsion of intestinal content.

Bortoff and Ghalib (1972) have very recently demonstrated propagated contractions in cat jejunal wall from which mucosa and submucosa had been previously removed. They also cite experiments demonstrating peristaltic activity in cat jejunal preparations treated with tetrodotoxin. They conclude that peristalsis appears to be basically myogenic rather than neurogenic. We see no discrepancy between these findings and our results of chemical stimulation of only the mucosa in conscious chronic intact dogs. No doubt these mechanisms as well as hormonal influences are simultaneously active.

We believe that the mucosal reflex is of great physiologica significance. Because of its extreme sensitivity to stimuli normally available in the intestinal contents, it has an adaptive potential not possessed by any other proposed mechanism. It may prove to be a dominant factor in normal propulsion.

SUMMARY

Simultaneous changes in intraluminal pressure at four levels in the upper small intestine in response to intraluminal injection of chemical solutions of physiological significance were recorded in seven chronic, unanesthetized dogs. Four animals were neurally intact, three had bilateral supradiaphragmatic vagal section, two of the latter had bilateral splanchnic section. Test solutions included 0.075 N HCl, autogenous bile, 2% K oleate, 2% Na desoxycholate, and 2% Ivory soap; these were delivered between the upper two and lower two levels in 0.2 or 0.5 ml amounts. Typical responses were characterized by pressure increase proximal and decrease distal to the site of stimulation, with decremental conduction of the increase orally and of the decrease caudally. Salt solutions and buffers with a wide range of osmolar and hydrogen ion concentrations were tested in like manner and found to be ineffective within the ranges comprising the test materials. No differences were attributable to area of upper small intestine studied nor to neural status of subjects. These findings confirm the occurrence of the intrinsic mucosal reflex and, with other available evidence, suggest that the reflex may be the basic physiologic mechanism of propulsive motility in the small intestine.

REFERENCES

Alvarez,W.C., 1914.
Functional variations in contractions of different parts of the small intestine.
Am. J. Physiol. 35:177.

Alvarez,W.C., 1948.
An introduction to gastroenterology.
Fourth edition, New York, Hoeber.

Alvarez,W.C., and Hosoi,K., 1930.
Conduction in different parts of the small intestine.
Am. J. Physiol. 94:448.

Alvarez,W.C., and Starkweather,E., 1918.
The metabolic gradient underlying intestinal peristalsis.
Am. J. Physiol. 46:186.

Alvarez,W.C. and Zimmerman,A., 1927.
The absence of inhibition ahead of peristaltic rushes.
Am. J. Physiol. 83:52.

Auer,J., and Krueger,H.,
Experimental study of antiperistaltic and peristaltic motor and inhibitory phenomena.
Am. J. Physiol. 148:350.

Baldwin,M.V., and Thomas,J.E., 1969.
Effect of mucosal stimuli on intraluminal pressure in the small intestine (abstr).
Fed. Proc. 28:717.

Baldwin,M.V., and Thomas,J.E., 1969.
Osmolar and pH sensitivity of some intestinal mucosal receptors (abstr).
The Physiologist 12:165.

Baldwin,M.V., and Thomas,J.E., 1970.
Role of the intrinsic plexuses in propulsive motility of the small intestine (abstr).
Gastroenterology 58:924.

Bayliss,W.M., and Starling,E.H., 1899.
The movements and innervation of the small intestine.
J. Physiol. (London) 24:99.

Bennett,M.R., Burnstock,G., Holman,M.E., 1966.
Transmission from intramural inhibitory nerves to the smooth muscle of the guinea-pig taenia coli.
J. Physiol. (London) 182:541.

Bortoff,A., and Ghalib,E., 1972.
Temporal relationship between electrical and mechanical activity of longitudinal and circular muscle during intestinal peristalsis.
Am. J. Dig. Dis. 17:317.

Burnstock,G., Campbell,G., Rand,M.J., 1966.
The inhibitory innervation of the taenia of the guinea-pig caecum.
J. Physiol. (London) 182:504.

Cannon,W.B., 1912.
Peristalsis, segmentation, and the myenteric reflex.
Am. J. Physiol. 30:114.

Code,C.F., 1968.
A concept of control of gastrointestinal motility, in Handbook of Physiology: Alimentary Canal.
Vol. V, Sec. 6, pg. 2891.
Edited by C.F. Code and W. Heidel.

Crema,A., and Frigo,G.M., 1969.
On the nervous mechanism controlling the peristaltic reflex of the colon (abstr).
Rendic,R.R. Gastroenterology 1 (Supp):150.

Day,M.D., and Warren,P.R., 1968.
A pharmacological analysis of the responses to transmural stimulation in isolated intestinal preparation.
Br. J. Pharmacol. 32:227.

Forster,A.C., and Hertzman,A.B., 1938.
Studies on the activity of circular and longitudinal muscle of extra-peritonealized ileum in a human subject.
Am. J. Physiol. 123:68.

Ganter,G., 1923.
Experimentelle untersuchungen uber die peristaltik des menschlichen dunndarmes.
Arch. f. d. ges Physiol. 201:100.

Ginzel,K.H., 1959.
Investigations concerning the initiation of the

peristaltic reflex in the guinea-pig ileum.
J. Physiol. (London) 148:75.
Hasselbrach,R., and Thomas,J.E.
Control of intestinal rhythmic contractions by a duodenal pacemaker.
Am. J. Physiol. 201:955.
Henderson,V.E., 1928.
Mechanism of intestinal peristalsis.
Am. J. Physiol. 86:82.
Hukuhara,T., Yamagami,M., Nakayama,S., 1958.
On the intestinal intrinsic reflexes.
Jap. J. Physiol. 8:9.
Kosterlitz,H.W., and Robinson,J.A., 1959.
Reflex contractions of the longitudinal muscle coat of the isolated guinea-pig ileum.
J. Physiol. (London) 146:369.
Kuntz,A., 1922-3.
On the occurrence of reflex arcs in the myenteric and sub-mucous plexuses.
Anat. Rec. 24:193.
Linz,H., Blomer,A., Sux,A., 1971.
Analysis of the propulsive movements of the small intestine. Cineradiographic and experimental studies.
Am. J. Dig. Dis. 16:1107.
Meltzer,S.J., and Auer,J., 1907.
Peristaltic rush.
Am. J. Physiol. 20:259.
Nakayama,S., and Nanba,R., 1961.
Electrophysiological studies on the intestinal intrinsic reflex.
Jap. J. Physiol. 11:499.
Posey,E.L.,Jr., and Bargen,J.A., 1951.
Observations of normal and abnormal human intestinal motor function.
Am. J. Med. Sci. 221:10.
Ritchie,J.A., Truelove,S.C., Ardran,G.M., et al, 1969.
Propulsion and retropulsion of normal colonic contents (abstr).
Rendic R.R. Gastroenterology 1 (Suppl):153.
Schofield,G.C., 1960.
Experimental studies on the innervation of the mu-

cous membrane of the gut.
Brain 83:490.

Szurszewski, J.H.
A migrating electric complex of the canine small intestine.
Am. J. Physiol. 217:1757.

Thomas, J.E., 1941.
An improved cannula for gastric and intestinal fistulas.
Proc. Soc. Exp. Biol. Med. 46:260.

Thomas, J.E., 1951.
Methods for study of external secretory function of the pancreas, in Methods in Medical Research.
Vol. 4, pg. 149.
Edited by M.B. Visscher.

Thomas, J.E., 1951.
Myenteric reflex in dog's duodenum (abstr).
Fed. Proc. 10:136.

Thomas, J.E., 1955.
The gradient theory versus the reflex theory of intestinal peristalsis.
Am. J. Gastroenterology 23:13.

Thomas, J.E. and Baldwin, M.V., 1969.
The intestinal "mucosal reflex" in the unanesthetized dog (abstr).
Rendic R.R. Gastroenterology 1 (Suppl):144.

Thomas, J.E., and Friedman, M.H.F., 1961.
The normal physiology of the digestive system in Handbuch der Allgemeinen Pathologie.
Berlin, Springer-Verlag.

Torsoli, A., Ramorine, M.L., Ammaturo, M.V., et al, 1969.
Mass movements and intracolonic pressures (abstr).
Rendic R.R. Gastroenterology 1 (Suppl):150.

Trendelenburg, P., 1917.
Physiologische und pharmakologische versuche uber die dunndarmperistaltik.
Naunym Schiedeberg's Arch. Exp. Path. 81:55.

White, H.L., Rainey, W.R., Monaghan, B., et al., 1934.
Observations on the nervous control of the ileocaecal sphincter and on intestinal movements in an unanesthetized human subject.
Am. J. Physiol. 108:449.

CHOLEDOCHODUODENAL JUNCTION

Martin F. Tansy and Francis M. Kendall

INTRODUCTION

Under normal conditions the flow of bile, from its source within the liver to its issue into the duodenum, is subject to the influence of two structures situated along the path of flow. These, the gall-bladder and the choledochoduodenal junction, not only affect the actual movement of bile but,by their combined activities, modify the character of the secretion as well. Though considerable experimental interest has centered on the anatomical region which bears the name of the choledochoduodenal junction, to date there is but slight accord concerning either the function or the possible significance of this region as part of a regulatory system.

The idea that there is a sphincter at the choledochoduodenal junction has been held since the time of Francis Glisson in 1681. In the year 1887, however, Ruggero Oddi took a closer look at the structure of the choledochoduodenal junction. He used two methods: maceration, and, sectioning and microscopic examination. With the maceration method he examined and described the sphincter muscle of the dog, sheep, ox, and hog. Oddi did not attempt to demonstrate the sphincter muscle in man by this method. He also studied serial cross-sections of the choledochoduodenal junction of the dog and other animals. Although he states that he has studied sections of the human bile duct, and that he found sphincter fibers around the end of the bile duct, his published research deals entirely with tissues derived from animals. The dog, together with the sheep, are the species upon which Oddi really based his description: ". . . a more or less pronounced bed of circular fibers encircling the choledochal canal—which one is able to consider as almost completely independent if one excepts some slender loops which lose themselves between the fibers proper of the intestine."

The association of Oddi's name to this structure was explained in 1937 in Boyden's account of this region when he wrote that "Oddi's name has been applied to it not because he was the first to examine it microscopically—that distinction belongs to the American anatomist Simon H. Gage—but because he was the first (1) to measure its resistance, (2) to show that removal of the gallbladder caused marked dilatation of the bile ducts, and (3) to postulate that dysfunction of this occluding apparatus might explain certain morbid affections of the biliary tract." Boyden's explanation for the immortalization of Oddi is thus justified by the fact that while Gage described the structure some eight years before Oddi published the original paper, Oddi attempted to pin down its function. Thus, Gage may have been the unlucky victim of history because the signal event which separated the two in time was the appearance of Claude Bernard's philosophical concept of the constancy of the internal environment.

The historical turning point was marked by a shift from descriptions of structures and functions as ends in themselves, to descriptions whose underlying reasons for existence was that the functions of various structures were in fact necessary. Thus, physiology in general entered a new era which led eventually to Walter Cannon's principle of homeostasis which in turn led to the present emphasis on the study of the regulation and control of function. In the particular case of the choledochoduodenal junction, the research impetus took two parallel pathways: an anatomical description of structure and an experimental determination of function. Both approaches implicity assumed that the extrahepatic biliary system had some sort of function and both sought to describe it. Viewed in totality from a modern viewpoint, both approaches can be described as efforts to provide the information required to identify a physical system. The most striking shortcoming of the work in this area appears to be that today the realization of a physical system is almost as far away as it was in Oddi's time. The principle reason appears to be that observations were made, on the basis of a philosophical necessity, that a homeostatic system must exist and not as the results of systematic attempts to determine whether in fact a set of formal observations could be used to infer the necessity of the existence of such a system.

THE SO-CALLED SPHINCTER OF ODDI

Is there a Distinct Sphincter Entity?

In reviewing an extensive literature concerning the choledochoduodenal junction we have formed the opinion that an encirclement of the intramural portion of the common duct by muscle does indeed occur in the vicinity of the exterior duodenal wall. However, there is no agreement as to whether these fibers constitute a discrete sphincter. Boyden (1937) explained the impasse with respect to the acceptance of sphincteric function on two basic grounds: (1) no accepted demonstration of the histologic independence of these fibers has been made, and (2) it has been impossible to demonstrate functional independence of these muscle fibers. In addition, generalization across species lines has not been possible because a muscular ring has not been successfully demonstrated in all species.

The most popular of the early experimental animals was the dog. This species is the one which provided the bulk of Oddi's observations. Interestingly enough, the dog also happens to be one noteworthy example of a species where the very presence of a physical entity which is capable of sphincteric action has been strongly questioned. Indeed, since Oddi's time, there have been several excellent histological studies by many workers, among whom may be mentioned Auster and Crohn (1922), Halpert, Rewbridge and Healey (1933) and most recently Bhatnagar, Samuel and Goyal (1972a). These have provided good reason to question whether in fact a sphincter does exist as a structural entity in the case of the dog. In general, it may be safely stated that even at this relatively late date, no agreement exists concerning this point.

The original, and still the most complete, descriptions of the structures associated with the terminal portion of the canine common bile duct are attributable to William Hendrickson (1898). His drawings of a series of cross sections of the common duct, which began at the entrance to the intestinal wall and continued serially to the inner portion of the duodenum, are most illuminating (figure 1). In short, these drawings indicate that as the common duct passes through the duodenal wall, a ring of surrounding duodenal

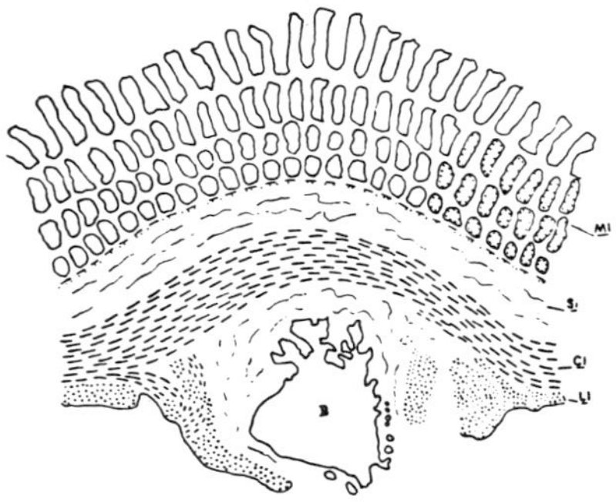

At entrance of common bile-duct into the intestinal wall of dog. x30

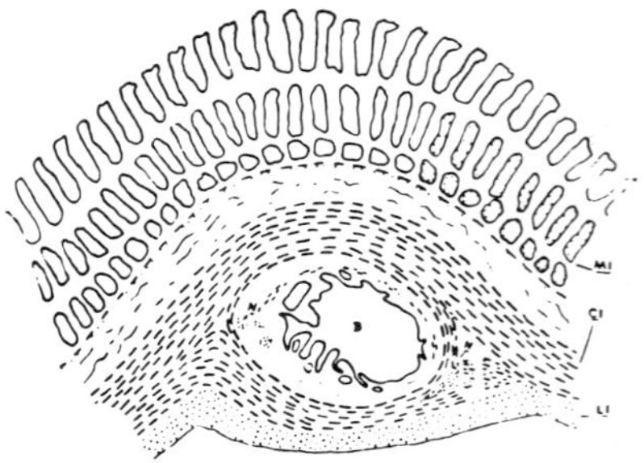

Near middle of duodenal portion of common bile-duct of dog. x30

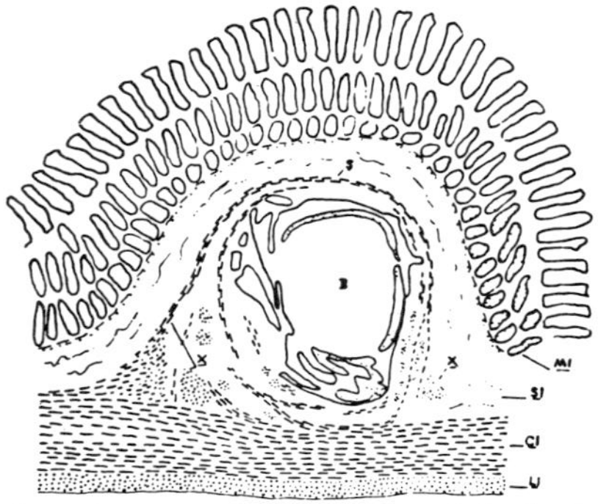

Somewhat removed from orifice of duodenal portion of common bile-duct of dog. x30

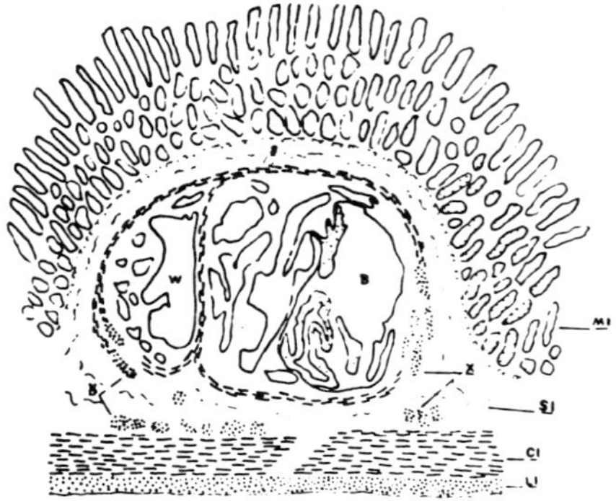

Near orifice of duodenal portion of common bile-duct of dog. x30

Figure 1

Fig. 1. Composite photograph of a series of line drawings of cross sections through the intramural portion of the canine common bile duct. Legend: MI, Mucous membrane; SI, Submucosa; CI, Circular muscle; LI, Longitudinal muscle; B, Common bile duct; N, Common bile duct muscle bundles; S, Sphincter fibers; X, Detached sphincter fibers; W, Duct of Wirsung. (From W. Hendrickson, Johns Hopkins Hospital Bulletin 9: 221, 1898).

---

muscle becomes progressively less well-defined and a rudimentray and incomplete muscular ring at the terminal duct soon becomes apparent. In this connection, it is of interest to mention that in certain of the experiments reported by Boyden (1937), it was found that there was no ampulla of Vater in the dog and, therefore, no papillary sphincter except for a few terminal rings of muscle about both the bile and pancreatic ducts. In subsequent experiments, Eichhorn and Boyden (1955) concluded that in the dog the developmental relationship between the intestinal musculature and the sphincteric muscle is so intimate as to almost defy analysis. First, the sphincteric muscle differentiates from mesenchyme as a series of isolated bands. Second, instead of completing the wall of a slit-like passage, the bundles of muscle curve around the bile duct in oblique C-shaped contours to join the tunica muscularis of the intestine. It should be added that this muscular arrangement to a very large degree makes the discharge of bile dependent upon the activity of the duodenum.

Nature of Sphincter Resistance

The fact that microscopic observations upon preparations made from dogs indicated that the muscle fibers at the mouth of the common duct were scanty, widely separated and diffuse, and at no time continuous, would indicate that at this portion of the duct a discrete muscular control by the sphincter proprius of ductal dynamics is probably impossible. Yet, in 1888, Oddi estimated that this sphincter offered a resistance of 50 mm Hg to fluids entering the lumen of the intestine. Archibald (1919) obtained data in agreement with this. Mann (1919) carried out extensive studies in six species of animals possessing a gallbladder and recorded a minimal resistance of 75 to 100 mm H_2O. Jacobsen and Gydesen (1922) found a resistance in dogs of 90 to 210 mm H_2O. On the other hand, Cole (1925) encountered 40 to 100 mm H_2O resistance in dogs. The range of values reported indicates the presence of at least one uncontrolled factor in these studies. In any event, these findings would seem to attribute to the sphincter a physiological significance out of proportion to the anatomical structure described (Burgett, 1925).

A functional argument in support of this contention can be advanced on the basis of three different approaches to the problem in the literature. Burgett (1926) severed the canine intramural duct proximal to the opening and relocated the cut end to another position in the mucosa. He reported that within 6 to 8 weeks following the procedure "ductal resistance" was essentially normal and appeared to be dependent basically on intestinal tonus. Much later, Brown et al. (1956), performed transduodenal sphincterotomies in dogs. They reported that "ductal resistence" decreased immediately following the procedures but returned to essentially preoperative levels within 6 to 8 weeks. Judd and Mann (1917) in a paper on the effect of cholecystectomy reported that following the removal of the gallbladder in the dog, the extrahepatic biliary ducts dilated within sixty days. On the other hand, the authors found that in those animals in which the muscle fibers were dissected free from the intramural portion of the duct at the time the gallbladder was removed, dilatation of the duct did not occur. This, they felt, would point strongly toward the seat of the resistance lying in that portion of the duct within the duodenal wall. The very recent work of Bhatnagar et al. (1972b) is in entire accord on this point.

Innervation of Common Bile Duct and Sphincter

Considerable emphasis has been placed in the literature on the presence of an extensive nerve plexus around the common bile duct. The inference is that there exists some nervous control over the action of the sphincter. It is interesting to note that in 1894 Oddi himself advanced a claim for independent nervous control of the canine sphincter. He proposed that a nervous center which mediated this control resided in the spinal cord opposite to the first lumbar vertebra.

Another ancient dictum states that the sphincter of Oddi receives both sympathetic and parasympathetic innervation. We cannot find experimental support for this assertion. The story goes that a reciprocal relationship exists whereby sympathetic activity produces sphincteric contraction while parasympathetic activity produces relaxation. The parasympathetic theory is often attributed to the contention of Westphal (1923), among others, that vagal stimulation produces gallbladder contraction and relaxation of the sphincter of Oddi. The sympathetic school is still heavily dependent upon the early report of Doyan (1894) that the splanchnic nerves produced an increase in the tone of the canine sphincter of Oddi.

In this connection it should be pointed out that Meltzer (1917) postulated a reciprocal action between the gallbladder and the sphincter. Meltzer suggested that inasmuch as the sphincter of Oddi must relax when the gallbladder contracts, if bile is to be extruded into the duodenum, the activities of these two parts of the biliary tract must be co-ordinated and under the "law of contrary innervation." This is a prime example of the type of tedious teleology which has consistently undermined any serious attempt at system identification. In regard to the reciprocal innervation of the sphincteric mechanism suggested by Meltzer, Alvarez (1940), in his legendary text on gastroenterology, indicates that "First, it was recognized by physiologists that there was little real evidence in favor of Meltzer's idea. He relied for confirmation of his "hunch" mainly on the work of Doyon, but that observer had used a poor technic and his results were discredited, particularly by the work of Bainbridge and Dale, and Oddi (1897)." Alvarez was not convinced either.

During the intervening years the idea of a reciprocal reflex relationship between the gallbladder and the sphincter of Oddi has been considered to be improbable, particularly if such a relationship depended on either vagal or splanchnic pathways. More recently Wyatt (1967) published evidence which suggests that a reflex effect upon the sphincteric region may result from the delivery of electrical and mechanical stimuli to the neck of the canine gallbladder. The reflex was mediated via a pathway through the coeliac ganglion that was independent of both vagal and splanchnic integrity. To date, there has been no further evidence leading from this observation which would support a functional significance much less a reciprocal relationship to anything else. The details of Wyatt's work do, however, provide good reason for caution with respect to the physical manipulation of the bile ducts during experimentation.

Hormonal Regulation

The difficulties and disagreements which arose as the results of attempts to demonstrate a neurally-mediated control of extrahepatic biliary function were among the factors which produced an interest in hormonally-produced effects. Cholecystokinin is known to produce contraction of the gallbladder and supposedly also produces relaxation of the sphincter of Oddi. However, the sphincteric effects of cholecystokinin are also accompanied by alterations in the activity of the duodenal musculature. More recently, it has been shown that the intravenous administration of cholecystokinin causes relaxation of the duodenal musculature of the cat, notably in the region of the ampulla (Persson and Ekman, 1972).

Interpretation of the literature which pertains to hormonal effects is difficult for two reasons: (1) Earlier investigations used crude extracts which may have possessed musculotropic effects which are quite different from those of the more highly refined C-terminal octapeptide CCK-PZ which has been used more recently. (2) The result obtained can be dependent on both the physical method of measuring the effect as well as the actual location of the measurement site. More on this latter point later.

Introduction of an agent via a route that permits widespread systemic action is an incorrect procedure if the purpose is to determine whether a highly discrete and localized effect occurs in situ. The same objection may be advanced with respect to the systemic administration of other agents, such as morphine or epinephrine, especially when the in vivo and in vitro sphincteric effects are already known to be different. Recently, Persson (1971) advanced evidence showing that in vivo morphine is active locally on the cat choledochoduodenal junction but inactive when added to the bath fluid of the isolated feline sphincter of Oddi. On the other hand, isolated spiral strips cut from the terminal bile duct respond to epinephrine by contracting (Crema and Benzi, 1960). However, when the terminal bile duct remains surrounded by the wall of the duodenum into which it is inserted, the action of intravenous epinephrine seems to depend on the tone and motility of the duodenum (Benzi et al., 1964).

An example of an early drug study is that of Winkelstein and Aschner in 1924. These authors used dogs and reported that the subcutaneous administration of pilocarpine increased ductal resistance while the administration of adrenalin and atropine by the same route decreased ductal resistance. They attributed their observations to the operation of the sphincter of Oddi. Shortly thereafter, Burgett (1926) reported that he produced the same effects with the same drugs, administered in the same way, but with dogs whose common bile ducts had been surgically re-inserted through the duodenal wall at a new location. He was, therefore, skeptical about a discrete sphincter effect. Winkelstein and Aschner's experiment has been essentially duplicated countless times during succeeding years. The results have been confirmed numerous times, and the various authors have continued to attribute their observations to the operation of a discrete sphincteric mechanism in spite of Burgett's evidence.

SPHINCTERIC ACTION

Determination

Central to the problem of defining the nature of sphincteric action is the use of a physical system of measurement which will permit repeatable estimates to be made of a given phenomenon. As is generally recognized, sphincters tend to be unstable systems in that for the most part they are either open or closed. When considering the mechanical response of any biological tissue it is also prudent to keep in mind that the viscoelastic properties of soft tissues always present the possibility that the mechanical responses of these systems will be nonlinear, at least to the extent that a given dynamic response will be a unique reaction to a particular forcing function. Thus, a combination of tissue nonlinearity and the essential nonlinearity of sphincteric action spell double trouble, a fact which is well attested to when the serious reader tries to make sense out of the large body of literature which has accumulated on this subject.

Quite a few interesting techniques have been used to observe or estimate sphincteric action. Examples include direct visualization by means of a duodenal cannula (Shore et al., 1971), measures of fluid flow when the common duct was infused by a constant pressure source (Wyatt, 1967), and the converse of measuring perfusion pressure changes produced as a consequence of a constant flow system (Liedberg and Halabi, 1970). And of course, there have been numerous in vitro studies of the effects of drugs upon the sphincteric tissues of quite a few different species.

A venerable estimate of sphincteric function has consisted of a series of measurements of sphincteric opening pressures. The strength of the opening pressure technique lies in the fact that, if performed carefully, a very repeatable system results which has the virtue of eliminating the consequences of most of the inherently nonlinear effects which were previously alluded to.

The physical factors which may act to influence sphincteric opening pressures may in some cases be consequences of uncontrolled physiological activity. As examples we may cite such ongoing phenomena as respiration, intra-abdominal pressure changes produced by muscular activity other than respiration, concurrent gastroduodenal motility, the presence or absence of gastric and duodenal drainage, the integrity of the extrahepatic biliary ducts, and the irritability of the anatomical structures of interest that has resulted from mechanical trauma during preparation. Another factor which may be suspected of influencing the actual physiological systems at a fundamental level would be the prior history of the experimental animal (e.g. fasted, dehydrated, debilitated). When viewed in this totality, it becomes understandable why Hopton (1973) was moved to remark that experiments of this nature ". . . were insufficiently controlled or else not comparable in terms of their results." To which we might add that this state of affairs really renders a true appreciation of a review of this subject to be impossible: The reader must, of necessity, refer to each specific reference cited in order to make a highly critical evaluation of his own as to whether the results cited are believable, comparable, or applicable to his particular interest.

It is significant as Wyatt (1967) points out that a Marriott bottle with a drop chamber inserted in its outflow tract, containing normal saline at room temperature as a perfusate, is not without its faults as a device for obtaining perfusion at constant pressure. This is a factor which warrants serious consideration. By a simple expedient of conducting both control and experimental opening pressure determinations with the same values of pressure rise rate, we eliminated the nonrepeatability of estimation which frequently occurred when we attempted to perform the same experiment with manual control of the pressure ramp. We also eliminated the problem of trying to obtain repeatable estimates of the flow resistance of an inherently unstable system. As a result of initial experiments (Tansy et al., 1973a), we empirically determined that a pressure ramp value of 7 cm per second was satisfactory for our purposes. This value was in substantial agreement with that utilized by Berci and Johnson (1965) and Wyatt (1967).

Sphincter Opening Pressures

We have recently presented evidence that the normal opening pressure of the sphincter of Oddi in the anesthetized dog with intact vagosympathetic trunks varied between 13 and 26 cm of saline, with an average of 19 cm (Tansy et al., 1973b). Under comparable experimental conditions other workers (Wyatt, 1967; Dardik et al., 1970) have obtained data in approximate agreement with this range. One might add too that these figures are also reasonably close to those already reported for the conscious dog (Crispin et al., 1970).

One of our specific objectives was to determine whether vagal integrity could be inferred to affect the intrinsic mean opening pressure of the sphincter of Oddi. The earlier literature reveals that considerable attention was paid to this question. Briefly, the literature indicates that vagotomy caused increases (Williams and Huang, 1969), decreases (Schein et al., 1969), and no effects (Stassa and Grafe, 1968), upon sphincteric opening pressures in the dog. In a recent review of this subject, Hopton (1973) was moved to declare that: "It is evident from these apparently contradictory results that the various investigators have been conducting experiments which were insufficiently controlled, or else not comparable in terms of results." We feel obliged to support this opinion. Table 1 lists the mean sphincteric opening pressures that were measured in 16 dogs in an initial control state and following prompt cervical vagotomy. In all instances, the control values were obtained subsequent to surgical preparation and prior to the performance of any other experimental procedures. Vagotomy followed the last control measurement. The salient facts reflected by these data may be summarized as follows: This series in its entirety is representative of the conclusion of other workers in that significant increases, significant decreases and non-significant changes are reflected. Examination of this table also suggests that the tendency of the trials to show a reduced standard deviation in measured opening pressures may represent a manifestation of the well known physiological observation that vagotomy produces at least a transitory gastrointestinal atonia. If this reduction in motor activity is in fact responsible for this observation, then

Table 1: Comparison of Mean Opening Pressure of the Choledochoduodenal Junction before and after Vagotomy

Dog No.	Baseline O.P.	Post Vagotomy O.P.
33837	19.9±3.2(12)	22.4±2.8(12)*
10091	26.3±4.0(13)	14.9±1.1(7)*
36201	21.1±3.8(18)	20.8±2.2(12)
72101	20.9±3.9(12)	19.8±2.1(6)
37600	15.1±3.2(12)	15.3±1.9(7)
67491	18.8±5.9(13)	19.7±4.5(7)
36557	23.2±7.5(19)	24.2±7.6(10)
38230	18.3±4.7(12)	16.8±2.5(12)
38251	18.6±2.5(12)	13.8±1.6(6)*
36672	14.5±3.7(15)	15.7±1.5(12)
11880	12.9±2.1(12)	16.1±4.8(14)*
11321	16.9±2.1(12)	16.5±2.4(11)
11411	23.8±2.1(12)	23.4±2.3(25)
37789	20.0±4.1(12)	17.9±2.6(15)
11949	17.8±3.4(12)	18.2±7.2(12)
39593	14.5±2.6(13)	13.0±2.1(11)
Range	12.9 - 26.3	13.0 - 24.2

O.P. – Opening pressure measurements in centimeters of water; ± standard deviation; ( ) number of observations. Same in all tables.
*Indicates significant change in mean opening pressure.

the dependence of sphincteric opening pressure upon the muscular tone of the duodenum would partially explain the variable results which have been reported by others. In any event, the data strongly suggest that the vagus nerves do not exert a direct control over the tone of the canine sphincter of Oddi (Tandy et al., 1973c).

Influence of Nerve Stimulation on Opening Pressure

Another one of our specific objectives in the same study was to determine if stimulation of various nerves could be inferred to influence the mean opening pressure of the sphincter. Table 2 summarizes the mean sphincteric opening pressures that were associated with control states and which were measured during stimulation of the dorsal and ventral abdominal vagi at the level of the diaphragm. As can be seen in the table, we were not able to conclude that any one of the various stimulus parameters was associated with a significant change in mean opening pressure. These observations with respect to the effects of peripheral vagal stimulation are in agreement with Hopton and White (1971) who also used a heroic combination of 209 electrical stimulus combinations and concluded that the vagal branches do not have a direct effect on the rhythmical activity of the sphincter of Oddi. Although not depicted, various combinations of electrical stimulus parameters applied to the central ends of the vagosympathetic trunks failed to be associated with significant changes in mean sphincteric opening pressures. Similarly, we were not able to demonstrate a significant change in mean sphincteric opening pressure during peripheral electrical stimulation of the right greater splanchnic nerve. In sum, we feel that our observations obligate us to support Alvarez (1940) who also stated that: "Actually a review of practically everything written on the innervation of the bile tract left me in 1927 with the same impression that Carlson had gained in 1925; namely, that the result of stimulating the nerves to this region were so slight, so transient, and so variable that no one should attempt to build theories on them." We have not found anything since then that appears to seriously compromise that statement.

LOCAL CIRCULATION DYNAMICS AND SPHINCTER ACTION

Relation between Blood Pressure and Sphincter Resistance

Table 2

Effect of Peripheral Vagal Stimulation on the Opening Pressures at the Choledochoduodenal Junction

Dog No.	Baseline O.P.	D.A.P.V. O.P.	Baseline O.P.	V.A.P.V. O.P.
		6 volts - 12 Hertz		
11091	19.5±8.9(8)	22.3±7.9(6)	14.8±1.0(7)	15.2±1.8(5)
		6 volts - 200 Hertz		
11091	19.5±8.9(8)	17.8±2.2(6)	19.5±9.0(8)	16.7±4.6(3)
		10 volts - 6 Hertz		
14652	15.3±4.8(12)	18.2±3.7(12)	15.3±4.8(12)	17.5±3.3(12)
		15 volts - 15 Hertz		
2806	33.8±4.6(12)	35.0±4.3(12)	33.8±4.6(12)	33.7±7.3(13)
		20 volts - 15 Hertz		
33521	18.1±2.8(12)	18.7±5.3(12)	18.1±2.8(12)	19.6±3.7(12)
2806	19.6±3.6(12)	18.5±5.3(14)	17.0±3.9(4)	17.0±5.1(14)
		30 volts - 20 Hertz		
33837	22.4±2.8(12)	21.3±3.3(12)	22.4±2.8(12)	24.7±3.2(11)
1168	34.9±5.2(13)	34.6±8.3(7)		
31122	23.6±7.4(28)	30.2±1.3(6)	23.6±7.4(28)	25.4±1.1(7)
		40 volts - 15 Hertz		
35117	22.6±2.6(12)	20.0±0(3)	22.6±2.6(12)	24.0±3.5(3)

D.A.P.V. – Dorsal Abdominal Peripheral Vagus stimulation; V.A.P.V. – Ventral Abdominal Peripheral Vagus stimulation. Mean experimental values are not significantly different from mean control values in all cases.

During our initial investigations, we observed that the inhalation of amyl nitrite vapor produced an immediate and profound but extremely transitory reduction in mean sphincteric opening pressures. One of the consequences of the inhalation of amyl nitrite vapor is also a severe reduction in mean arterial pressure. Consequently, we decided to investigate the possible effects produced by changes in circulatory parameters which were not accompanied by possible direct effects of amyl nitrite upon the choledochoduodenal junction (Tansy et al., 1973d).

Significant reduction in sphincteric opening pressures were observed in our experiments during reductions in femoral arterial pressure which were produced by occluding either the abdominal vena cava or the aorta at the level of the diaphragm. Opening pressures tended to return to control values within a few minutes after the cessation of the occlusion procedures. Such hemodynamic influences on sphincteric opening pressures are reflected in the recordings sequentially depicted in figure 2. As can be seen from this figure, arterial pressure was reduced consequent to a series of rapid arterial hemorrhages. It can be readily seen that the loss of blood volume was accompanied by a progressive diminution of sphincteric opening pressures. This figure also reveals that the opening pressures gradually increased during and subsequent to infusion of the withdrawn blood.

The consequences of increased blood volume are depicted in figure 3. A systemic venous infusion of saline resulted in an increase in femoral and mesenteric arterial pressures. Ductal opening pressures were in turn markedly elevated. Shortly after the infusion was complete, the ductal opening pressures had returned to control values. Norepinephrine was then introduced into the terminal duct and maintained in stasis for 15 minutes following which time another systemic venous saline infusion was performed. During this latter procedure another series of opening pressures were determined. Arterial pressures increased as a result of the infusion but ductal opening pressures did not increase despite the fact that the norepinephrine had been flushed from the duct. Other workers have obtained data in agreement with our observations. Benzi et al., (1964) showed, in four cats, that the intravenous infusion of 10 ml. per kilogram of Tyrode solution decreased the rate of flow through the bile duct and slightly increased the blood pressure. Their work, however, did not provide a causal relationship between vascular and ductal effects, much less an explanation or postulate concerning the mechanism of such a relationship. These authors merely recalled that the importance of the vascular component has been emphasized by Arianoff (1959).

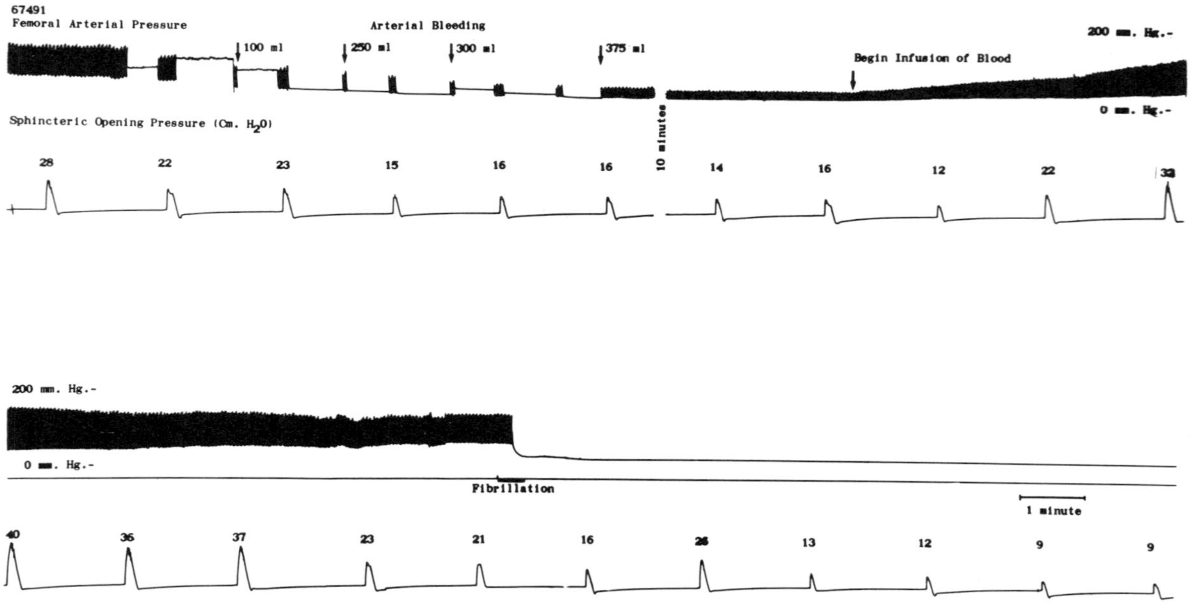

Fig. 2. This figure depicts the change in systemic arterial pressure and sphincteric opening pressures which were associated with reductions and increases in cardiovascular fluid volume. The lower trace shows an observed post mortem decline in sphincteric opening pressures.

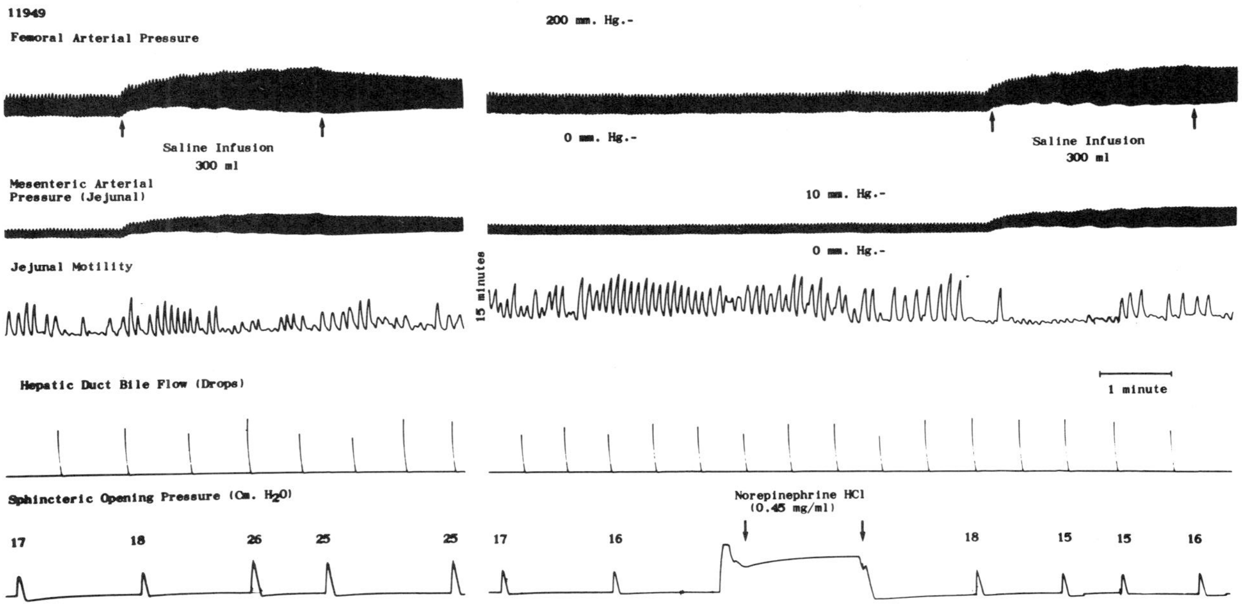

Fig. 3. Polygram depicting the time course of femoral arterial pressure, mesenteric arterial pressure, bile flow rate, and ductal opening pressures, during rapid (100 ml/min) saline infusion into a femoral vein prior to and subsequent to the intraductal administration of norepinephrine. The fortuitous cessation of jejunal motor activity which is depicted is not considered to be associated with the administration of the drug. The pressure limb rise and plateau configuration seen in this and the next figure represent the system pressure during the introduction and subsequent stasis of a test agent (indicated by arrows). The drop in pressure limb represents the rapid washout of the small fluid volume and the reversal of the infusion pump.

Figure 4 depicts the ductal opening pressures which were observed following the intraductal introduction and stasis of histamine and norepinephrine. The top traces illustrate the characteristic increases in ductal opening pressures that were observed consequent to histamine administration. The center traces show that the histamine effect was abolished by the subsequent administration of norepinephrine, and the bottom traces illustrate our observation that the prior intraductal administration of norepinephrine successfully prevented an increase in ductal opening pressures subsequent to a dose of histamine which closely follows the former agent.

Hydraulic Nature of Sphincter Opening/Closing

The common thread which runs through our observation is hydraulic in nature. The ubiquitous similarity in the direction of change in venous blood pressure and ductal opening pressure indicates that the latter effect was probably produced by a hydraulic event. Thus, either increased venous blood pressure or the intraductal administration of histamine are associated with an increase in ductal opening pressure. The observation that the prior intraductal administration of norepinephrine prevents this response in either case suggests that the local mechanism which determines the value of opening pressure is vascular in nature. The lack of a change in systemic blood pressure and duodenal motility which can be associated either during or subsequent to intraductal drug administration also suggests that the mechanism is local.

The hydraulic contention is supported in part by the literature. In earlier experiments Dardik et al. (1970), were interested in evaluating possible neuroendocrine influences on the dynamics of the choledochal sphincter in the dog. While there are no experimental data to support the view, the authors conceded that vascular effects which were produced as a consequence of their experimental procedures could not be excluded as possible mechanisms which linked cause and effect. In this connection, it is of interest to mention that recent evidence, advanced by Gilsdorf, Urdaneta and Leonard (1970) on neuroeffector drug influences on biliary sphincter resistances in the awake cat, also suggests a vascular component. This group concluded that the triple response of ductal pressures occurring after intravenous epinephrine administration, i.e., an initial

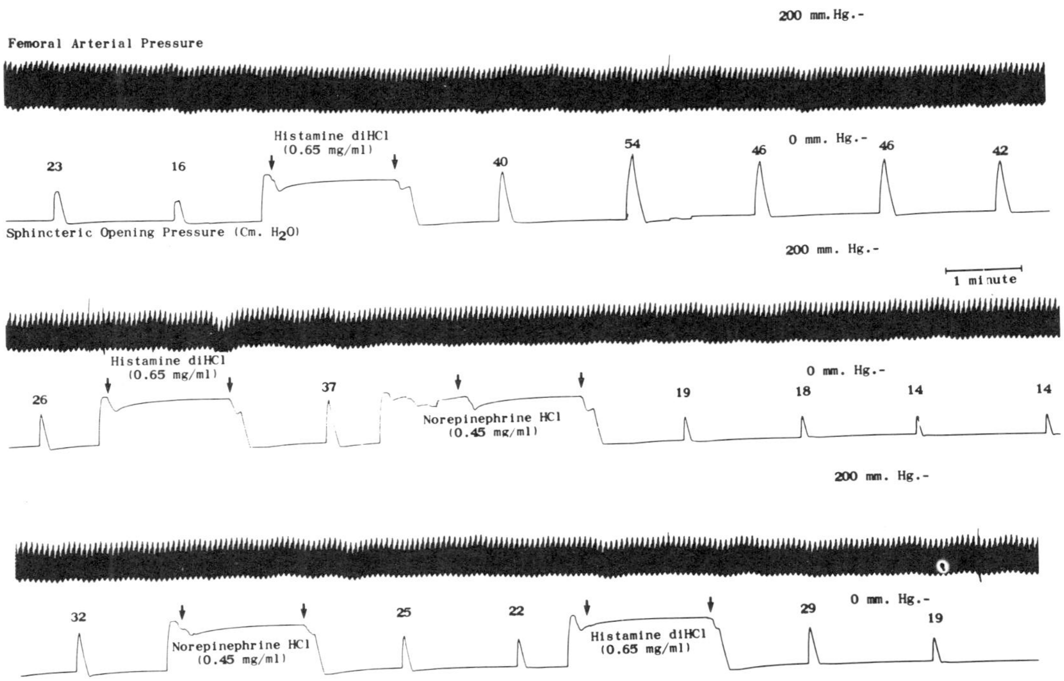

Fig. 4. Polygram showing ductal opening pressures which were measured subsequent to the intraductal administration of histamine and norepinephrine. The top traces show an increase in opening pressures subsequent to histamine. The center traces show that an intraductal administration of histamine produces a heightened ductal opening pressure which is reducted by norepinephrine. The bottom traces show that prior administration of norepinephrine apparently prevents an increase in ductal opening pressures following a prompt subsequent dose of histamine.

rise, a short fall, then the prolonged elevation, parallels the drug-induced blood pressure changes which they observed. They also reported that norepinephrine and isoproterenol produced a more unidirectional response and, like epinephrine, these changes were parallel to the observed cardiovascular pressure changes. Furthermore, apparent ductal resistance was reduced consequent to the intravenous administration of acetylcholine with the decrease paralleling the characteristic systemic hypotension. Yet, they simply concluded that sphincter constriction is mediated by alpha adrenergic agents and relaxation by beta adrenergic and cholinergic agents. Again, the possible significance of the altered circulatory events was disregarded.

It can be generally stated that those experiments which can be cited to advance claims of alterations in ductal dynamics as the result of various experimental procedures or the systemic application of some rather potent vasoactive agents, are either devoid of records which display the cardiovascular events which were associated with given experimental procedures, or were accompanied by records that frequently show that systemic blood pressure was indeed affected in one direction or another. Thus, the validity of the conclusions advanced in those reports which did not include cardiovascular data becomes questionable.

Role of Vasculature of Ductal Mucosa

A histological description of the mucosa of the terminal duct probably illuminates the observations which we made with respect to the marked elevation of mean opening pressures which we could produce by the intraductal administration of histamine, serotonin, and bethanechol (Tansy et al., 1973e). Bhatnagar, Samuel and Goyal (1972a) described the ductal mucosa as being generally of a type which is associated with a high degree of local vascularity.

The very repeatable nature of the observations which we made and the anatomically well-defined region of the duct where we placed our measurement catheters provided the necessary impetus for us to take a look at the microscopic anatomy of the choledochoduodenal junction for a structural explanation for our observations. Our results clearly indicated what we should expect to find and our expectations turned out to be well-founded.

Figure 5 is a longitudinal section through the choledochoduodenal

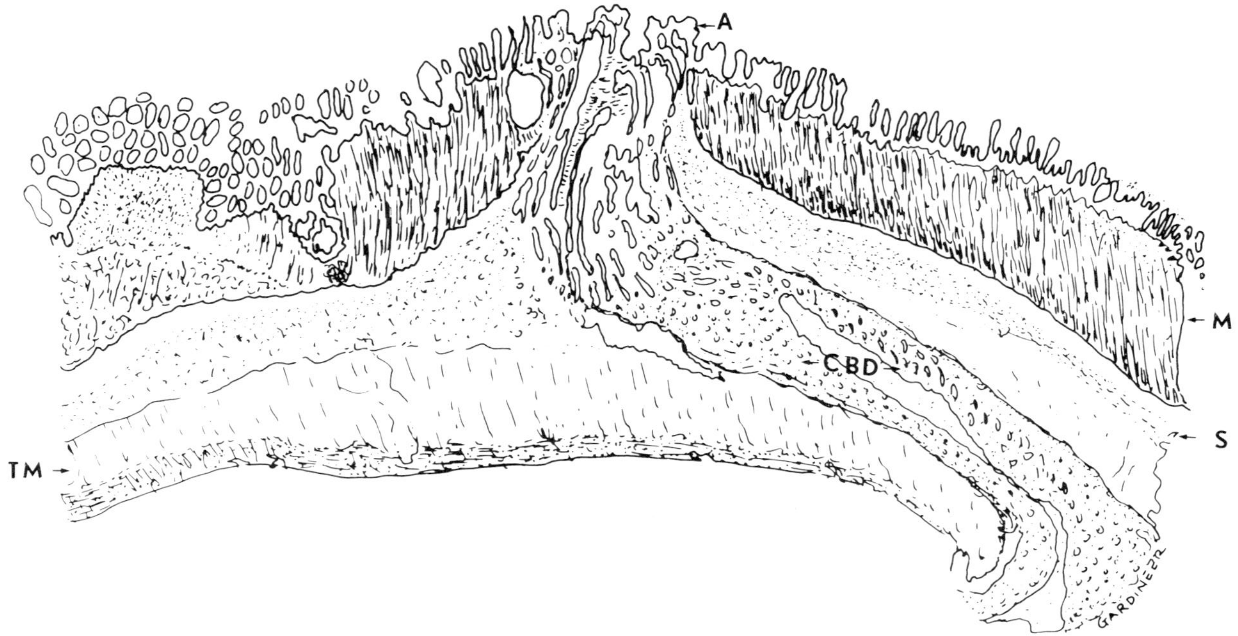

Fig. 5. Longitudinal section through the orifice of the terminal portion of the canine common bile duct. X2. This tissue was removed immediately following the intraductal administration and 1.5 minute stasis of 0.2 ml of histamine dihydrochloride (0.65 mg/ml). Note the heavily convoluted mucosal folds at the ductal orifice (ampulla) and the engorgement of the mucosal vasculature in this area. Legend: M, Mucosa; S, Submucosa; TM, Tunica muscularis; CBD, Common bile duct; A, Ampulla.

junction of a dog which had been subjected to a prior intraductal administration of histamine. The figure shows that the intramural portion of the common duct contains folds of mucosa which become progressively more numerous and convoluted as the duct approaches the orifice. A closer examination of these folds under high magnification reveals that they are heavily vascularized, and that these small vessels are engorged with red blood cells. The picture is one of vascular engorgement and not one of hemorrhage. It would appear that the antagonistic local effects of histamine and norepinephrine which we observed with respect to alterations in ductal opening pressures might very well be explained on the same basis as the increase in upper airway resistance which occurs in allergic rhinitis.

This structural explanation for our experimental results has really existed from antiquity (figure 1). These line drawings were made by Hendrickson in 1898 and they clearly show that the intraduodenal opening of the terminal duct is heavily filled with stippled areas which represent mucosal folds. In this region, the large ratio of intramural diameter to the thickness of the rudimentary and incomplete surrounding muscular ring would indicate that at this portion of the common duct a discrete muscular control of ductal dynamics is highly unlikely. It is at this terminal region where our opening pressure measurements were made. Therefore, it seems to be entirely likely that our results are best explained as functions of the vascularity of the mucosal folds rather than as results of the activity of the surrounding C-shaped musculus proprius. Thus, to the obvious factors which are known and accepted to influence the release of bile into the duodenum, such as respiration and duodenal motility, must now be added both the general cardiovascular status of the experimental animal and the degree of vascular engorgement of the intramural mucosal folds.

The anatomical details of the choledochoduodenal junction indicate that the physiological function of this region may be defined by both the physical properties and physiological activities of at least three discrete regions which are in series. The inferences which can be made from physical measurements of pressure and flow may in fact be determined by the location of the tip of the perfusing catheters. The lack of accurate specification of catheter tip location in much of the literature which pertains to this area may easily account for a great deal of the disagreement which exists with respect to function and control. The mucosal vascularity itself poses obvious hazards with respect to the consequences of over-enthusiastic cannulation procedures whose secondary purpose is to effect a hydraulic seal.

A final consideration is that of the equivalence of physical measurements. Until proven otherwise, it must be assumed that the dynamics of the intramural duct and its attendant structures are those of a nonlinear system. Therefore, attempts to describe ductal dynamics in terms of physical responses to different forcing functions can be expected to produce results which may or may not agree in direction but will certainly not agree quantitatively.

In view of the foregoing, the general confusion and disagreement concerning the physiological significance of the choledochoduodenal junction becomes understandable.

REFERENCES

Alvarez,E.C., 1940.
The mechanics of the gallbladder in An Introduction to Gastroenterology.
Paul B. Hoeber, Inc., New York, p. 440.

Archibald,E., 1919.
The experimental production of pancreatitis in animals as the result of the resistance of the common duct sphincter.
Surg. Gynecol. Obstet. 28:529.

Arianoff,A.A., 1959.
Des modificateurs de la tonicite des sphincters biliaries.
Acta. Chir. Belg., 58:108.

Auster,L.S., and Crohn,B.B., 1922.
Notes on studies in the physiology of the gallbladder.
Am. J. Med. Sci., 164:354.

Benzi,G., Berte,F., Crema,A., and Frigo,G.M., 1964.
Actions of sympathomimetic drugs on the smooth muscle at the junction of the bile duct and duodenum studies in situ.
Br. J. Pharmacol., 23:101.

Berci,G., and Johnson,N., 1965.
Functional studies of the extrahepatic biliary system in the dog by use of a controlled biliary fistula.
Ann. Surg., 161:286.

Bhatnagar,K.K., Samuel,K.C., and Goyal,R.A., 1972a.
The choledochoduodenal function and common bile duct: A morphological study in dogs.
Indian J. Med. Res., 60:636.

Bhatnagar,K.K., Samuel,K.C., and Goyal,R.A., 1972b.
An experimental study of biliary ducts in dogs after cholecystectomy.
Indian J. Med. Res., 60:1498.

Boyden,E.A., 1937.

The sphincter of Oddi in man and certain representative mammals.
Surgery, 1:25.

Brown,W.H., Earley,T., and Eiseman,B., 1956.
Common duct pressures following sphincterotomy.
Surg. Forum, 7:419.

Burget,G.E., 1925.
The regulation of the flow of bile.
Am. J. Physiol., 74:583.

Burget,G.E., 1926.
The regulation of the flow of bile. II. Effect of eliminating the sphincter of Oddi.
Am. J. Physiol., 79:130.

Cole,W.H., 1925.
Relation of gastric content to the physiology of the common duct sphincter.
Am. J. Physiol., 72:39.

Crenam,A., and Benzi,G., 1960.
Rilievi farmacologici sullo sfintere di Oddi.
Arch. Int. Pharmacodyn., 129:264.

Crispin,J.S., Wiseman,D.C.H., Gillespie,D.J., and Lind, J.F., 1970.
A direct manometric study of the canine choledochodenal junction.
Arch. Surg., 101:215.

Dardik,H., Gliedman,M.L., Christ,R., Koslow,A., and Schein,C.J., 1970.
Neuroendocrine influences on the dynamics of the choledochal sphincter.
Surg. Gynecol. Obstet., 131:675.

Doyon,M., 1894.
Del action exercee par le systeme nerveux sur l'appareil excreteur de la bile.
Arch. de physiol. norm. et path., 6:19.

Eichhorn,E.P., and Boyden,E.A., 1955.
The choledochoduodenal junction in the dog--a restudy of Oddi's sphincter.
Am. J. Anat., 97:431.

Gilsdorf,R.B., Urdaneta,L.F., and Leonard,A.S., 1970.
Neurocffector drug influences on pancreatic and biliary sphincter resistances in the awake cat.
Cur. Top. in Sur. Res., 2:41.

Halpert,B., Rewbridge,A.G., and Healey,C., 1933.
Effect of cholecystectomy on the biliary system. A morphologic study in the dog.
Arch. Surg., 26:589.

Hendrickson,W.F., 1898.
A study of the musculature of the entire extrahepatic biliary system including that of the duodenal portion of the common bile duct and the sphincter.
Bull. Johns Hopkins Hosp., 90:221.

Hopton,D.S., and White,T.T., 1971.
Effect of hepatic and celiac vagal stimulation on common bile duct pressure.
Am. J. Dig. Dis., 16:1095.

Hopton,D.S., 1973.
The influence of the vagus nerves on the biliary system.
Br. J. Surg., 60:216.

Jacobson,C., and Gydesen,C., 1922.
The function of the gallbladder in biliary flow.
Arch. Surg., 5:374.

Judd,E.S., and Mann,F.C., 1917.
The effect of removal of the gallbladder.
Surg. Gynecol. Obstet., 24:437.

Liedberg,G., and Halabi,M., 1970.
The effect of vagotomy on flow resistance at the choledochoduodenal junction. An experimental study in the anesthetized cat.
Acta. Chir. Scand., 136:208.

Mann,F.C., 1919.
A study of the toxicity of the sphincter at the duodenal end of the common bile duct.
J. Lab. Clin. Med., 5:107.

Meltzer,S.J., 1917.
The disturbance of the law of contrary innervation as a pathogenetic factor in the diseases of the bile ducts and the gall bladder.
Am. J. Med. Sci., 153:469.

Oddi,R., 1887.
D'une disposition a sphincter speciale de l'ouverture du canal choledoque.
Arch. Ital. Biol., 8:317.

Oddi,R., 1888.
Effetti dell estirpazione della cystifellea.
Bull, d. sc. med. Bologna, 21:194.

Oddi,R., 1894.
Di una speciale disposizione di sfintere allo sbocco.
Sperimentale, 48:180.

Persson,C.G.A., 1971.
The action of morphine on the cat choledochoduodenal tract.
Acta Pharmacol. Toxicol., 30:321.

Persson,C.G.A., and Ekman,M., 1972.
Effect of morphine, cholecystokinin, and sympathomimetics on the sphincter of Oddi and intramural pressure on cat duodenum.
Scand. J. Gastroent., 7:345.

Schein,C.J., Rosen,R.G., Warren,A., and Gliedman,M.L., 1969.
The effect of vagotomy on biliary pressure.
Surgery, 66:345.

Shore,J.M., Silverman,A., Siegel,M., and Bakal,M., 1971.
Direct observations of the canine sphincter of Oddi.
Ann. Surg., 174:264.

Stassa,G., and Grafe,W.R., 1968.
The cineradiographic evaluation of the biliary tract after drug therapy following cholecystectomy, sphincterotomy and vagotomy.
Radiology, 91:297.

Tansy,M.F., Innes,D.L., and Kendall,F.M., 1973a.
Estimation of the mean opening pressure of the sphincter of Oddi.
Clin. Res., 21:527.

Tansy,M.F., Innes,D.L., and Kendall,F.M., 1973b.
An evaluation of neural influences on the sphincter of Oddi in the dog.
Physiologist, 16:467.

Tansy,M.F., Innes,D.L., Martin,J.S., and Kendall,F.M., 1973c.
An evaluation of neural influences on the sphincter of Oddi in the dog.
Am. J. Dig. Dis., (submitted).

Tansy,M.F., Innes,D.L., Martin,J.S., and Kendall,F.M., 1973d.
Vascular influences on the dynamic stability of the choledochoduodenal junction.
Am. J. Dig. Dis., (submitted).

Tansy,M.F., Innes,D.L., Martin,J.S., and Kendall,F.M., 1973e.
The effects of various substances found in bile on the canine choledochoduodenal junction.
Arch. Int. Pharmacodyn., (submitted).

Westphal,K., 1923.
Muskelfunktion, nervensystem u. pathologie der gallenwege. I. Untersuchungen uber den schmerzanfall der gallenwege und seine austrahlenden reflexe.
Ztschr. f. Klin. Med., 96:22.

Williams,R.D., and Huang,T.T., 1969.
The effect of vagotomy on biliary pressure.
Surgery, 66:353.

Winkelstein,A., and Aschner,P.W., 1924.
The pressure factors in the biliary-duct system of the dog.
Am. J. Med. Sci., 168:812.

Wyatt,A.P., 1967.
The relationship of the sphincter of Oddi to the stomach, duodenum and gallbladder.
J. Physiol., (London), 193:225.

SESSION II.

GASTROINTESTINAL SECRETORY ACTIVITIES

BASIC MECHANISM OF HCl PRODUCTION

Warren S. Rehm

INTRODUCTION

This paper will be primarily concerned with the basic mechanisms of ion transport in the gastric mucosa. We start by briefly reviewing some well known facts. For the mammalian stomach the Cl^- concentration of gastric juice is about 170 mM, the H^+ concentration about 150 mM and the sum of the Na^+ and K^+ concentrations about 20 mM; other ions are present in only relatively small amounts (Babkin, 1950). It is established for the in vivo dog stomach and in general for the mammalian stomach that the nutrient or blood side is about 60 mv positive in an external circuit to the secretory or lumen side (Rehm, 1944). For the in vitro frog stomach the potential is about half of this (Davies, 1948). Since the Cl^- is transported against both a concentration gradient and an electrical gradient it is clear that the Cl^- is actively transported (Rehm, 1950; Hogben, 1955). Since the H^+ is produced at very high concentrations it can easily be shown that there must be a metabolic machine for the production of the H^+ (Rehm, 1972b). In other words, there must be a source of metabolic energy for the transport of both H^+ and Cl^-. In the mammalian stomach during moderate to high rates of secretion the Na^+ and K^+ are transported down their electrochemical potential gradients (Thull and Rehm, 1956). However, it should be noted that in the mammalian stomach during rest or at very low secretory rates Na^+ is actively transported from the secretory to the nutrient side (Bornstein et al., 1959; Cummins and Vaughan, 1963;

Kitahara et al., 1969).

Water transport is linked to ion transport and there is substantial evidence indicating that water is transported as a result of the osmotic gradient between the lumen and the interstitial fluid (Gilman and Cowgill, 1931, 1933; Thull and Rehm, 1956; Rehm et al., 1970). Under some conditions the secretion may be hypotonic but convincing explanations for the hypotonicity have been presented within the framework of the osmotic gradient theory of water transport (Rehm et al., 1970). The osmotic theory of water transport is well established.

Another important aspect of gastric ion transport is concerned with the acid-base balance of the cell. It has been shown that for every H^+ secreted into the lumen a HCO_3^- is transported into or appears in the interstitial fluid (Hanke, 1937; Davies, 1948; Teorell, 1951).

The methods used in studies of the electrophysiology of the gastric mucosae have been described elsewhere. Briefly, for the dog, a flap of stomach is placed in an appropriate lucite chamber in such a way as to maintain an intact blood supply and in general four electrodes are used; two for PD measurements and two for the application of electric current (Rehm, 1945; Rehm, 1956). A similar method is used for studies on in vitro stomachs (Davies, 1951; Forte, 1970). The methods for measuring the H^+ and Cl^- rates have been described many times and need not be reviewed here (Rehm, 1962).

The main questions arising in connection with the problem of the basic mechanism of HCl production are the following: 1) which cells secrete the ions and water? 2) which cellular membranes are the sites of the ion transport? 3) what is the energy source for the Cl^- and H^+ production? e.g., is the energy derived from ATP or from oxidation-reduction reactions? and 4) the most important of all: what is the detailed molecular mechanism of ion transport?

NATURE OF MOLECULAR MECHANISMS

According to a theory presented many years ago and referred to as the separate site theory, there is in the secretory membrane an array of H^+ pumps parallel to an array of Cl^- pumps, the pumps being linked by means of electrical coupling (Rehm, 1950). This separate site theory as shown in figure 1 is often referred to as the electrogenic theory of HCl secretion. By the term electrogenic I mean an active ion transport mechanism in which there is a net transport of

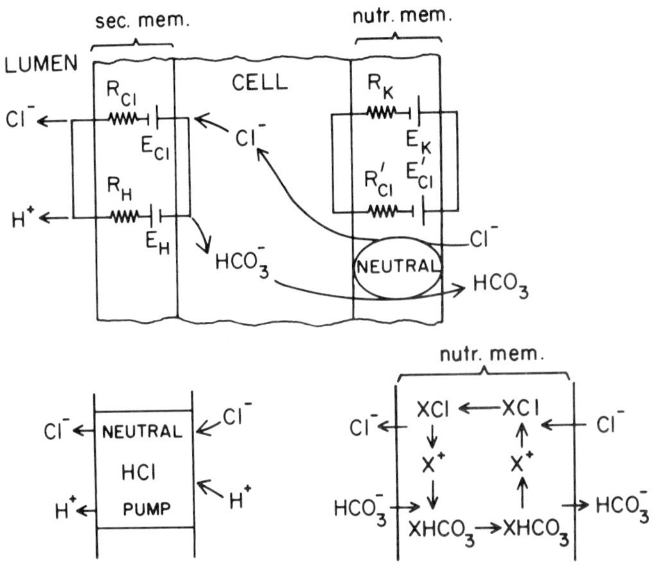

Fig. 1. Representation of the present state of our knowledge of the mechanisms of ion transport in the gastric mucosa. In the top the separate site theory is represented by equivalent circuits with Cl^- and H^+ electrogenic mechanisms in the secretory (sec) membrane. It also illustrates that the conductance of the nutrient (nutr) or submucosal-facing membrane is equal to the sum of the K^+ and Cl^- conductances (the sum of the conductances of all other ions – zero). The neutral exchange mechanism for HCO_3^- and that portion of the Cl^- transport equal to the H^+ secretory rate is indicated by the region labeled neutral. A detailed Cl^--HCO_3^- neutral carrier exchange mechanism is shown in the lower right. The lower left illustrates a neutral mechanism for HCl production which is still a viable possibility under standard conditions (i.e., with Cl^- bathing solutions). See text.

charge across the membrane at the site of the pump. This is in contrast to a neutral mechanism in which there is no net transport of charge at the pump site. With a neutral mechanism the transport of an anion, say Cl^-, from the cell to the lumen would be linked via the pump to the transport of another anion from the lumen back into the cell or to the transport of a cation into the lumen simultaneously with the Cl^-. Sometimes the word electrogenic is used to indicate a neutral mechanism which results in ion gradients between the cell and the bathing fluid which in turn is responsible for diffusion emfs across the membranes. I am not using the phrase electrogenic in this sense. I mean by electrogenic, a pump in which there is a net transport of charge per se and the pump itself is not neutral.

Solely on the basis of the fact that both H^+ and Cl^- are transported uphill the molecular mechanism could be neutral or could be electrogenic. In this connection it should be noted that we have established that the H^+ pump is electrogenic in the absence of Cl^- (sulfate bathing media) but with Cl^- media it is still possible that HCl is produced by a neutral mechanism (Rehm, 1965; Rehm and LeFevre, 1965). Detailed postulates of possible mechanisms for neutral and electrogenic mechanisms have been presented in recent papers and have been reviewed in recent symposia (Rehm, 1972a; Rehm, 1972b; Makhlouf and Rehm, in press). It is, of course, understood that an electrogenic ion transport mechanism can be represented by an emf in series with a resistance and that the potency of an electrogenic mechanism is proportional to the magnitude of its emf and inversely proportional to its resistance.

An important aspect of the problem of the nature of the molecular mechanisms for gastric ion transport is concerned with the transport of ions across the nutrient membrane (i.e., the membrane facing the blood side). It is well established that the rate of H^+ secretion is equal to the rate of HCO_3^- exit from the cell into the interstitial fluid. In work over the last ten years we have solved the problem of the nature of the mechanisms for ion transport in the nutrient membrane. The following is a brief resume of this aspect of the subject.

The conductance of the nutrient membrane is equal to the sum of the K^+ and Cl^- conductances (see fig. 1) and the sum of all other ion conductances for this membrane is essentially zero (Harris and Edelman, 1964; Spangler and Rehm, 1968). There are no conductance channels of appreciable magnitude for other ions such as HCO_3^-, H^+, OH^- and Na^+ (Sanders et al., 1972, Rehm et al., 1973). Since HCO_3^- transport is via a neutral mechanism most of the Cl^- must enter via a neutral mechanism, otherwise electroneutrality would be violated.

Another line of evidence has also led to the above conclusion. Work with Ba^{++} has shown that there is a neutral mechanism for Cl^- and HCO_3^- (Rehm, 1967; Pacifico et al., 1969). A neutral carrier exchange mechanism for these ions is depicted in figure 1. It should be noted that what has been shown is that a neutral mechanism (or mechanisms) is involved in a process, the end result of which is the entrance of Cl^- and exit of HCO_3^-; the actual neutral mechanism may not be an actual Cl^--HCO_3^- exchange as depicted in figure 1 (see Sanders et al., 1972 for details). It should be emphasized that the Cl^- can move across the nutrient membrane via a neutral mechanism and also via a conductive mechanism. It is somewhat ironic that what is referred to in the literature as "the neutral chloride" is that portion of the Cl^- transport that moves across the nutrient membrane via conductive channels. In the past it was implicitly assumed that the transport of Cl^- and HCO_3^- across the nutrient membrane was via conductive channels since the Cl^--HCO_3^- exchange across the red blood cell membrane was assumed to be via conductive channels. Following our demonstration that there is a neutral mechanism for Cl^- and HCO_3^- transport across the nutrient membrane it has been shown (Harris and Pressman, 1967; Hunter, 1967; Lassen, 1972) that the Cl^--HCO_3^- exchange mechanism for red blood cells is not via conductive channels but is also via a neutral exchange mechanism.

THE ENERGY SOURCE OF HCl PRODUCTION

On the basis of the original formulation of the separate site theory the energy for HCl production comes from oxidation reduction reactions (Rehm, 1950; Davies, 1951; Conway, 1953). On the other hand, an obvious possibility is that ATP provides the energy since it has been shown that ATP provides the energy for a number of active ion transport mechanisms. It is of interest to compare and contrast the evidence for ATP involvement in Na^+ transport with that for HCl production. In the squid axon it has been shown that, after depression of active Na^+ transport by dinitrophenol, injection of ATP into the axon restores active Na^+ transport (Caldwell et al., 1960). Obviously this type of experiment is not feasible in a tissue like gastric mucosa. In studies on other tissues other approaches have provided convincing evidence that ATP furnishes the energy for the uphill transport of Na^+. For example, in red blood cells it is possible to load the cells with ATP during hypotonic hemolysis and then following the restoration of isotonicity it has been shown that Na^+ transport is restored (Hoffman, 1962). Comparable experiments are in progress on the in vitro gastric mucosa of the frog. We have found that the frog mucosa can withstand markedly hypotonic fluids for periods of about a half hour (Sanders and Rehm, 1968; Sanders et al., 1970). Following the reduction of the total osmotic pressure of the bathing fluids to about 24 mOsM/1, acid secretion is reduced to zero but after restoration of isotonicity the H^+ rate returned. The time constant for diffusion of ions across the diffusion barrier in the in vitro frog mucosa is about one minute (Spangler and Rehm, 1968) so that under these conditions the mucosal cells bear the full brunt of the hypotonicity after a few minutes. By means of electron microscopy we demonstrated very marked swelling of the cells during the hypotonic period, yet astonishingly the cells return to normal appearance following the return to isotonic bathing media (unpublished work by Helander et al.). Our planned experiments are similar to those performed on the red blood cells, i.e., incorporation of ATP into the cells during hypotonic cytolysis and the restoration of isotonicity during metabolic inhibition.

One set of experiments (Rehm and LeFevre, 1965), however, which were designed to determine the role of ATP makes us pessimistic about the significance of the planned hypotonic experiments. In the Rehm-LeFevre experiments the gastric HCl mechanism was inhibited by dinitrophenol and after the H^+ secretion was reduced to zero we added massive amounts of ATP to the nutrient fluid. With massive amounts of ATP in the nutrient fluid some ATP might enter the cells and produce at least a modicum of H^+ secretion. We found that there was no restoration of the H^+ rate. We next used amounts of dinitrophenol which depressed the H^+ rate but not to zero. We postulated that with less damage to the mucosa exogenous ATP might produce a measurable increase in H^+ secretion. To our surprise we found that the H^+ rate, instead of increasing or not changing, decreased rapidly to zero. We then studied the effects of ATP in the absence of dinitrophenol and found that ATP added to the nutrient fluid is a good inhibitor of H^+ secretion (Sanders and Rehm, 1971a). Obvious possibilities of explaining this inhibition, such as changes in pH, Ca^{++} or Mg^{++} activities of the nutrient fluid were easily ruled out (Sanders and Rehm, 1971b). This inhibitory action of exogenous ATP on H^+ secretion makes it much more difficult to design intelligent experiments to test the ATP hypothesis. Furthermore Kidder (1973) has presented evidence that ATP enters the gastric cells under standard in vitro conditions.

Even though we have not shown that ATP is essential for H^+ secretion on the basis of experiments which were successful on squid axons and red blood cells, the discovery by Kasebaker and Durbin (1965) of a gastric ATPase is evidence for ATP involvement. These workers found an ATPase in gastric mucosa which did not respond to Na^+ and K^+ but was stimulated by HCO_3^- and inhibited by SCN^- The latter effect is of interest since it is well known that SCN^- rapidly and reversibly inhibits H^+ secretion (Rehm, 1962). However, further work with this ATPase (Blum et al., 1971) has shown it is not unique to the stomach and furthermore it is difficult in my opinion to present a viable scheme for HCl production on the basis of an ATPase which is stimulated by HCO_3^- (Rehm, 1972b). It is much easier to present a plausible scheme if it was the other way around, if the ATPase was stimulated by CO_2 and inhibited by HCO_3^-. Ganser and Forte (1973) have found a gastric ATPase stimulated by K^+ (and not influence by Na^+) which may be of importance but its possible role in HCl secretion has not been delineated.

It is apparent that the question of the role of ATP as the source of energy for gastric HCl production is at present unresolved. I should point out that even if it turns out that ATP provides the energy for HCl secretion this finding in itself does not enable us to determine the molecular nature of HCl secretion, i.e., whether it is neutral or electrogenic.

SITE OF SECRETION OF IONS AND H_2O

In the vertebrates lower than the mammals there is only one major cell type lining the tubules while in the mammal there are two major types, i.e., the parietal and chief cells (Helander, 1962; Ito, 1967). It is generally assumed that the chief cells secrete enzymes and the parietal cells HCl. In the lower vertebrates it is assumed that the tubular cells secrete HCl, water and the enzymes of gastric juice.

Many attempts have been made in the past from the time of Claude Bernard (1859) to determine the site of H^+ secretion by the use of pH indicators. A substantial body of literature seems to support the concept that the fluid in the canaliculi of the parietal cells and tubular lumen is essentially neutral and that acid is formed on the surface of the stomach (see Rehm, 1972a for references). However, we have shown that none of the indicator experiments

(White et al., 1956) have any meaning whatsoever from the point of view of determining the pH of the lumina. On the other hand, it has been shown on the basis of the osmotic theory of water transport that the H^+ and Cl^- must be osmotically active in the tubules so that the pH in the lumen must be essentially the same as that of the gastric juice (Rehm et al., 1970). Furthermore we have also shown that even if the parietal cells do not secrete H^+ the pH in the canaliculi must be essentially the same as that of the final secretion (Rehm, 1972a). This is all I wish to say about the indicator approach in the present paper. I would like to now turn to the implications of the separate site theory.

According to this theory in its simplest form, there is an array of electrogenic H^+ pumps in parallel with an array of Cl^- pumps in the secretory membranes of the parietal cells. Electrical neutrality would obviously be maintained by electrical coupling between the pumps. Now with separate sites for Cl^- and H^+ the question arises as to why the electrical coupling could not extend beyond the limits of a single cell; in other words could one cell type secrete Cl^- and other H^+? It seemed to us that the best way to grapple with this problem was to formulate a good working hypothesis. Parenthetically, I define a good hypothesis as one which can be easily disproved and contrariwise, a poor hypothesis is one not easily disproved. Our first hypothesis on the basis of this criterion was a good hypothesis. We first looked at the possibility that the surface cells secreted Cl^- and the parietal cells H^+ and the consequences of this hypothesis are illustrated in figure 2. An important finding in this analysis is that the surface cells are essentially impermeable to water in a net transport sense; that is, the application of an appreciable osmotic gradient across the surface cells does not result (in either the resting or secreting condition) in a significant net transport of water (Rehm et al., 1953). The fact that there is a large unilateral flux of water across the mucosal surface is seemingly in conflict with our results on net transport. Before proceeding further I would like to show that there is no essential conflict between the unilateral flux rate and the net transport rate. The next section can be regarded as parenthetical and following this interlude on water transport we will revert to our theme.

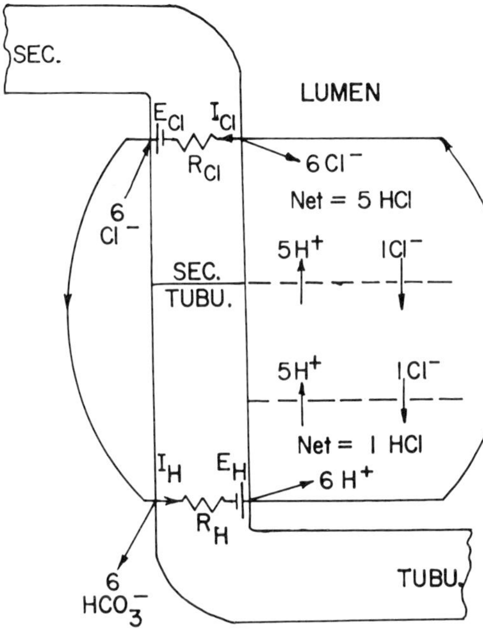

Fig. 2. Consequences of H^+ secretion by tubular and Cl^- by surface cells. Transference number for H^+ is five times that for Cl^-. Therefore, five sixths of HCl accumulates at the surface cell border. With only the tubular cells permeable to water, only one sixth of the secreted HCl is osmotically active; hence, secretion would be six times that of an isotonic fluid.

PREDICTIONS OF NET TRANSPORT OF WATER ACROSS THE SURFACE CELLS ON BASIS OF UNILATERAL WATER FLUXES

In this section we will show that within the framework of the assumption that water traverses the limiting secretory membranes of the surface cells by diffusion one would predict a unilateral flux rate of water about 200 times the net transport rate resulting from an osmotic gradient of about 300 mOsM.

On the basis of Fick's equation, the diffusion water is given by

$$Qw = -DA\frac{dC_w}{dX} \qquad (1)$$

or for unilateral flux rates

$$\vec{Q}_w = DA \frac{C_w}{\Delta X} \tag{2}$$

where Q_w and $\vec{Q}_w$ are the rates of water movement in moles per second, D is the diffusion coefficient of water (cm^2/sec), A is the area of the membrane and C_w is the concentration of water and X is the distance inward from the surface of the membrane. The concentration of water is given by

$$C_w = \frac{n_w}{V} \tag{3}$$

where n_w are the moles of water in the system and V is the volume of the system. V for distilled water equals $n_w \bar{V}_w$ where $\bar{V}_w$ is the partial molal volume of water, hence for pure water $C_w = 1/\bar{V}_w$ (C_w is in moles/cm^3 and $\bar{V}_w$ is in cm^3/mole) so equation (2) for pure water becomes

$$\vec{Q}_w = \frac{DA}{\Delta X} \frac{1}{\bar{V}_w} \tag{4}$$

Now for a solution, C_w is given by equation (3) where

$$V \simeq \bar{V}_w (n_w + n_s) \tag{5}$$

and n_s represents the number of moles of solute in the system and the simplifying assumptions are made that the solution is ideal and that $\bar{V}_w = \bar{V}_s$ where $\bar{V}_s$ is the partial molal volume of solute. So that for a solution C_w is given by the following equation

$$C_w = \frac{n_w}{\bar{V}_w (n_w + n_s)} \tag{6}$$

The net flow of water, say from distilled water to blood (a solution that 300 mOsM), would be given as follows

$$Q_{net} = \vec{Q}_w - \overleftarrow{Q}_w \tag{7}$$

and by the use of equations (2), (3), (4) and (6) we have

$$Q_{net} = \frac{DA}{\Delta X \bar{V}_w}\left[1 - \frac{n_w}{n_w + n_s}\right] \qquad (8)$$

which reduces to

$$Q_{net} = \frac{DA}{\Delta X \bar{V}_w}\left[\frac{n_s}{n_w + n_s}\right] \qquad (9)$$

Now we wish to determine the ratio of unilateral movement of water to net movement and by using equations (4) and (9) we have

$$\frac{\overrightarrow{Q}_w}{Q_{net}} \simeq \frac{n_w + n_s}{n_s}$$

With n_s = 0.3 mole and n_w – 55.5 moles $\overrightarrow{Q}_w/Q_{net}$ = 186. Therefore we predict that the unilateral flux rate would be approximately 200 times the net transport rate when the osmotic gradient is 300 mOsM/l. The net transport rate for an osmotic gradient of 300 mOsM from the lumen to the blood is approximately 0.04 ml hr^{-1} cm^{-2} (Rehm et al., 1953) and the unilateral flux is around 200 times this (Cope et al., 1943; Code et al., 1963). The experiments performed for the determination of the unilateral flux rates were not designed to eliminate the role of unstirred layers so they are only approximate. Furthermore there is considerable variations in the values for net transport rates so all that can be done at present is to show that the findings are compatible with the postulate that water moves across the limiting membranes of the surface cells by diffusion. Therefore there is no real discrepancy between the unilateral flux and the net transport rates. When we compare the net transport of water during secretion (in the units of ml hr^{-1} cm^{-2} per unit of osmotic gradient) with the water permeability of the surface cells, which in these units is about 0.00013 ml hr^{-1} cm^{-2} per/mOsM (0.04/300), we find that the water permeability of the surface cells would have to be over a thousand fold greater to account for the water of secretion [i.e., during secretion the water permeability is approximately 0.3 ml hr^{-1} cm^{-2} per mOsM (where the area is the macroscopic area of the mucosa)].

HYPOTHESIS THAT SURFACE CELLS SECRETE Cl^- AND PARIETAL CELLS H^+

On the basis of the above analysis it is clear that the water of secretion comes from the tubular cells. Now examination of figure 2 reveals that with Cl^- secreted by the surface cells and H^+ by the parietal cells, the electrical current coupling between the emfs results in current flow in the indicated direction and since the transference number of H^+ is about 5 times that for Cl^-, 5/6 of the HCl would accumulate at the border of the surface cells and only 1/6 in the tubules (Rehm et al., 1953). Hence only 1/6 of the HCl would result in water transport with the consequence that the final secretion would be expected to be about 1 molar. This is absurd and we conclude that this form of the separate site theory is clearly not a viable one. As I pointed out above, this was good working hypothesis since it was easily disproved.

Now if we turn it around, so to speak, and have H^+ secreted by the surface cells and Cl^- and water by the parietal cells we find that this is a much more difficult hypothesis to disprove. This is shown in figure 3 and by similar reasoning it follows that 5/6 of the HCl would accumulate in the tubules and result in water transport with the consequence that the final secretion would be about 20 per cent greater than the osmotic pressure of the interstitial fluid. Now, by means of ad hoc postulates that do not seem completely absurd, one can obtain a model in which the final secretion would be about that which is observed experimentally (Rehm et al., 1953). The idea that the surface cells secreted Cl^- and the parietal cells H^+ did not seem completely absurd to most of my colleagues but when we turned it around then we were in for trouble. In fact, the suggestion that the surface cells secreted H^+ almost resulted in my expulsion from the very prestigious Parietal Cell Club.

Although we felt that the idea that the surface cells secreted H^+ was not to be taken seriously we would like to disprove it. About this time Earl Thomas called my attention to the glycine findings of Teorell (1939–40). Earl Thomas was quite skeptical of the Teorell claim that the primary acidity of gastric juice was about 0.46 normal. However, he did not dismiss the Teorell findings out of hand and he looked for possible small systematic errors which could account for the rather startling findings. As most of you know Teorell got mad

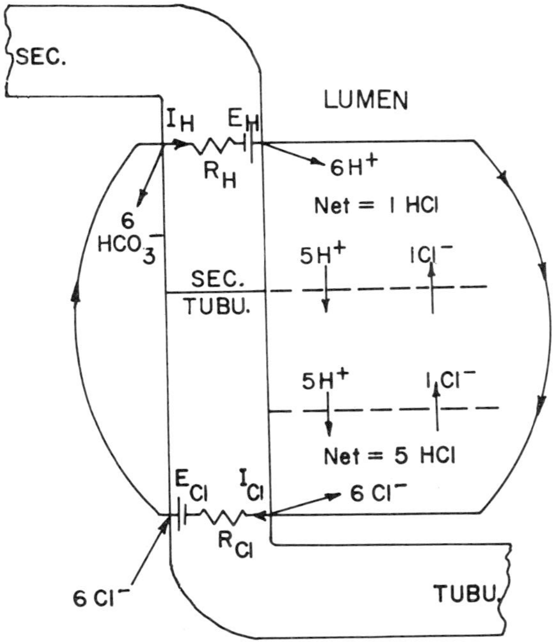

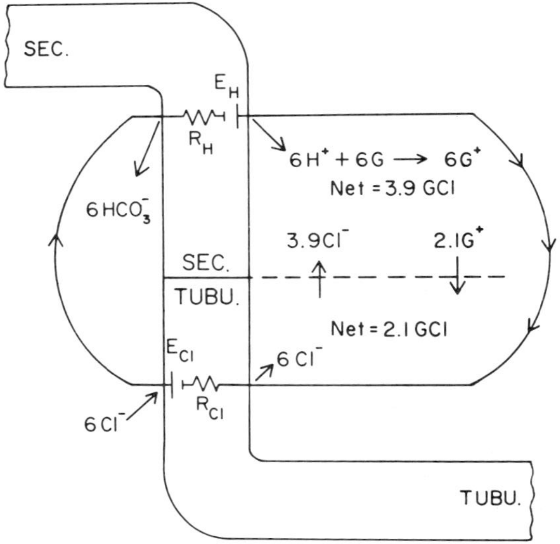

Fig. 3. (Left) Consequences of H^+ being secreted by surface cells: five sixths of the HCl would accumulate at the tubular border and the final secretion would be about 0.19M HCl.

Fig. 4. (Right) Consequences of essentially all of the secreted H^+ combining with glycine; the amount of glycine chloride accumulating in the tubules would result in a calculated H^+ concentration of secretion of 0.46N. See text.

because no one took his findings seriously and he started publishing in German. This didn't satisfy him, so he repeated and confirmed his glycine results a number of years after the original publication (Linde et al., 1947). The glycine findings were subsequently confirmed by Heinz (1951) working in Gregory's laboratory.

Now what did Teorell find? He found that with glycine on the secretory side the calculated H^+ concentration approached 0.46 normal as the secretory rate approached zero. Teorell's idea was that glycine would trap the H^+ so as to minimize the back diffusion of H^+. Now the hypothesis that the surface cells secrete H^+ and the parietal cells Cl^- without any other postulates predicts at very low secretory rates in the presence of glycine a calculated H^+ concentration of 0.46 normal. This is illustrated in figure 4. At low secretory rates practically all the H^+ would be in the form of glycine ions and so the problem becomes: what are the transference numbers of the glycine ion and Cl^-? It turns out that with the values found in standard references, calculation of the amount of glycine Cl^- accumulating in the tubules compared to the total amount of H^+ secreted yields a calculated value of 0.46 normal (Rehm et al., 1953).

I would like to make it clear that I am not holding Earl Thomas responsible for our suggestion that the surface cells secrete H^+ ions, this would be a sacrilege to his memory. However I would like to point out that I've had many delightful discussions with Earl Thomas and always found them fruitful.

Subsequently Canosa and I (Canosa and Rehm, 1968), on the basis of our microelectrode findings on the dog stomach, argued that the resistance linking the surface cells and the parietal cells is too high to be compatible with the idea that one ion is produced by the surface cells and the other by the parietal cells. However, as with all microelectrode data on epithelial tissues it is difficult to establish rigorously conclusions based on such data. The glycine date and the recent findings of Moody and Durbin (1965) can be explained, in my opinion, on the basis of the ratio of the amount of HCl that diffuses out of the tubules without resulting in osmotic movement of water to the total amount of HCl secreted. As the secretory rate approaches zero the rate of HCl which moves out by simple diffusion becomes relatively larger. So whether rightly or wrongly, we no longer are exploring the hypothesis that the surface cells secrete H^+

and the parietal cells Cl^- and water. Now if we look at another pair of cells, i.e., the chief and parietal cells,and if one postulates that the chief cells secreted one of the ions and the parietal cells the other ion, then this hypothesis is a poor one, i.e., it is very difficult to disprove, at least within the framework of our present experimental techniques. We have hopes that with recent development with our microelectrode studies (O'Callaghan et al., 1973) together with our square wave studies (Noyes and Rehm, 1970) we will be able at least for the frog gastric mucosa to dissect in a biophysical sense the caracteristics of the limiting membranes of both the surface cells and the tubular cells. However,the problem with respect to the mammalian stomach seems awfully formidable.

I would like to raise the question in the minds of this audience as to why you believe that the parietal cells secrete HCl. You might reply that a very acid secretion is an almost unique phenomenon in biology and the parietal cells are unique. You might elaborate: parietal cells are not found in other tissues so the uniqueness of HCl secretion and the uniqueness of the parietal cells argues strongly in favor of the conclusion that the acid secretion is produced by the parietal cells.

Apropos of this point I would like to tell you about some work by Oschman and Berridge (1970). They found a tissue with cells indistinguishable from parietal cells. These cells have intracellular canaliculi, foldings of the luminal membrane, lateral interdigitations, staining properties and mitochrondia just like the parietal cells of the mammalian mucosa. Now this may come as a shock to you: these cells are found in the salivary gland of the blow fly larvae and they produce an essentially isotonic KCl secretion. I leave as a homework problem the problem of the decision as to which cell (or cells) secrete which ions in the gastric mucosa.

REFERENCES

Babkin,B.P., 1950.
Secretory mechanisms of the digestive glands, ed.2. Hoeber Publishers, New York and London.

Bernard,C., 1859.
Lecons sur les properties physiologiques et les alterations pathologiques de liquides-de l'organisme. Paris.

Blum,A.L., Shah,G., St. Pierre,T., Helander,H.F., Sung, C.P., Wiebelhaus,V.D., and Sachs,G., 1971.
Properties of soluble ATPase of gastric mucosa II effect of HCO_3.
Biochem. Biophys. Acta. 249:101.

Bornstein,A.M., Dennis,W.H., and Rehm,W.S., 1959.
Movement of water, sodium, chloride and hydrogen ion across the resting stomach.
Am. J. Physiol., 197:332.

Caldwell,P.C., Hodgkin,A.L., Keynes,R.D., and Shaw,T.I., 1960.
The effects of injecting "energy-rich" phosphate compounds on the active transport of ions in the giant axons of Laligo.
J. Physiol. (London), 152:561.

Canosa,C., and Rehm,W.S., 1968.
Microelectrode studies on dog's gastric mucosa.
Biophys. J., 8:415.

Code,S.F., Higgins,J.A., Moll,J.C., Orvis,A.L., and Scholer,J.F., 1963.
The influence of acid on the gastric absorption of H_2O, sodium and potassium.
J. Physiol. (London), 166:110.

Conway,E.J., 1953.
The biochemistry of gastric acid secretion.
Charles C. Thomas, Publisher, Springfield, Ill.

Cope,O., Blatt,H., and Bull,M.R., 1943.
Gastric secretion III, the absorption of heavy water from pouches of the body and antrum of the stomach of the dog.
J. Clin. Investigation, 22:111.

Cummins,J.T., and Vaughan,B.E., 1963.
Relation of sodium to the bioelectric mucosa.
Biochem. J., 42:609.
Davies,R.E., 1951.
The mechanism of hydrochloric adic production by the stomach.
Biol. Rev., 26:87.
Forte,J.G., 1970.
Hydrochloric acid secretion by gastric mucosa, in Bittar E.E., Membranes and Ion Transport, Vol. 3, John Wiley and Sons, Inc.
Ganser,A.L., and Forte,J.G., 1973.
K+ stimulated ATPase in purified microsomes of bull frog oxyntic cells.
Biochem. Biophys. Acta., 307:169.
Gilman,A., and Cowgill,G.R., 1931.
Osmotic relations of blood and glandular secretions. I. The regulatory action of total blood electrolytes on the concentration of gastric chlorides.
Am. J. Physiol., 99-172.
Gilman,A., and Cowgill,G.R., 1933.
Osmotic relations between blood and body fluids.
Am. J. Physiol., 103:143.
Hanke,M.E., 1937.
The acid-base and energy metabolism of the stomach and pancreas.
Science, 85:54.
Harris,E.J., and Pressman,B.C., 1967.
Obligate cation exchanges in red cells.
Nature, 216:918.
Harris,J.B., and Edelman,I.S., 1964.
Chemical concentration gradients and electrical properties of gastric mucosa.
Am. J. Physiol., 206:769.
Heinz,E., 1951.
Uber die primare aziditat der magensaure.
Biochem. Biophys. Acta., 6:434.
Helander,H.F., 1962.
Ultrastructure of the fundus glands of the mouse gastric mucosa.
J. Ultrastruct. Res. 4 (Suppl):1.

Hoffman,J.F., 1962.
Cation transport and structure of the red-cell plasma membrane.
Circulation 26:1201.
Hogben,C.A.M., 1955.
Biological aspects of active chloride transport, in Shanes,A.M., Electrolytes in Biological Systems, pg. 176.
American Physiological Society, Washington,D.C.
Hunter,F.R., 1967.
Facilitated diffusion in the chloride shift in human erythrocytes.
Biochem. Biophys. Acta. 135:784.
Its,S., 1967.
Anatomic structure of the gastric mucosa, in Code, C.F.,Handbook of Physiology: Alimentary Canal.
American Physiology Society, Washington,D.C.
Volume 2, Section 6, pg. 705.
Kasbekar,D.K., and Durbin,R.P., 1965.
An adenosine triphosphatase from frog gastric mucosa.
Am. J. Physiol. 105:472.
Kidder,G.W. III, 1973.
Purine nucleotide entry, exit and interconversions in bull frog gastric mucosa.
Am. J. Physiol. 224:809.
Kitahara,S., Fox,K.R., and Hogben,C.A.M., 1969.
Acid secretion Na^+ absorption, and the origin of the potential difference across isolated mammalian stomachs.
Am. J. Dig. Dis. 14:221.
Lassen,U.V., 1972.
Membrane potential and membrane resistance of red cell in Astrup, P. and Rorth,M., Oxygen Affinity of Hemoglobin and Red Cell Acid-Base Status.
Academic Press, New York.
Linde,S., Teorell,T., and Obrink,K.J., 1947.
Experiments on the primary acidity of gastric ju juice.
Acta. Physiol. Scandinav. 14:220.
Makhlouf,G.M., and Rehm,W.S.
Gastric secretion, amphibia, chemical zoology.

Academic Press, New York.
Vol. 9 (In Press).

Moody,F.G., and Durbin,R.P., 1965.
Effects of glycine and other instillates on concentration of gastric acid.
Am. J. Physiol. 209:122.

Noyes,D.H., and Rehm,W.S., 1970.
Voltage response of the frog gastric mucosa to direct current.
Am. J. Physiol. 219:184.

O'Callaghan,J., Sanders,S.S., Shoemaker,R.L., and Rehm, W.S., 1973.
Site of action of Ba^{++} on in vitro gastric mucosa with microelectrode technique.
Physiologist 16:411

Oschman,J.L., and Berridge,M.J., 1970.
Structural and function aspects of salivary fluid secretion in calliphora.
Tissue and Cell 2:281.

Pacifico,A.D., Schwartz,M., MacKrell,T.N., Spangler,S. G., Sanders,S.S., and Rehm,W.S., 1969.
Reversal by potassium of an effect of barium on the frog gastric mucosa.
Am. J. Physiol. 216:536.

Rehm,W.S., 1944.
The effect of histamine and HCl on gastric secretion and potential.
Am. J. Physiol. 141:537.

Rehm,W.S., 1945.
The effect of electric current on gastric secretion and potential.
Am. J. Physiol. 144:115.

Rehm,W.S., 1950.
A theory of the formation of HCl by the stomach.
Gastroenterology 14:401.

Rehm,W.S., 1956.
Effect of electric current on gastric hydrogen ion and chloride ion secretion.
Am. J. Physiol. 185:325.

Rehm,W.S., 1962.
Acid secretion, resistance, short-circuit current and voltage-clamping on frog's stomach.
Am. J. Physiol. 203:63.

Rehm,W.S., 1965.
Electrophysiology of the gastric mucosa in Cl-free solutions.
Fed. Proc. 24:1387.

Rehm,W.S., 1967.
Membrane conductivity and ion transport in gastric mucosa.
Fed. Proc. 26:1303.

Rehm,W.S., 1972a.
Some aspects of the problem of gastric hydrochloric acid secretion.
Arch. Intern. Med. 129:270.

Rehm,W.S., 1972b.
Proton transport in Hokin,L.E., Metabolic Pathways, Vol. VI.
Academic Press, New York and London.

Rehm,W.S., and LeFevre,M.E., 1965.
Effect of dinitrophenol on potential resistance, and H+-rate of frog stomach.
Am. J. Physiol. 208:922.

Rehm,W.S., Schlesinger,H.S., and Dennis,W.H., 1953.
Effect of osmotic gradients on water transport hydrogen ion and chloride ion production in the resting and secreting stomach.
Am. J. Physiol., 175:473.

Rehm,W.S., Butler,C.F., Spangler,S.G., and Sanders, S.S., 1970.
A model to explain uphill water transport in the mammalian stomach.
J. Theor. Biology, 27:433.

Rehm,W.S., Sanders,S.S., Shoemaker,R.L., O'Callaghan, J., Tarvin,J.T., and Friday,E.A., 1973.
Proton conductance of cell membranes.
J. Theor. Biology, 39:131.

Sanders,S.S., and Rehm,W.S., 1968.
Effect of hypotonic solutions on in vitro frog gastric mucosa.
Biophys. J., 8:WF8.

Sanders,S.S., and Rehm,W.S., 1971a.
Inhibition by exogenous ATP of H+ secretion in frog gastric mucosa.
Biophys. Soc. Abs., 11:79a.

Sanders,S.S., and Rehm,W.S., 1971b.
Studies on the role of Ca++ in the ATP inhibition of H+ secretion in rana pipiens' stomach.
Fed. Proc., 30:477.

Sanders,S.S., Shanbour,L.L., and Rehm,W.S., 1970.
Resistance changes of in vitro frog gastric mucosa bathed in very hypotonic fluids.
Biophys. Soc. Abs., 10:32a.

Sanders,S.S., O'Callaghan,J., Butler,C.F., and Rehm, W.S., 1972.
Conductance of submucosal facing membrane of frog gastric mucosa.
Am. J. Physiol., 222:1348.

Spangler,S.G., and Rehm,W.S., 1968.
Potential responses of nutrient membrane of frog's stomach to stop changes in external K+ and Cl- concentrations.
Biophys. J., 8:1211.

Teorell,T., 1939-1940.
On the primary acidity of the gastric juice.
J. Physiol., 97:308.

Teorell,T., 1951.
The acid-base balance of the secreting isolated gastric mucosa.
J. Physiol., 114:267.

Thull,N.B., and Rehm,W.S., 1956.
Composition and osmolarity of gastric juice as a function of plasma osmolarity.
Am. J. Physiol., 185:317.

White,T.D., Swigart,R.H., and Rehm,W.S., 1956.
Limitations on the use of indicators for determination of activity in the gastric lumina.
Am. J. Physiol., 184:453.

REGULATION OF GASTRIC SECRETION

Basil I. Hirschowitz

INTRODUCTION

The intact stomach functions at several levels of organization more complex than the individual secretory cells. This hierachy comprises multiples of each of several cell types, and the juxta-position of different cells with differing functions but possibly interdepedent controls, on a framework of submucosa and muscularis which maintains cellular and mucosal orientation. More importantly the intact state provides circulation of blood and lymph, and hormonal and nervous control, interaction and feedback.

The several secretory functions of the stomach comprise water and electrolytes on the one hand and organic molecules (pepsinogens, mucins, intrinsic factor) on the other. These may be secreted by one cell type in some species and by two or three different cells in others.

The control of mucin secretion or of intrinsic factor secretion is outside the scope of this symposium and there is little known about the physiological controls of either.

In mammals, pepsinogen and electrolyte are secreted from two different cells. Control of secretion has been extensively studied in man, dog, cat and rat with occasional studies in other species such as the pig, the monkey and the ferret. Generally man and pig have similar controls and the dog and cat resemble each other. In the latter group, in which there is no basal secretion, the two cell types (peptic and oxyntic) can be independently affected by stimuli and inhibitors under a number of different conditions (Hirschowitz, 1967; Hirschowitz, 1967). Some agents may have opposite effects, e.g. secretin may inhibit H^+ while stimulating pepsinogen secretion (Nakajima et al., 1969; Brooks and Grossman, 1971; Stening et al., 1969; Johnson and Grossman, 1971); insulin only inhibits electrolyte secretion, and histamine maximally stimulates H^+ secretion while at the same time inhibiting pepsinogen secretion. Vagal stimuli have an equal stimulating effect on both acid and pepsinogen secretion while gastrin has an intermediate effect, stimulating pepsin secretion but less strongly than does vagal secretion (Hirschowitz, 1967; Hirschowitz, 1967). Figure 1 summarizes these relations.

In man, in whom gastric secretion also exhibits a clear response to vagal stimulation, the secretion by the oxyntic and peptic cells can not be nearly as easily differentially affected as in dog and cat. Thus histamine, gastrin and vagal stimuli all stimulate pepsin secretion as they do acid secretion. Though with these, as with secretin and CCK there may be considerable differences in the relative stimulation of pepsin and of H^+, there is no circumstance in which opposite actions can be obtained on the two cell types in man, as it can in the dog. The same is true for the rat.

In most reptiles, amphibia and birds, acid(i.e. electrolytes and water) and pepsinogen are secreted by the same cell. The one exception among commonly studied species is the frog where the peptic cells are localized in the lower esophagus and the acid and mucin secreting cells are in the stomach. The chicken is the one submammalian species which has been best studied in the intact state under various conditions of stimulation and inhibition (Ruoff and Sweing, 1970; Long, 1967; Burhol and Hirschowitz, 1970; Burhol, 1971). Using the stimulants histamine, pentagastrin, urecholine, pancreozymin and the inhibitors secretin and atropine in dose response studies in the gastric fistula chickens (Burhol, 1971) H^+ and pepsin outputs always were affected in the same direction, i.e. they were both stimulated or inhibited together with only minor differences in the ratio of H^+ to pepsin with the various agents. Secretin was especially interesting in that, unlike in the dog and cat where pepsinogen secretion is stimulated while H^+ secretion is inhibited (Nakajima et al., 1969; Brooks and Grossman, 1971; Stening and Grossman, 1969; Johnson and Grossman, 1971), both H^+ and pepsinogen were equally depressed.

It is thus obvious that one cannot speak of gastric secretion

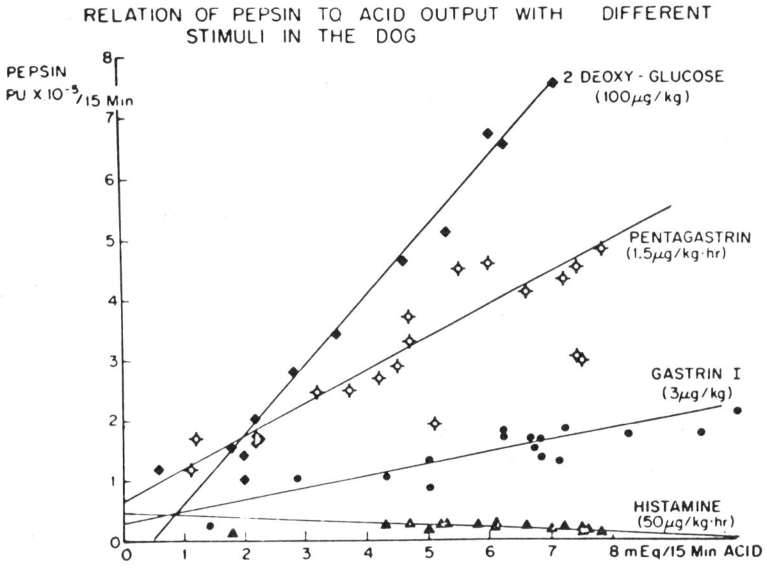

Fig. 1. Relative effects of the 3 major types of gastric stimuli on H^+ and pepsin secretion in the fistula dog. Each point is the coordinate for a 15 min sample during the infusion of each of the stimuli at one near-maximla dose.

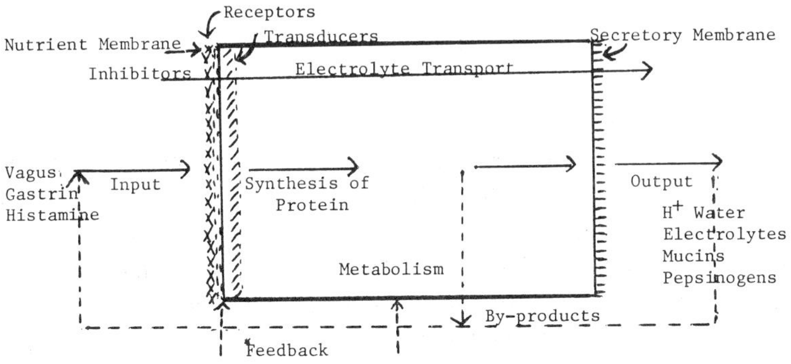

Fig. 2. System diagram showing the various points at which gastric secretion can be regulated or modified. Not shown are inhibitors which can act at different sites in the system.

without defining the secretant, the species, and the condition under which it was obtained, and relating the effect on one cell type to the other. Coupling of function could thus come about from having a common secretory cell as in the submammal or from a common stimulus like the vagus in the mammal, or from other, as yet unidentified means of communication from one mucosal cell type to another.

REGULATION OF GASTRIC SECRETION

The quantity and composition of gastric secretion represents the net effect of interaction of stimuli, inhibitors, feedback mechanisms, and inherent rate limiting steps in the secretory cells and their membranes.

These factors may be represented by a systems diagram (fig. 2)

There are obviously several control points in this system which could be extensively discussed. This presentation will largely confine itself to the receptor systems of the parietal cell (and to a lesser extent the peptic cell) in the light of data available from the dog stomach, including apparent interactions between stimuli or their receptors. Since current evidence is fragmentary, models of these receptors must be tentative and limited. With this clearly understood, I will propose a working model for receptors of the stimuli of H^+ secretion by the parietal cell. Brief mention will also be made of other polypeptides which affect gastric secretion and of the role of blood flow in this regulation.

STIMULI

Gastric secretion of acid and pepsinogen is stimulated by three groups of agents—histamine, gastrin and acetylcholine and some of their analogs. Given appropriate quantitative collection techniques (Hirschowitz, 1968a;Hirschowitz, 1968b;Hirschowitz and Hutchison, 1973) the response of the intact stomach to stimuli can be studied quantitatively and this information can be analyzed kinetically so as to provide numerical values for V^{max} rates of secretion, the amount of drug giving 50% maximum output (K_m) and the threshold dose for drug (Hutchison and Hirschowitz, 1969). Such studies have been performed in man, dogs, cats and chicken with intact stomachs and with various surgical preparations, and are beginning to provide the necessary quantitative data for direct comparison of stimuli and of stomachs.

The Vagus

The vagus is clearly capable of maximally stimulating both acid and pepsin secretion. It is also evident that the vagus plays an additional role in modifying the action of hormones and histamine on the stomach and fact has found major application in the treatment of peptic ulcer by vagotomy. Whether the vagus is also involved in inhibition is much less certain.

Stimulation of Vagus

The gastric vagus in the intact animal can be stimulated by reducing the concentration of metabolizable glucose in a specific center in the hypothalamus (Himsworth, 1970; Himsworth and Colin-Jones, 1969; Hirschowitz and Sachs, 1965). This can be done by insulin hypoglycemia, or by administering into the cerebral center directly (Himsworth, 1970) non-metabolizable sugars such as 2-deoxyglucose or 3 methyglucose. When given intravenously, these analogs are transported into the vagal nuclei and reduce the intracellular concentration of metabolizable glucose (Hirschowitz and Sachs, 1965; Hirschowitz and Robbins, 1966). Other sugars with much weaker action include fructose (Hirschowitz and Sachs, 1965) and xylose (Hirschowitz, unpublished), presumably acting by reducing entry of glucose into the vagal centers and arginine (Hirschowitz, unpublished), acting by an unknown mechanism. Most of those also have other homeostatic effects including, under various conditions, stimulation of hypothalamic, pituitary, islet and adrenal hormone secretion (Himsworth, 1970), but the effect on the vagus seems to be primary and independent of other hormone release. Understanding the action of insulin hypoglycemia is further complicated by other and presumably direct actions of insulin on cell membranes, including the powerful inhibition of acid and electrolyte, ($H^+$and K^+) secretion (Hirschowitz and Robbins, 1966).

However, it is not likely that the cytoglucopenic mechanism is a normal control system for vagal stimulation of gastric electrolyte and pepsin secretion, and the neuro-physiological control mechanisms for the physiological stimulation of the secretory vagus by hunger, habit, appetite or Pavlovian reflex have not been elucidated.

Vagal interactions

From experiments in which, during stimulation by gastrin or histamine the cholinergic influence is removed or blocked e.g. by vagotomy (fig. 3) or atropine administration (fig. 4) and from experiments in which cholinergic agents such as Urecholine are infused as background during stimulation by other agents (fig.5), an important role for acetylcholine emerges.

This role is seen as one of modulation of the receptors for histamine or gastrin whereby removal of acetylcholine (a-ch) makes the histamine receptor less responsive and addition of a-ch,e.g. by background infusion,makes the receptor more responsive to other stimuli. These two actions are represented in the dose response curve by shifts to the right ("competitive" inhibition) or to the left (synergism) or by the term v in the Michaelis equation:

$$\frac{1}{V} = \frac{(K_m)}{(V_m)} \cdot \frac{(\ 1\ )}{(y\ .\ S)} + \frac{1}{V_m} \qquad (1)$$

(V_m = maximum calculated response, K_m the dose of drug giving 50% of V_m)

where V = response and S = dose of drug or hormone being modulated by changes in acetylcholine at the receptor and y is proportional to the amount of acetylcholine. The evidence for this concept is discussed in detail elsewhere (Hirschowitz and Hutchison 1973) and is illustrated in figure 6.

A background of urecholine not only decreases the K_m but also increases the V^{max} (fig. 5). This phenomenon is called potentiation and may be explained by the presence of cholinergic receptors which may themselves result in H^+ secretion but which are not normally receptive to histamine—so called spare receptors. Potentiation may be described in the Michaelis equation by another term x so that equation 1 now has the form:

$$\frac{1}{V} = \frac{K_m}{(V_m + x)} \cdot \frac{1}{(y\ .\ S)} + \frac{1}{(V_m + x)} \qquad (2)$$

where x is a function of the amount of cholinergic background, and V_m is the calculated maximum output in response to drug S. By the

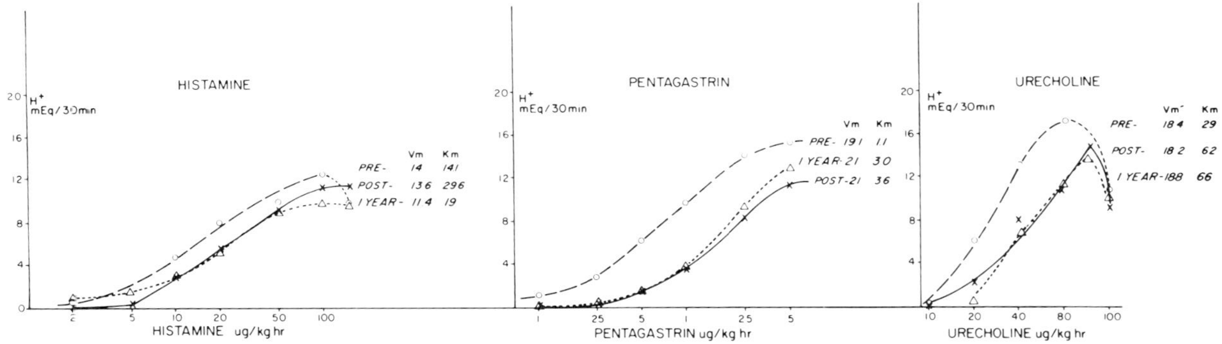

Fig. 5. Effect of denervation of the fundus (highly selective vagotomy) in 3 dogs on dose responses to histamine, pentagastrin and to urecholine, showing competitive inhibition—i.e. V_{max} unchanged, K_m increased. At this time the dogs were unresponsive to vagal stimulation by 2-deoxy-glucose.

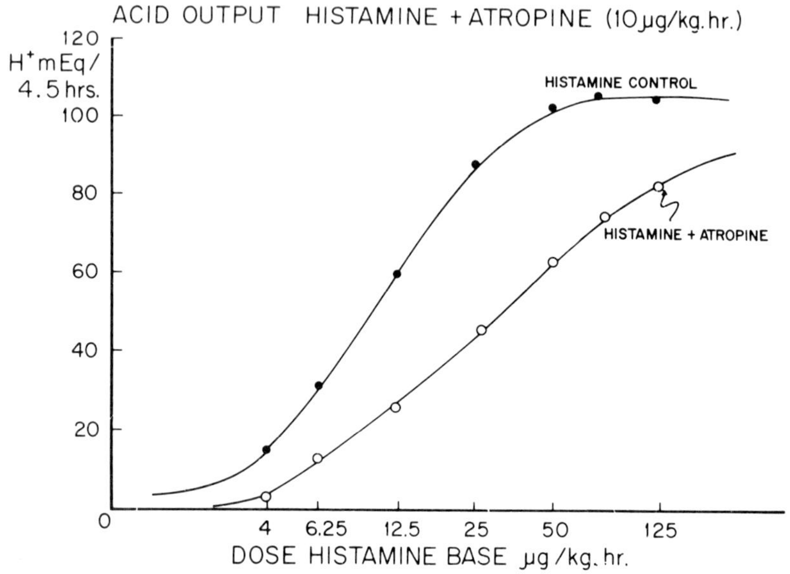

Fig. 4. Competitive inhibition of histamine by atropine given as background in the dose of 10 ug/kg. hr. V_{max} unchanged, curve shifted to the right (K_m increased).

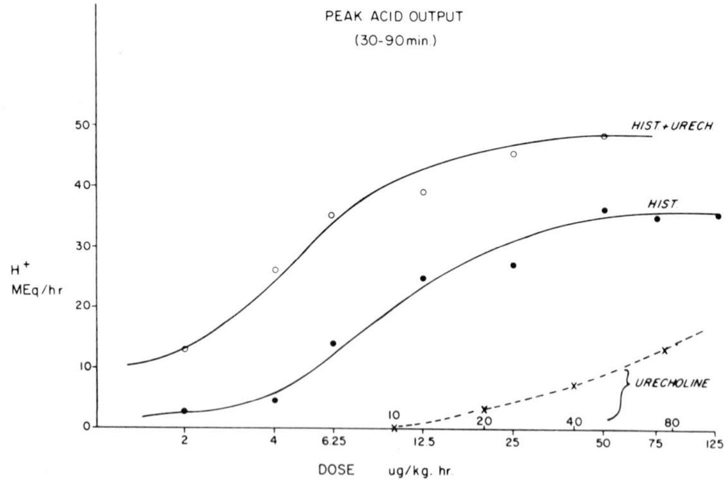

Fig. 5. Three dose response curves in fistula dogs with histamine alone, urecholine alone and histamine with background urecholine (40 ug/kg. hr) showing synergism - curve shifted to left and potentiation-curve shifted up.

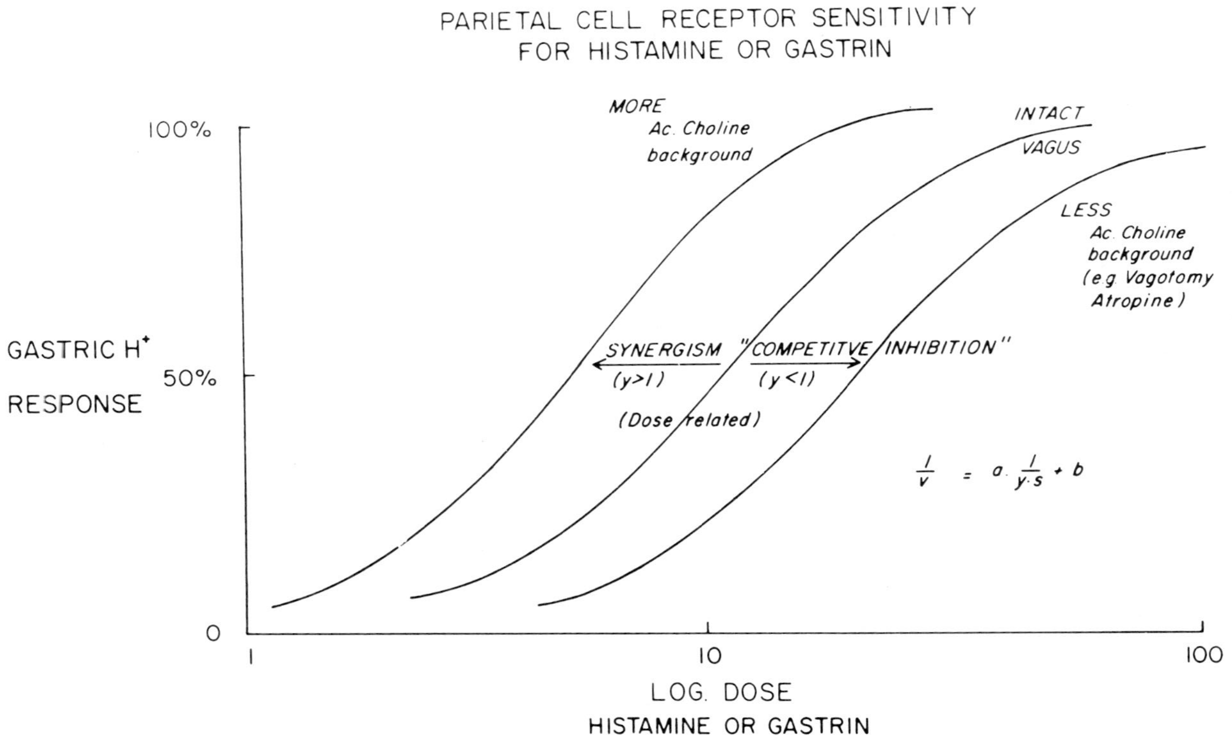

Fig. 6. Graphic illustration of synergism and of competitive inhibition as a function of activity of the cholinergic receptor acting on histamine or gastrin stimulation.

hypothesis proposed here x can only be positive for the effect of vagus on other stimuli, and (V_m + x) the calculated maximal output for the stimulus combination (y . S).

In the normal physiology synergism between acetylcholine and gastrin allows for the relatively small amount of gastrin released from the antrum by vagal activity to stimulate gastric H^+ secretion from the "primed" fundus (Grossman, 1970).

Other Functions of Vagus

While the vagus appears to be the major control mechanism for gastric antral motility and emptying, only a minor or negligible literature exists on the possible role of the vagus in the secretion of mucins or intrinsic factor, in gastric mucosal regeneration or in regulating gastric blood flow, in inhibitory reflexes or hormonal inhibition of acid secretion.

HISTAMINE

Though histamine is obviously involved in acid secretion, its precise physiologic role has not yet been identified. Histamine has actions on other tissues—smooth muscle, adrenal medulla and brain, and these are blocked by "conventional" antihistamines, whereas the gastric effect is not (Roch, 1961). Black and his colleagues (Black, 1973) have shown that the gastric histamine receptor is different from the others and have not only synthesized specific antagonists for this receptor (designated H-2), but have also studied two histamine analogs one of which (4-Methyl histamine) is much more specific for the H-2 receptor, and another (2-Methyl histamine) which is much more active in the other tissues (H-1 receptors).

We have studied a series of active histamine analogs in the dog with regard to both H^+ and pepsin secretion (Hirschowitz and Hutchison, 1973). These studies show that the peptic and parietal cell do not share receptor characteristics in the dog.

These compounds are histamine, 2 chain analogs—n-methyl histamine and n-dimethyl histamine, and 3 ring analogs betazole, triazole and 4-methyl-histamine.

From the dose response curves for H^+ output the chain methyl analogs have the same characteristics as does histamine—with the same K_m and V_{max}. In a separate group of animals 4-methyl histamine was also found to have essentially the same characteristics (V_{max} and K_m) as histamine (Hirschowitz et al., 1974). Triazole is less potent and betazole much less so than histamine.

Pepsin secretion is stimulated more by triazole and betazole in the dog than by the other analogs, indicating differences in the receptor systems for histamine between these two cells. Further difference between the two cells is shown by the lack of inhibition of pepsin secretion by the specific H-2 histamine antagonist Metiamide. In fact, in some circumstances, e.g. during cholinergic stimulation, Metiamide may even stimulate pepsin secretion while inhibiting acid secretion (Hirschowitz, 1973).

Because of the lack of stimulation or even inhibition of pepsin secretion by histamine (Hirschowitz, 1968) we have proposed elsewhere (Hirschowitz and Sachs, 1968; Hirschowitz and Sachs, 1969) that histamine is unlikely to be the mediator for gastrin or cholinergic stimulation of gastric secretion, at least in the dog.

GASTRIN

In the dog gastrin is a potent H^+ stimulus and a moderate stimulus of pepsin secretion. Its effects are "competitively" inhibited by vagotomy to about the same extent as are those of histamine (fig. 3). However, gastrin stimulation is extremely sensitive to atropine inhibition, (Hirschowitz and Sachs, 1969), almost as much as are cholinergic stimuli, but much less so than histamine. This suggests that gastrin receptors are not only modulated by acetylcholine, as is histamine, but may in fact share the cholinergic receptor. Since it is also inhibited by burimamide, the histamine H-2 antagonist, (Black, 1973) we would have to conclude that gastrin also shared the histamine receptor. Further evidence for the latter is the failure to find either synergism or potentiation, but only additive effects when pentagastrin is given as background to histamine (Hirschowitz, 1973). This may be described by the modified Michaelis equation:

$$\frac{1}{V} = \frac{(K_m)}{(V_m)} \quad \frac{1}{(S + Z)} + \frac{1}{V_m} \tag{3}$$

where S is the dose of histamine and Z the histamine equivalent of the gastrin background.

The control of gastrin secretion and the many other actions of gastrin are discussed elsewhere in this symposium.

Receptor Models

A tentative receptor model for the parietal cell in the dog is that there are 2 types of receptors, histamine (H-2) and cholinergic (muscarinic), each being distinct for its primary agonist. Gastrin is seen as binding to both and thus its action can be inhibited by specific antagonists to either. Furthermore the cholinergic stimuli or their receptor play a major secondary role in modulating the other receptor. No specific data are available yet on whether histamine has an equivalent role in the function of the acetylcholine receptor.

OTHER POLYPEPTIDES

The unravelling of the peptide structure of the gastrointestinal hormones has led to a number of studies of structure-funciton relationships. The identity of the C-terminal pentapeptide-amide structure of gastrins I or II from all species, cholecystokinin (now known to be identical to pancreozymin, hence CCK-PZ) and caerulein extracted from the skin of the frog Hyla caerulea explains the similar actions of these agents on gastric secretion and adjacent organs (Johnson et al., 1970) in various species in vivo and in some cases in vitro (Nakajima et al., 1971).

CCK-PZand Caerulein

In the dog and in man CCK-PZ and caerulein stimulate gastric acid and pepsin secretion but only to about 50% as high at maximum rates as does gastrin, whereas in the cat and rat CCK stimulates to the same maximum. When tested together, CCK competitively inhibits gastrin stimulation of secretion in man and dog but not in the cat or rat. Desulfated caerulein is a several-times potent gastric or gall bladder stimulant than natural caerulein (Johnson et al., 1970) but is not an inhibitor of gastrin stimulated secretion in the dog (Johnson and Grossman, 1971). This anomaly does not fit the ready explanation for the apparently competitive inhibition of gastrin-stimulation by CCK-PZ. Further CCK-PZ but not secretin, has been found to be an inhibitor of H^+ secretion in vitro in the amphibian mucosa

(Nakajima et al., 1971). When CCK or caerulein are tested against histamine-stimulated secretion in the dog (innervated or denervated), there is no inhibition but rather, at intermediate doses of histamine an additive response (Stening et al., 1969), as for pentagastrin (Hirschowitz, 1973). These peptides thus seem to have specificity for binding sites, rather than for the secretory cells in their inhibition of secretion by the stomach. These findings are of singular interest since none of over 600 analogs of gastrin prepared by Morely exhibited any inhibitory action against gastrin (Morley, 1968a; Morley, 1968b).

Secretin

Among many upper gastrointestinal and vascular effects, secretin inhibits methacholine or gastrin-stimulated acid secretion non-competitively in the dog and man but not in the cat nor does it significantly inhibit histamine-stimulated secretion in any species (Nakajima et al., 1969; Brooks and Grossman, 1971; Stening et al., 1969). At the same time in dog and in man secretin is a potent pepsigogue, even in the presence of histamine-stimulation as well as in the cat where it does not inhibit acid secretion. These actions can be reproduced by endogenous release of secretin from the duodenum by acid perfusion (Morley, 1968; Johnston and Duthie, 1969). In the chicken, however, secretin inhibits both H^+ and pepsin secretion equally (Burhol, 1971).

The inhibition of histamine-stimulated acid secretion by fat in the duodenum exceeds the action of exogenous secretion of CCK (Johnston and Duthie, 1969; Gregory, 1967; Johnson and Grossman, 1969) and suggests that secretin may not be the inhibitory hormone of the intestine (enterogastrone) (Uvnas, 1970) — other polypeptides such as G.I.P. may fit the role.

Glucagon

Glucagon, structurally related to secretin, has much more disputed actions on the stomach (Grossman, 1970) — at high doses it appears to be a partial inhibitor of weaker stimulation by either gastrin or feeding, but like secretin does not reduce histamine-stimulated acid secretion in most reported experiments (Dotevall et al., 1969).

Insulin

Insulin is the only known hormone which is capable of complete inhibition of either near maximal gastrin, histamine or vagally stimulated gastric H^+ and electrolyte secretion in the innervated or denervated dog stomach. The inhibition is independent of hypoglycemia or of vagus stimulation (Hirschowitz, 1966) and is not reproduced by 2-deoxy-D-glucose (Hirschowitz and Sachs, 1965), a powerful stimulant acting like hypoglycemia on the gastric secretory vagus. Inhibition is dose related, being evident at doses of 0.3 units/kg and maximal at doses $\gtrsim$ 0.9 units/kg. It is not related to its glucagon impurity and cannot be reproduced by glucagon (40 ug/kg) injection (Hirschowitz and Robbins, 1966). Unlike inhibition secondary to reduction in blood flow, there are major and specific changes in composition of gastric juice viz. reduced $[H^+]$, increased $[Na^+]$, and reduction in $[K^+]$ to levels below plasma concentration. The volume of gastric juice is reduced proportionately to the concentration of K^+ in gastric juice (Hirschowitz, 1966; Hirschowitz and Sachs, 1967). This inhibition is further different from other (hormone) inhibitors in that its effect can be immediately and specifically reversed by the intravenous injection of K^+ or Rb^+ (Hirschowitz and Sachs, 1967) but not by Cs^+, Li^+, Na^+, NH_4^+, Ca^{++}, Mg^{++} or Cl^-. Reversal is evident at an intravenous dose of KCl or RbCl of 0.5 mEq/kg given in 5 minutes, is complete at a dose of 1 mEq/kg and the inhibition can be prevented by the intravenous preloading of 1–2mEq/kg. hr.

An action of insulin has been shown in the *in vitro* guines pig gastric mucosa (Hirschowitz and Robbins, 1966) with reduction in both H^+ and I_{sc} but not in amphibian mucosa.

There is no ready explanation for this action of insulin among its many others, but it does appear to be primary, rather than a secondary, homeostatic response to some other action of insulin, such as hypoglycemia. Insulin could be involved in physiological feedback control of acid secretion, but is not likely to do this normally acting alone. The potent insulin-stimulating effects or gastrin, secretin and CCK (Unger et al., 1967) may be important in this regard. No experiments have as yet been done to determine whether insulin could potentiate the inhibitory actions of each of the other hormones, CCK-PZ, secretin or glucagon on gastric electrolyte secretion, nor whether inhibition by the other hormones is reversible by K^+.

BLOOD FLOW IN REGULATION OF GASTRIC SECRETION

The intact stomach differs perhaps as much as anything from the isolated or in vitro gastric mucosa in possessing and depending upon the circulation of blood for the supply of oxygen, water, ions (esp. Cl and K); to bring these and the stimulant as close to the secretory cells as possible and by removing HCO_3^--laden, Cl^--depleted blood, to control the composition of the extracellular fluid bathing the gastric cells. Thus both the total blood flow and the partition of this blood between the mucosa and submucosa are likely to be important in the situation where blood flow may be rate-limiting to gastric secretion. In conscious dogs both histamine and gastrin increase gastric mucosa blood flow with increasing secretion but not total blood flow in Heidenhain pouches (Swan and Jacobson, 1967). For the same rate of H^+ secretion, histamine increases mucosal blood flow more (Swan and Jacobson, 1967). On the other hand, vagal stimulation of gastric secretion concurrently increases both total arterial and mucosal blood flow in the innervated stomach, and all parameters are reduced by atropine or by pentobarbital (Jacobson and Chang, 1969). Intraduodenal fat reduces aminopyrine clearance proportionately less than H^+ secretion, showing that the inhibitory effect is not circulatory (Bochenek et al., 1971). In direct studies of blood flow and secretion in a flap of dog stomach (Moody, 1967) blood flow is always increased with increased secretion, but with inhibition, e.g. by thiocyanate, may remain increased while H^+ secretion is reduced.

The three major gastric stimuli—histamine, gastrin and vagus—also have direct concurrent actions on mesenteric and mucosal blood flow; by the same token there are inhibitors such as atropine which act by simultaneously blocking vagal or cholinergic stimuli at the mucosa and the blood vessels, i.e. the equivalent of simultaneous withdrawal of the stimulus to both. There are other inhibitors in vivo such as pitressin (Blum, 1971; Bell and Battersby, 1969) and norepinephrine (Cowley and Code, 1970) which have no action on the gastric mucosa in vitro, but have a significant primary direct effect on splanchnic and gastric blood vessels (Bell and Battersby, 1969). Thus blood flow may be rate limiting to acid secretion, but is usually in great excess for even maximum rates of secretion (Blum, 1971).

Since H^+ ions are formed *de novo*, and free water is extracted from the interstitial fluid for this secretion, the interstitial fluid would soon become so hypertonic and alkaline that the cells would be damaged and secretion would cease. An increase in mucosal blood flow is, therefore, important in maintaining gastric mucosal homeostasis (Hirschowitz, 1968a, 1968b, 1968d; Altamirano et al., 1969). This maintenance of a relatively stable environment for the gastric mucosal cells may explain why the intact mucosa would function for so much longer and at a higher rate than the *in vitro* gastric mucosa, where, even with the muscle layer stripped, the diffusion pathway is several times longer than from the secreting cells to the capillaries.

REFERENCES

Altamirano,M.,Izaquirre,E.and Milgram,E., 1969.
Osmotic concentration of the gastric juice of dogs.
Amer. J. Physiol. 202:283.

Bell,P.R.F. and Battersby,C., 1969.
Effect of vasopressin (pitressin) on gastric mucosal blood flow measured by clearance of krypton.
Surgery 66:510.

Black,J.W., 1973.
Definitions and antagonisms and Histamine H-2 receptors.
Nature 236:385.

Blum,A.L., 1971.
Kinetics of inhibition of canine gastric secretion by vasopressin.
Gastroenterology 61:461.

Bochenek,W.,Long,J.F. and Balint,J.A., 1971.
Relationship of aminopyrine clearance to gastric secretion after feeding and feeding plus fat.
Amer. J. Physiol. 220:945.

Brooks,A.M. and Grossman,M.I., 1971.
Effect of secretin and cholecystokinin on pentagastrin-stimulated gastric secretion in man.
Gastroenterology 59:114.

Burhol,P.G., 1971.
Gastric secretion in chickens.
Scand. J. Gastroent. 6, Suppl. 11, pp. 1.

Burhol,P.G. and Hirschowitz,B.I., 1970.
Single subcutaneous doses of histamine and pentagastrin in gastric fustula chickens.
Amer. J. Physiol. 218:1671.

Cowley,D.J. and Code,C.F., 1970.
Effects of secretory inhibitors on mucosal blood flow in nonsecreting stomach of conscious dogs.
Amer. J. Physiol. 218:270.

Dotevall,G., Kock,N.P. and Walan,A., 1969.
Inhibition of pentagastrin induced gastric acid secretion in man by glucagon given intravenously.
Scand. J. Gastroent. 4:713.

Emas,S. and Grossman, M.I., 1967.
Comparison of gastric secretion in conscious dogs and cats.
Gastroenterology 52:29.
Gregory,R.A., 1967.
"Enterogastrone", in Gastric Secretion, Mechanisms and Control. Edit by Schnitka,T.K., et al.
Pergamon Press, Oxford.
Grossman,M.I., 1970.
Hormone-hormone and vagus-hormone interactions, on gastric acid secretion, in Frontiers in Gastrointestinal Hormone Research.
Nobel Symposium XVI Stockholm.
Himsworth,R.L., 1970.
Hypothalamic control of adrenaline secretion in response to insufficient glucose.
J. Physiol. (Lond.) 206:411.
Himsworth,R.L. and Colin-Jones,D.G., 1969.
Factors which determine the gastric secretory response to 2-deoxy-D-glucose.
Gut 10:1015.
Hirschowitz, B.I., 1966.
Characteristics of inhibition of gastric electrolyte secretion by insulin.
Am. J. Dig. Dis. 11:183.
Hirschowitz,B.I., 1967a.
The control of pepsinogen secretion.
New York Acad. Sci. 140:709.
Hirschowitz,B.I., 1967b.
The secretion of pepsinogen in Handbook of Physiology - Alimentary Canal, Edit by C.F. Code.
Amer. Physiol. Soc., Washington, D.C.
Hirschowitz,B.I., 1968a.
Histamine dose responses in gastric fistula dogs - decreasing secretion with time.
Gastroent. 54:523.
Hirschowitz,B.I., 1968b.
Restoration of homeostasis during histamine-stimulated gastric secretion.
Gastroent. 54:898.
Hirschowitz,B.I., 1968c.
Apparent kinetics of histamine dose responsive gas-

tric water and electrolyte secretion in the dog.
Gastroenterology 54:514.
Hirschowitz,B.I., 1968d.
Homeostatic consequences of gastric water, acid and electrolyte secretion in the dog.
Gastroenterology 54:887.
Hirschowitz,B.I., 1973.
Effects of burimamide and metiamide on gastric acid and pepsin secretion in the dog.
Proc. London Conference on H_2 Receptors (In Press).
Hirschowitz,B.I. and Gibson,R. and Hutchison,G.A., 1974.
Stimulation of acid and pepsin secretion in the fistula dog by 4(5) methyl histamine, a specific H-2 agonist.
Amer. J. Dig. Dis. (In Press).
Hirschowitz,B.I. and Hutchison,G.A., 1973a.
A working hypothesis for urecholine effects on histamine stimulation of gastric secretion.
Scand. J. Gastroent. 8:569.
Hirschowitz,B.I. and Hutchison,G.A., 1973b.
Gastric H^+, Cl^-, and pepsin secretion in dogs with histamine, betazole, triazole and n-methyl histamines.
Am. J. Physiol. (In Press).
Hirschowitz,B.I. and Robbins,R.C., 1966.
Direct inhibition of gastric electrolyte secretion by insulin independently of hypoglycemia or the vagus.
Amer. J. Dig. Dis. 11:199.
Hirschowitz,B.I. and Sachs,G., 1965.
Vagal gastric secretory stimulation by 2-deoxy-D-glucose.
Amer. J. Physiol. 209:452.
Hirschowitz,B.I. and Sachs,G., 1967.
Insulin-inhibition of gastric secretion: reversal by rubidium.
Amer. J. Physiol. 213:1401.
Hirschowitz,B.I. and Sachs,G., 1968.
Gastrin I, pentagrastrin and histamine in the fistula dog.
Fed. Proc. 27:1318.
Hirschowitz,B.I. and Sachs,G., 1969.

Atropine inhibition of insulin-, histamine-, and pentagastrin stimulated gastric and pepsin secretion in the dog.
Gastroenterology 56:693.

Hirschowitz,B.I., Sachs,G. and Hutchison,G.A., 1973.
Lack of potentiation or synergism between histamine and pentagastrin in the fustula dog.
Amer. J. Physiol. 224:509.

Hutchison,G.A. and Hirschowitz,B.I., 1969.
Two models of gastric H, Na, K and Cl secretion in the dog using histamine and pentagastrin.
Amer. J. Physiol. 216:487.

Jacobson,E.D. and Chang,A.C.K., 1969.
Comparison of gastrin and histamine on gastric mucosal blood flow.
Proc. Soc. Exp. Biol. & Med. 130:484.

Johnson,L.R. and Grossman,M.I., 1969.
Effects of fat, secretin and cholecystokinin on histamine-stimulated gastric secretion.
Amer. J. Physiol. 216:1176.

Johnson,L.R. and Grossman,M.I., 1971.
Intestinal hormones as inhibitor of gastric secretion.
Gastroenterology 60:120.

Johnson,L.R. Stening,G.F. and Grossman,M.I., 1970.
Effect of sulfation on the gastrointestinal actions of caerulein.
Gastroenterology 58:208.

Johnston,D. and Duthie,H.L., 1969.
Effect of fat in the duodenum on gastric acid secretion before and after vagotomy in man.
Scand. J. Gastroent. 4:561.

Long,J.F., 1967.
Gastric secretion in unanesthetized chicken.
Amer. J. Physiol. 212:1303.

Moody,F.G., 1967.
Gastric blood flow and acid secretion during direct intraarterial histamine administration.
Gastroenterology 52:216.

Morley,J.S., 1968a.
Structure-function relationships in gastrin-like peptides.
Proc. Roy. Soc. B. 170:97.

Morley, J.S., 1968b.
Structure-activity relationship.
Fed. Proc. 27:1314.
Nakajima,S., Hirschowitz,B.I., Shoemaker,R.L. and Sachs,G., 1971.
Inhibition of gastric acid secretion in vitro by C-terminal octapeptide of cholecystokinin.
Amer. J. Physiol. 221:1009.
Nakajima,S., Nakamura,M., and Magee,D.R., 1969.
Effect of gastric secretion on gastric acid and pepsin secretion in response to various stimuli.
Amer. J. Physiol. 216:87.
Roch e Silva,M., 1961.
On the nature of the receptors for histamine.
Chemotherapia 3:544.
Ruoff,H.J. and Sewing,K.F., 1970.
Histamin, Histidendicarboxylase und Gastrin im oberen Verdauungstrakt des Huhns.
Nauny-Schmiedenberg Arch. Pharmak. 265:301.
Stening,G.F., Johnson,L.R. and Grossman,M.I., 1969a.
Effect of secretin on acid and pepsin secretion in cats and dogs.
Gastroenterology 56:468.
Stening,G.F., Johnson,L.R. and Grossman,M.I., 1969b.
Effect of cholecystokinin and caerulein on gastrin and histamine-evoked gastric secretion.
Gastroenterology 57:44.
Swan,K.G. and Jacobson,E.D., 1967.
Gastric blood flow and secretion in conscious dogs.
Amer. J. Physiol. 212:891.
Unger,R.H., Ketterer,H. and Dupree,H., Elsentraut,A.M., 1967.
The effects of secretin, pancreozymin, and gastrin on insulin and glucagon secretion in anesthetized dogs.
J. Clin. Invest. 46:630.
Uvnas B., 1970.
Bulbogastrone.
Brohee Lecture, 4th World Congress of Gastroenterology. Copenhagen, Denmark.

HISTAMINE H_2-RECEPTOR ANTAGONISTS AND GASTRIC SECRETION

M. E. Parsons and J. W. Black

INTRODUCTION

Histamine is a potent stimulant of gastric acid secretion in all species that have been studied, including man, but its possible role in the normal physiological control of secretion has always been controversial. McIntosh (1938) proposed that histamine in the gastric mucosa might be the local common mediator for physiological stimulation of secretion. His evidence was mainly circumstantial but studies on histamine formation and metabolism led Code(1965) to reiterate this hypothesis. The hypothesis implies that the normal controls for stimulation of secretion, that is via the vagus nerve and endogenous gastrin, act through a histamine link. If this is the case then a specific inhibitor for this action of histamine would be of great value in the understanding of the physiology of gastric acid secretion and possibly in its control.

However, conventional antihistamines such as mepyramine, even in high concentrations, fail to inhibit histamine-stimulated gastric secretion. They also fail to inhibit the effect of histamine in increasing heart rate and in inhibiting contractions of the rat uterus. This led to the classification of histamine receptors into two types (Ash and Schild, 1966; Black et al., 1972), H_1-receptors that can be blocked by mepyramine and related antihistamines and H_2-receptors which are refractory to mepyramine. Histamine-stimulated gastric secretion is mediated by the H_2-histamine receptor and we have developed the specific competitive antagonists, burimamide and metiamide, for this receptor (Black et al., 1972, 1973).

The evidence that inhibition of histamine-stimulated gastric acid secretion is the result of the blockade of H_2-histamine receptors has been presented previously (Black et al., 1972; Parsons, 1973) and the present paper starts with this assumption and deals with the interaction of metiamide with gastric secretion stimulated by histamine, pentagastrin and the stable choline ester, carbachol. The experiments reported here were all performed in our laboratory but details of other investigations using metiamide will be published in the Proceedings of a Symposium on Histamine H_2-Receptor Antagonists held in London on October 1st and 2nd, 1973.

Gastric secretion was studied in three preparations: the lumen perfused stomach of the anesthetized rat (Ghosh and Schild, 1958; Parsons, 1969), a similar preparation using the anesthetized cat, and the conscious Heidenhain pouch dog.

EXPERIMENTAL RESULT

In the rat preparation intravenous infusion of 0.25 u mol/kg/min histamine produced approximately 70% of maximal acid secretion, the dose required for maximal secretion proving to be too toxic for long-term administration. Using this rate of infusion a secretory plateau is obtained in 30–45 minutes and can be maintained at a fairly constant level for 2–3 hours. Using single intravenous injections of metiamide during the plateau the dose-response relationship inhibition, based on peak change in H^+ secretion, was established in a group of 35 rats and the inhibitory ED_{50} was found to be 1.6 (1.2–2.2) umol/kg.

A more detailed study was carried out using single intravenous injections of histamine and an intravenous infusion of metiamide 0.1 u mol/kg/min. Each of a group of nine rats received 0.5, 1.0 and 2.0 u mol/kg of histamine intravenously, the order of allocation being determined by three 3 x 3 Latin squares. Then the infusion of metiamide was started and a single dose of histamine (1 u mol/kg) was given repeatedly until stable inhibition was achieved. Each rat then received 4.0, 8.0 and 16.0 u mol/kg of histamine, the order of allocation being determined by a further three 3 x 3 Latin squares. The dose-response curves were based on peak changes in H^+ output and are shown in figure 1. Statistical analysis showed that the curves were linear, parallel and displaced by a dose ratio of 7.0. Metiamide

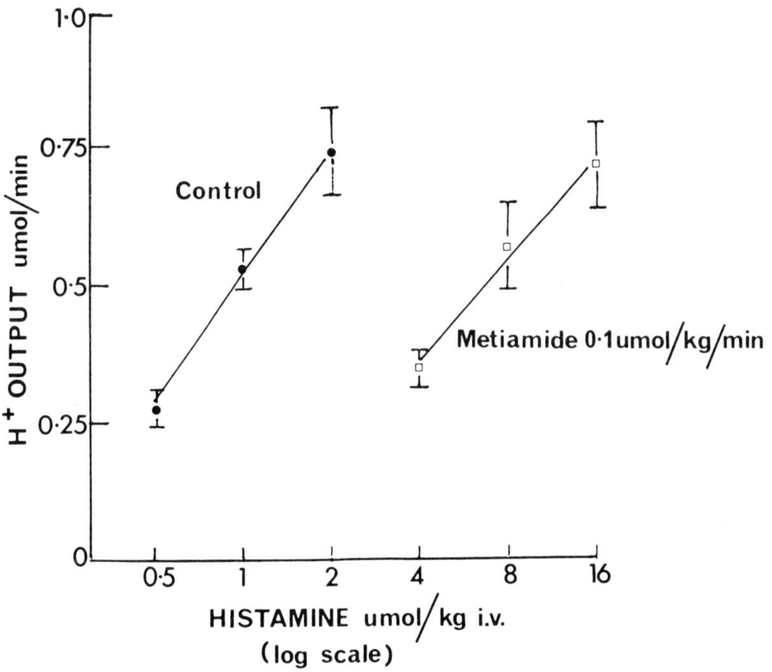

Fig. 1. Rat gastric secretion: The effect of an intravenous infusion of metiamide on the secretory responses to single intravenous injections of histamine.

is thus an effective surmountable inhibitor of histamine-stimulated gastric secretion in the anesthetized rat.

The specificity of the inhibition is indicated by the failure of metiamide to inhibit dibutyryl cyclic-AMP-stimulated secretion. Dibutyryl cyclic-AMP infused intravenously at a rate of 2.0 mg/kg/min stimulates gastric secretion in the anesthetized rat and an intravenous injection of metiamide 4 umol/kg, (that is, twice the ED_{50} for inhibition of histamine-stimulated gastric secretion) produced no inhibition. In the same preparation a dose of 16 umol/kg of pyridene-2-thioacetamide, an analogue of the Searle "antigastrin", produced marked inhibition. This dose had been previously shown to be approximately equipotent to 4 u mol/kg of metiamide in inhibiting histamine-stimulated secretion. These results show that metiamide at dose levels which cause marked inhibition of histamine-stimulated secretion does not do so by some unspecified suppression of the secretory process, since it is ineffective against dibutyryl cyclic-AMP.

However, when similar studies to those described for histamine were carried out using pentagastrin 1 u g/kg/min as the secretory stimulant, metiamide caused inhibition which was quantitatively, and in time-course, similar to that seen against histamine. The inhibitory ED_{50} against pentagastrin was found to be 2.4 (1.9–3.0) umol/kg which is very si nilar to that obtained against histamine, and shows that metiamide is an effective inhibitor of pentagastrin-stimulated secretion in the rat.

Doses of metiamide which caused marked inhibition of histamine- and pentagastrin-stimulated secretion were ineffective against secretion evoked by the stable choline ester, carbachol 0.5 ug/kg/min, (figure2). However, high doses of metiamide (above 64 umol/kg) did produce some inhibition of cholinergically evoked secretion.

That the inhibition of histamine-stimulated gastric secretion by metiamide is not restricted to the rat was shown by studies carried out using a stomach lumen perfusion technique in the anesthetized cat. Near maximal secretion stimulated by histamine infused at a rate of 0.05 umol/kg/min was inhibited by metiamide in a dose-dependent manner and the inhibitory ED_{50} of 1.2 umol/kg is not significantly different from that obtained in the rat.

The studies described so far were carried out in anesthetized animals–could they be extended to the conscious Heidenhain pouch dog?

Complete dose-response curves to graded rates of histamine administration were established in each of six dogs and a dose of 20 u mol/h was chosen as suitable for establishing a maximal rate of secretion in any dog. Histamine infused at this rate produced a secretory response which reached a plateau after 1–1.5 hours and this rate of secretion could be maintained for 5–6 hours. The inhibitory effect of three doses of metiamide 2.0, 4.0 and 8.0 u mol/kg given by rapid intravenous injection during a maximal plateau response to histamine were studied. In these and subsequent studies % inhibition was calculated from the acid output in the 15 minute sample immediately prior to metiamide administration and the acid output in the sample at peak inhibition. From 21 experiments the inhibitory ED_{50} in the dog was found to be 3.1 (2.0–4.9) u mol/kg which is not significantly different from the value found in the rat. These results indicate that metiamide is an effective inhibitor of histamine-stimulated secretion in the dog.

Further studies were carried out using a single intravenous injec-

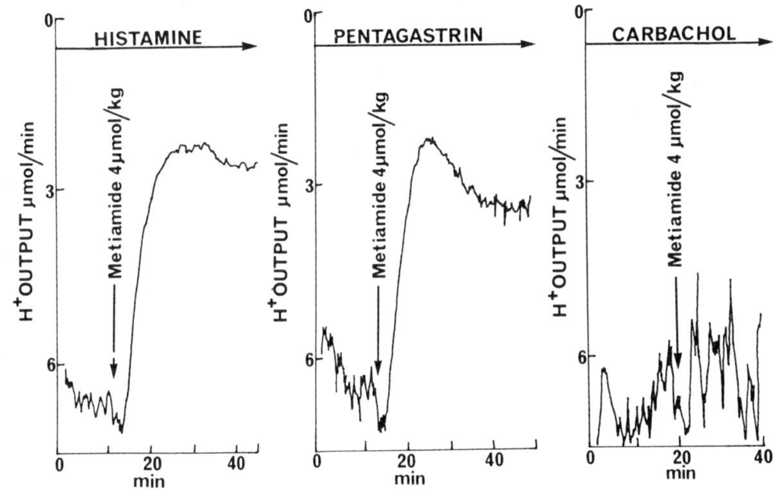

Fig. 2. Dog gastric secretion: The effect of a single intravenous injection of metiamide on the secretory response to four dose levels of histamine infusion.

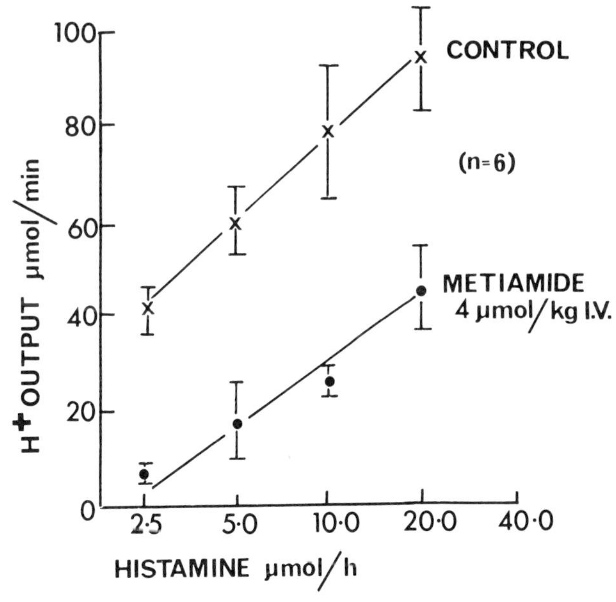

Fig. 3. Dog gastric secretion: The effect of a single intravenous injection of metiamide on the secretory response to three dose levels of pentagastrin infusion.

tion of metiamide 4.0 umol/kg against the secretory plateau to four dose levels of histamine infusion 2.5, 5.0, 10.0 and 20.0 u mol/h, all the secretory levels being studied in each of six dogs. The dose-response curves are shown in figure 3, the control curve being based on the acid output immediately prior to metiamide injection and the treated curve on the lowest level of acid output obtained after metiamide. Statistical analysis showed that the two curves were linear and parallel, indicating that metiamide is a surmountable inhibitor of histamine-stimulated gastric secretion in the dog.

Similar studies were carried out in the same group of dogs using pentagastrin as the stimulant. Initial dose-response studies indicated that an intravenous infusion of pentagastrin 8 u g/kg/h produced maximal secretion in any dog, and using this rate of infusion the effect of intravenous injection of metiamide 2.0, 4.0 and 8.0 u mol/kg were studied during the plateau response. From 17 experiments the inhibitory ED_{50} was found to be 6.1 (1.4–26.9) u mol/kg which is not significantly different from that obtained against histamine but the confidence region for pentagastrin is very wide.

Using single intravenous injection of metiamide 4.0 u mol/kg against the secretory plateau to three dose levels of pentagastrin infusion 0.5, 1.0 and 2.0 u g/kg/h in each of the six dogs, dose-response curves were established as described for histamine above, (fig. 4). Statistical analysis showed that the two curves were linear and parallel indicating that metiamide is a surmountable inhibitor of pentagastrin-stimulated gastric secretion in the dog.

Preliminary studies using maximal carbachol-stimulated secretion (carbachol 100 u g/h) showed that, unlike in the rat, metiamide by rapid intravenous injection was an effective inhibitor of cholinergically evoked secretion, a dose of 8 u mol/kg intravenously producing 65.0 $\pm$ 3.5% inhibition (n = 6). Using this dose against the secretory plateau stimulated by three rates of carbachol infusion 25, 50 and 100 u g/h resulted in the dose-response curves shown in figure 5. Statistical analysis showed that although the two dose-response curves were linear, metiamide did not produce a parallel displacement in contrast to the results found with histamine and pentagastrin.

To study the inhibitory action of metiamide under nearer equilibrium conditions, the effects of intravenous infusions of the antagonist were tested against intravenous infusions of the agonist. Control dose-response curves were established to the agonist using stepwise doubling increments in the rate of intravenous infusion in

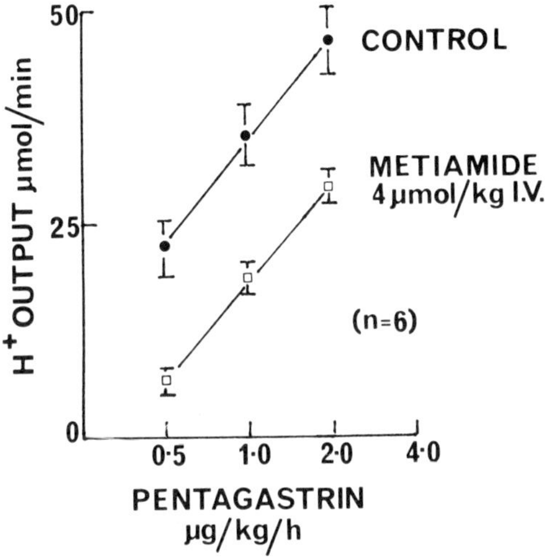

Fig. 4. Dog gastric secretion: The effect of a single intravenous injection of metiamide on the secretory response to three dose levels of pentagastrin infusion.

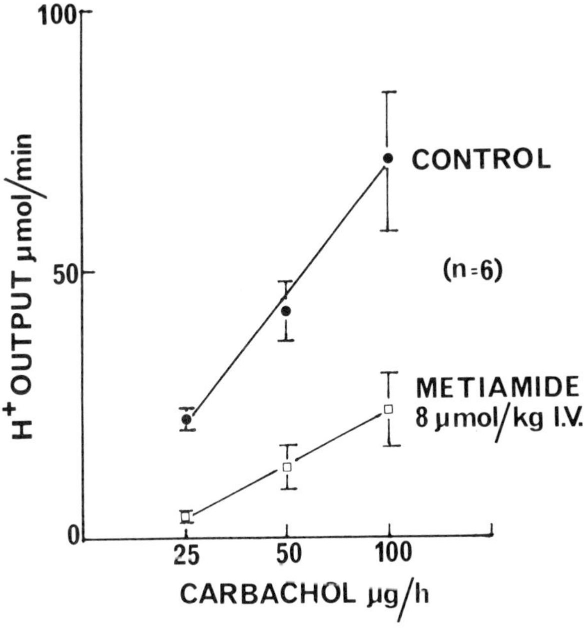

Fig. 5. Dog gastric secretion: The effect of a single intravenous injection of metiamide on the secretory response to three dose levels of carbachol infusion.

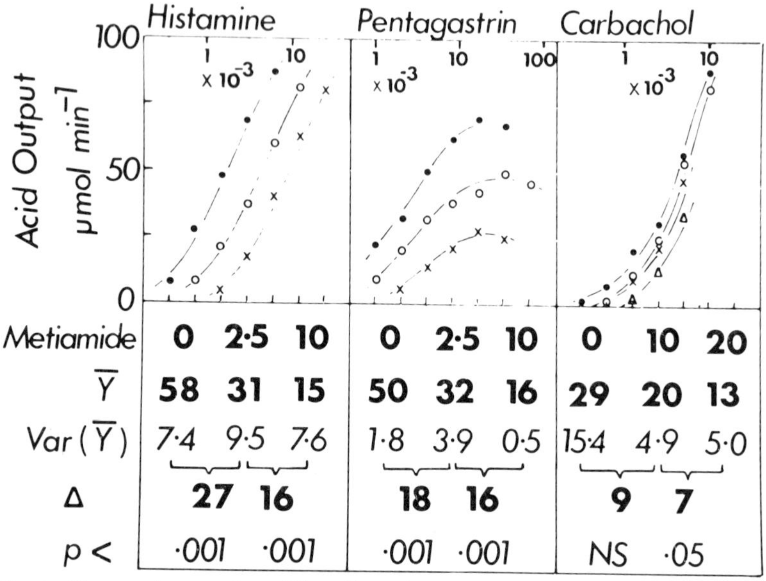

Fig. 6. Dog gastric secretion: The effect of intravenous infusions of metiamide on the secretory responses to intravenous infusions of histamine, pentagastrin and carbachol. A test of significance for the difference between the dose-response curves was based on estimates of the overall mean (Y) and the variance (var $\bar{Y}$) for each curve. The same number of (corresponding) doses was used in each of curves, four for histamine, five for pentagastrin and four for carbachol.

the dose range for histamine of 1—16 umol/h, for pentagastrin 0.5—16 ug/kg/h and for carbachol 6—200 ug/h, the infusion rate being changed every hour and the mean of the last two 15 minute readings being used to calculate the curves. Figure 6 shows the mean control curves for each agonist from six experiments in six different dogs. The treated curves were established in the same way except that a continuous intravenous infusion of metiamide at rates of either 2.5, 10.0 or 20.0 umol/kg/h was started 45 min before the commencement of the agonist and continued throughout the experiment.

DISCUSSION

Both infusion rates of metiamide produced a significant shift of the histamine dose-response curve to the right. Further statistical analysis showed that the three curves were linear and parallel over the range of the top four doses and there was not depression of the maximum. Taking off dose-ratios from individual experiments and plotting log (DR-1) against log (infusion concentration of metiamide) (Arunlakshana and Schild, 1959; Waud, 1968) gave a linear regression with a slope of 0.95 (0.63–1.27) which is not significantly different from unity although the precision of the analysis is not high. These results can be interpreted as showing metaimide to be a competitive antagonist of histamine-stimulated gastric acid secretion in the dog.

Against carbachol-stimulated secretion metiamide in doses up to 10 umol/kg/h, which had marked effects against histamine-stimulated secretion, had no significant inhibitory activity, but at 20 u mol/kg/h significant displacement of the dose-response curve was achieved. The high infusion rate of carbachol (200 ug/h) was not studied extensively in the presence of metiamide at 10 and 20 umol/kg/h but when it was a marked reduction in the maximum response occurred. This was invariably accompanied by side-effects such as vomiting which renders the biological significance of the results doubtful.

These results could be explained if carbachol stimulated gastric secretion by two separate pathways—one a direct action on a cholinergic receptor in the gastric mucosa (unsusceptible to metiamide) and the other an indirect one via gastrin released from the antrum which could be blocked by metiamide. This would explain why carbachol was a little more difficult to inhibit than the other agonists. The discrepancies between the dog and the rat, where cholinergically-stimulated secretion is much more resistant to inhibition, could also be explained by the fact that in our acute rat preparation the antral area is heavily ligated and carbachol may have a predominently direct action. The use of preparations in which the sources of endogenous gastrin have been excluded would help to solve this problem.

Considering the pentagastrin dose-response curves, statistical analysis showed that metiamide is producing significant displacement of the dose-response curve with the same doses and to a similar extent as found with histamine. However, the maximum responses are also depressed, a phenomenon normally associated with non-competitive inhibition which would suggest that metiamide was not blocking pentagastrin through the same interaction with H_2-receptors as described for histamine.

Interpretation is complicated by the known inhibitory effects of pentagastrin on histamine-stimulated gastric secretion in the dog. A model has been proposed (Black, 1973) in which there are two receptors for pentagastrin, one excitatory and one inhibitory and metiamide only competes for the excitatory receptor. If competitive displacement of the agonist element is produced without interfering with the inhibitory one, curves can be obtained which closely resemble those shown in figure 6. That is, we appear to have non-competitive interaction when there is a competitive basis for it. Testing in other species where pentagastrin does not have an inhibitory effect may help to answer this problem. It is also arguable if one should necessarily expect a one to one relationship between the amount of pentagastrin injected and the amount of histamine released and hence the curves for pentagastrin in the presence of metiamide may not necessarily mirror those found with histamine.

Since metiamide has high specific activity, low toxicity and good oral bioavailability, evaluation of its therapeutic potential in man has been started. Early studies in human volunteers (Black et al., 1973) showed that metiamide given by intravenous infusion or orally was an effective inhibitor of maximal histamine and pentagastrin-stimulated gastric acid secretion. Clinical investigations have now commenced both in the U. K. and the U. S. A.

CONCLUSION

We have previously provided evidence that metiamide inhibits histamine-stimulated gastric secretion by blockade of histamine H_2-receptors (Parsons, 1973). In the present paper we have shown that pentagastrin-, and to a lesser extent, carbachol-stimulated secretion can also be inhibited by metiamide. The simplest hypothesis is that it does so by blocking histamine H_2-receptors, but more experimental work of the type suggested in this paper will be required to comfirm the hypothesis.

REFERENCES

Arunlakshana,V., and Schild,H.O., 1959.
Some quantitative uses of drug antagonists.
Br. J. Pharmac. Chemother., 14:48.

Ash,A.S.F., and Schild,H.O., 1966.
Receptors mediating some actions of histamine.
Br. J. Pharmacol., 27:427.

Black,J.W., 1973.
H_2-Receptors, in International Symposium.
Smith Kline & French Laboratories Ltd., (London), (In Press).

Black,J.W., Duncan,W.A.M., Durant,G.J., Ganellin,C.R., and Parsons,M.E., 1972.
Definition and antagonism of histamine H_2-Receptors.
Nature, (London), 236:385.

Black,J.W., Duncan,W.A.M., Emmett,J.C., Ganellin,C.R., Hesselbo,T., Parsons,M.E., and Wyllie,J., 1973.
Metiamide - an orally active histamine H_2-receptor antagonist. Agents and Actions.
(In Press).

Code,C.F., 1965.
Histamine and Gastric Secretion - a later look, 1955 - 1965.
Fed. Proc., 24:1311.

Ghosh,M.N., and Schild,H.O., 1958.
Continous recording of acid gastric in the rat.
Br. J. Pharmacol., 13:54.

McIntosh,F.C., 1938.
Histamine as a normal stimulant of gastric secretion.
J. Exp. Physiol., 28:87.

Parsons,M.E., 1969.
Quantitative studies of drug-induced acid gastric secretion.
Ph.D. Thesis, University of London.

Parsons,M.E., 1973.
H_2-Receptors, in International Symposium.
Smith Kline & French Laboratories Ltd., (London), (In Press).

Waud,D.R., 1968.
Pharmacological receptors.
Pharmacol. Rev., 20:49.

HORMONAL CONTROL OF SECRETION

Leonard R. Johnson

INTRODUCTION

Four steps are required to establish the existence of a gastrointestinal hormone. First, one must demonstrate—physiologically—that a stimulus applied to one part of the digestive tract changes the activity in another part. Second, the effect must persist after all nervous connections between the two parts of the tract have been severed. Third, from the site of application of the stimulus, one must isolate a substance which, when injected into the blood stream, mimics the effect of the stimulus. Fourth, one must identify the substance chemically and confirm its structure by synthesis. Ideally, one should also demonstrate that the stimulus releases the particular substance identified in the preceding steps. At this point in time three gastrointestinal hormones have been identified and their roles elucidated. They are gastrin, cholecystokinin (CCK), and secretin. In addition to these, several other peptides are candidates for hormonal status. GIP (gastric inhibitory peptide) and VIP (vasoactive intestinal peptide) have been isolated from intestinal mucosa and their actions determined. It is not yet known, however, whether they are released physiologically. Pancreatic glucagon has a number of effects on the gastrointestinal tract which presumably are shared by gut glucagon or enteroglucagon. Enteroglucagon, however, has not yet been isolated.

TYPES OF ACTIONS

As pure and synthetic preparations of the three gastrointestinal hormones were made available to investigators during the past decade, they were unexpectedly found to affect a wide variety of targets. These actions are not limited to classical ones on secretion and motility, but include absorption, metabolism and hormone release. The various categories of actions found to be affected by the gastrointestinal hormones are listed in table 1. The remainder of this discussion will deal only with the first three—those involving secretion. The trophic actions are included because it is now known that gastrin is required to maintain the functional and structural integrity of the gastric mucosa and probably the duodenum and pancreas as well (Johnson, 1974).

Table 1

Actions of GI Hormones

Water and Electrolyte Secretion
Stomach, Pancreas, Liver, Gut
Enzyme Secretion
Stomach, Pancreas
Trophic Effects
Stomach, Pancreas, Gut
Endocrine Secretion
GI hormones, Insulin, Glucagon, Calcitonin
Motility
Stomach, Gut, Sphincters
Intestinal Absorption
Water, Electrolytes, Nutrients

Two basic problems have emerged which complicate the assessment of the importance of any particular action of an individual hormone. First, is it a physiological action? Second, does it occur in all species or is it particular to one or two?

Physiological Versus Pharmacological

Several years ago Grossman (1968) proposed two guidelines for ascertaining whether an effect of one of the gastrointestinal hormones is physiological: (1) the effect should occur in response to a dose of the hormone which does not exceed the maximal dose for the primary action of the hormone, and (2) the effect should be reproduced by endogenous release of the hormone. Since the advent of radioimmunoassays for gastrointestinal hormones it has become apparent that while these criteria are necessary they are certainly not rigid enough. Instead of using a dose, in criterion one, which does not exceed maximal, a dose should be used which does not raise serum levels of the hormone past those which normally occur in response to a meal. For example, 4 units secretin/kg-hr produces maximal pancreatic secretion in the dog. The threshold below which acid causes secretin release from the duodenum is pH 4.5 (Meyer et al., 1970). During the response to a meal duodenal pH drops below 4.5 for only a short time and even then does not usually go below pH 3.0, the pH needed for maximal secretin release. Meyer and Grossman have calculated that serum secretin levels attained physiologically probably never excede 0.25–0.50 unit/kg-hr. The high pancreatic bicarbonate-volume response following a meal is due to the potentiating effects of CCK on small amounts of secretin (Meyer et al., 1971).

As Grossman (1974) has recently pointed out, a better guide to the amount of hormone release during a meal would be the D_{50}, that is the dose required for half maximal response, rather than that producing near the maximal response. In the dog, for example, the dose of gastrin which causes near maximal acid secretion is 4 times greater than the D_{50} (Johnson and Grossman, 1969).

Further compounding the "dose" problem is the fact that many investigators often administer gastrointestinal hormones as single intravenous shots. Following a meal the maximal increase in serum gastrin is about 100 pg/ml. If one gives a rapid injection of 125 ug gastrin/kg, a dose which is near threshold for some so-called physiological actions of gastrin, the increment in serum gastrin is 1500 pg/ml (Grossman, 1974). Continuous intravenous infusions, rather than single bolus injections should, therefore, be used when trying to ascertain the significance of a particular effect of one of the gut hormones.

Species Differences

Most everyone is by now aware that many of the secretory effects of gut hormones do not pertain to all species. The best examples of this are the effects of secretin and CCK on gastric acid secretion. In the dog secretin is a potent inhibitor of gastrin stimulated acid secretion (Johnson and Grossman, 1968). Secretin exhibits the same inhibitory effect on gastrin stimulated secretion in the rat. It is considerably less effective in man and virtually ineffective in the cat. CCK is a strong competitive inhibitor of gastrin stimulated secretion in the dog (Johnson and Grossman, 1970). At the opposite extreme, CCK is a full agonist in the cat, equipotent to gastrin in stimulating acid secretion (Deveney and Way, 1973). It is obvious that one must be careful in drawing conclusions about the effects of the gastrointestinal hormones in one species based on data collected from another.

Effects of Gut Hormones on Secretion

The effects of the three gastrointestinal hormones on salt, water and enzyme secretion are tabulated in table 2. The primary actions of these hormones—stimulation of gastric acid secretion by gastrin, stimulation of pancreatic enzyme secretion by CCK, and stimulation of pancreatic fluid and electrolyte secretion by secretin—are widely recognized and led to the discovery of the hormones. Each of the three hormones, however, affects both types of secretion from all parts of the tract. What is the significance of these other actions?

Table 2

Effects of GI Hormones on Water, Salt and Enzyme Secretion

Water-Salt Secretion	Gastrin	CCK	Secretin
Stomach	S^+	S	I
Pancreas	S	S	S^+
Liver	S	S	S
Small Intestine	S	S	S
Enzyme Secretion			
Stomach	S	S	S
Pancreas	S^+	S^+	S

S = stimulates; I = inhibits; $^+$ = a major physiological effect.

The stimulation of pancreatic enzyme secretion occurs early in the response to a meal. Preshaw, Cooke and Grossman (1965) demonstrated that vagal release of gastrin during the cephalic phase and antral stimulation of gastrin release during the gastric phase of secretion accounted for the stimulation. Thus, in addition to stimulating acid secretion gastrin is responsible for part of the pancreatic enzyme response to a meal.

Besides stimulating pancreatic enzyme secretion, CCK plays a physiologically significant role in the stimulation of water and bicarbonate from the pancreas. Although a weak stimulator by its self, CCK strongly potentiates the effects of small amounts of secretin (Meyer et al., 1971). Likewise, secretin potentiates the stimulation of pancreatic enzyme secretion, and these combined actions appear to be highly significant physiologically.

Secretin is no doubt a significant inhibitor of acid secretion in the dog, for this effect occurs at doses below the threshold dose for pancreatic secretion (Johnson and Grossman, 1969a). However, the significance of this action in other species is doubtful. Secretin is the most potent choleretic of the gastrointestinal hormones and this may be an important action of this hormone.

The stimulation of pepsin secretion by gastrointestinal hormones is probably of only minor if any physiological significance. This statement is made in light of the fact that acid itself stimulates pepsin secretion when it comes in contact with the gastric mucosa, accounting for much of the pepsin response to gastrin and secretin (Johnson, 1972). The remainder of the actions of the various hormones listed in table 2 are probably only of pharmacological significance.

STRUCTURE—ACTIVITY RELATIONSHIPS

The gastrointestinal hormones and related peptides can be divided into two structurally similar groups.

Gastrin, CCK and the related decapeptide, caerulein, make up one group of structural homologues (table 3). The smallest peptide fragments having gastrin-like activity also have CCK-like activity, indicating that the active portions of the hormones are identical. A peptide is more closely related to gastrin if its potency for stimulating gastric acid secretion is much greater than its ability to cause the gallbladder to contract. CCK and peptides more closely related to it are more potent cholecystogogues. The smaller active peptides such as the tri-, tetra-, and pentapeptides are more closely related to gastrin. Potency does not shift to the CCK side until 7 amino acids are present from the C-terminal end. Table 3 shows that gastrin-contains a tyrosyl residue in position 6 and CCK in position 7. Except for some in vitro situations it makes no difference in the activity of gastrin whether it is sulfated or not. In CCK the tyrosyl residue is in position 7, and it is always sulfated. If the sulfate is removed from CCK or caerulein a peptide having gastrin-like activity results (Johnson et al., 1970). Therefore, if the tyrosyl residue is in position 6 from the C-terminal end or if it is unsulfated, gastrin-like activity results. Sulfated and in position 7, CCK-like activity predominates in the residue.

Table 3

Gastrin Related Heptapeptides

	7	6	5	4	3	2	1	
Gastrin II	–ALA–	TYR–	GLY–	TRP–	MET–	ASP–	PHE–	NH_2
		| HSO_3						
CCK	–TYR–	MET–	GLY–	TRP–	MET–	ASP–	PHE–	NH_2
	| HSO							
Caerulein	–TYR–	THR–	GLY–	TRP–	MET–	ASP–	PHE–	NH_2
	| HSO_3							

The tetrapeptide amide of gastrin possesses the full range of biological activities of the whole molecule and is about one-twelfth as potent as the parent hormone (Gregory and Tracy, 1964). Until recently, it was believed that smaller fragments were totally void of activity. Lin (1972), however, has shown that the C-terminal tri-peptide has activity, although only one two-thousandth of that of the tetrapeptide. This information is of no physiological significance; but coupled with the fact that none of the side group of the tetra-peptide have been shown to be indispensable for biological activity, it indicates that there is no one "active site" on the molecule. One can shorten the gastrin molecule by 5 amino acids (starting from the

N-terminus) before encountering a loss in activity. Further removal of residues further decreases activity; thus there are probably a series of sites on the receptor which recognize different portions of the hormone. Potency is determined by the number of sites occupied—providing, of course, that at least the tripeptide amide is present.

The secretin family of peptides consists of four members: secretin, glucagon, GIP and VIP (table 4). These peptides contain from 27 to 43 amino acid residues and homologies occur throughout the entire molecules. Secretin has 27 amino acids, and unlike gastrin and its homologues, contains no active fragment. All 27 amino acids are required for activity; substitution for any one of them renders the molecule inactive. Glucagon has been isolated from man, cow, and hog; no difference in the amino acid sequency from the three species was discovered (Bromer et al., 1971). Fragments of GIP have not been studied. Some fragments of VIP have small amounts of vascular effects (Bodanszky et al., 1973). Secretin has been isolated only from the hog. It will be interesting to see if secretins from additional species differ. It is doubtful, however, that they will, for secretin is a miniature helix and the entire primary structure is probably necessary to maintain this conformation.

Table 4

Secretin and Related Peptides

Peptide	Length	Identity With Secretin
Secretin	27	—
Glucagon	29	14
GIP	43	9
VIP	28	9

REGULATION OF HORMONE RELEASE

The various factors which act from within the digestive tract to influence the release of gut hormones are summarized in table 5. Gastrin is released by antral distension, shortchain amino acids such as glycine and alanine and by ethanol and propanol. Release of gastrin is inhibited when the antral pH drops below 3.5. Csendes and

Grossman (1972) have recently reported that D- and L-isomers of alanine and serine were equally effective gastrin releasers. This finding contrasts with studies of the CCK release mechanism which can be activated only by L-amino acids. CCK is released from the mucosa of the upper small intestine by fatty acids as well as amino acids. Hydrogen ion itself is a weak releaser of CCK and it is doubtful whether it plays a role under normal circumstances. Meyer and Grossman have calculated that the ratio of secretin to CCK released by acid is about 24 to 1. The strongest releaser of secretin is hydrogen ion. The threshold for secretin release by acid occurs at pH 4.5. Between pH 4.5 and 3.0 there is a rapid rise in pancreatic secretion. Lowering the pH below 3.0 does not increase secretin release, providing the amount of titratable acid entering the gut is held constant. Below pH 3.0 secretin release and pancreatic bicarbonate secretion are related only to the amount of titratable acid entering the gut per unit time (Meyer and Grossman, 1970). Meyer (in press) has also recently found that fatty acids given as soap micelles or in bile acid micelles release secretin. The physiological significance of the contribution of secretin release stimulated by fat remains to be evaluated.

Table 5

Release of GI Hormones by Luminal Factors

	Gastrin	CCK	Secretin
Distension	S	—	—
Fat	0	S	S
Protein	S	S	0
Carbohydrate	0	0	0
Acid	I	0	S

S = stimulates; I = inhibits; 0 = no effect

Recently the relationship between gut hormones and endocrinology in general has been emphasized by the discoveries that gastrointestinal hormones release insulin and glucagon (table 6). Glucagon and secretin, on the other hand, inhibit antral gastrin release (Becker et al., 1973). The opposite occurs in patients having Zollinger-Ellison Syndrome, for tumor gastrin release is stimulated by both secretin and glucagon. This knowledge has proven clinically useful in diagnosing Zollinger-Ellison Syndrome in patients not having excessively high serum gastrin levels.

Table 6

Release of GI Hormones by Hormones

	Gastrin	CCK	Secretin	Glucagon
Release of				
Gastrin	—	—	I	I
Secretin	S	—	—	—
Glucagon	0	S	0	—
Insulin	S	S	S	S

S = stimulates; I = inhibits; 0 = no effect

TROPHIC ACTIONS

In 1969 Johnson, Aures and Yuen reported that gastrin stimulated protein synthesis in gastric and duodenal mucosa. This effect was confined to tissues of the gastrointestinal tract, and it did not depend on acid secretion. We hypothesized that gastrin was a trophic hormone for certain gastrointestinal tissues. During the past few years gastrin has been shown to stimulate all aspects of the growth response in the pancreas and gastric and duodenal mucosa (table 7). This material has recently been reviewed in detail (Johnson, 1974). Many of the responses to gastrin listed in table 7 can be caused by a single dose near the maximal acid secretion dose. While this does not alone satisfy our criteria for a physiological response, one must remember that growth occurs over a protracted time period and is the result of a number of continual or repeating factors influencing cell division. The fact, then, that a single dose of gastrin increases DNA synthesis 400% is especially significant (Johnson and Guthrie, 1974). The physiological significance of this

Table 7

Trophic Effects of GI Hormones

Action	Gastrin	CCK	Secretin
Growth			
Oxyntic Mucosa	S	—	I
Duodenal Mucosa	S	—	0
Pancreas	S	S	0
Protein Synthesis			
Oxyntic Mucosa	S	—	—
Duodenal Mucosa	S	—	—
Pancreas	S	S	0
RNA Synthesis			
Oxyntic Mucosa	S		
Duodenal Mucosa	S		
Pancreas	S		
DNA Synthesis			
Oxyntic Mucosa	S	—	I
Duodenal Mucosa	S	—	0
Pancreas	S	S	—
Ileal Mucosa	S	—	0
Cell Division			
Oxyntic Mucosa	S	—	—
Duodenal Mucosa	S	—	—

S = stimulates; I = inhibits; 0 = no effect

point is illustrated by the rapid loss of weight, RNA and DNA from the oxyntic gland and duodenal mucosa following antrectomy in the rat (Johnson and Chandler, 1973). Three injections of pentagastrin during the 24 hr before killing rats, which had undergone antrectomy 30 days previously, restored the RNA and DNA values to near normal levels. Miller, Jacobson, and Johnson (1973) demonstrated that the growth promoting effects of gastrin occurred when the hormone was administered *in vitro* to cultures of duodenal and gastric mucosal cells. At this point it seems fair to conclude that gastrin is necessary for the normal growth and development of gastrointestinal mucosa.

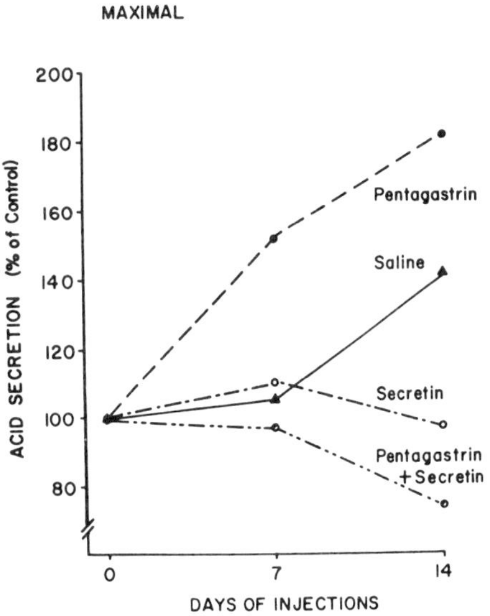

Fig. 1. Acid outputs in response to a single subcutaneous injection of a maximal dose of pentagastrin before, and on the 7th and 14th days after, beginning injections, three times daily of pentagastrin (250 ug/kg), saline, secretin (100 unit/kg), or pentagastrin plus. (From Stanley et al., 1972, by permission of Gastroenterology).

Any substance regulating the growth of a particular tissue will, of course, have a profound effect on its function as well. This is aptly illustrated in figure 1 which depicts the maximal secretory capacities of several groups of rats over a 2 week period. Control animals were injected every day with saline and progressed normally. Gastrin injected animals increased their secretory capacities significantly over the control group. Secretin appears to inhibit growth of the oxyntic gland region, for it prevented the increase due to gastrin and the increase due to normal growth of the animals (Stanley et al., 1972). Parietal cell counts were directly related to maximal acid outputs in all groups.

Mayston and Barrowman (1971) were the first to demonstrate the trophic effect of gastrin on the pancreas. As a result they hypothesized that it was a required growth hormone for the pancreas in the same manner as had been suggested for the stomach. Since the actions of gastrin and CCK are qualitatively identical it was not surprising that Mainz, Black and Webster (1973) reported that CCK stimulated pancreatic DNA synthesis. Thus, all three of the gut hormones are probably involved in regulating the growth and development of gastrointestinal tract. It is possible that these functions may even eclipse in importance their short term effects on secretion.

REFERENCES

Becker,H.D., Reeder,D.D., and Thompson,J.C., 1973.
Effect of glucagon on circulating gastrin.
Gastroenterology 65:28.

Bodanszky,M., Klausner,Y.S., and Said,S.I., 1973.
Biological activities of synthetic peptides corresponding to fragments of and to the entire sequence of the vasoactive intestinal peptide.
Proc. Nat. Acad. Sci. U.S.A. 70:383.

Bromer,W.W., Boucher,M.E., and Koffenberger,J.E., 1971.
Amino acid sequence of bovine glucagon.
J. Biol. Chem. 246:2822.

Csendes,A., and Grossman,M.I., 1972.
D- and L- isomers of serine and alanine equally effective as releasers of gastrin.
Experientia, 28:1306.

Deveney,K., and Way,L.W., 1972.
Effect of fat in the duodenum on gastric acid secretion in cats.
Gastroenterology 62:405.

Grossman,M.I., 1968.
Physiological role of gastrin.
Fed. Proc. 27:1312.

Grossman,M.I., 1974.
Gastrointestinal hormones: spectrum of actions and structure - activity relations, in Chey, W.Y. Symposium on recent advances in gastrointestinal hormone research (In Press).

Johnson,L.R., 1973.
Regulation of pepsin secretion by topical acid in the stomach.
Am. J. Physiol. 223:847.

Johnson,L.R., 1974.
Gut hormones on growth of gastric mucosa, in Chey, W.Y. Symposium on recent advances in gastrointestinal hormone research (In Press).

Johnson,L.R., and Chandler,A.M., 1973.
RNA and DNA of gastric and duodenal mucosa in antrectomized and gastrin treated rats.
Am. J. Physiol. 224:937.

Johnson,L.R., and Grossman, M.I., 1968.
Secretion: the enterogastrone released by acid in the duodenum.
Am. J. Physiol. 215:885.
Johnson,L.R., and Grossman,M.I., 1969.
Potentiation of gastric acid response in the dog.
Gastroenterology 56:687.
Johnson,L.R., and Grossman,M.I., 1969a.
Characteristics of inhibition of gastric secretion by secretin.
Am. J. Physiol. 217:1401.
Johnson,L.R. and Grossman,M.I., 1970.
Analysis of inhibition of acid secretion by cholecystokinin in dogs.
Am. J. Physiol. 218:550.
Johnson,L.R., and Guthrie,P.D., 1974.
Mucosal DNA synthesis: a short term index of the trophic action of gastrin.
Gastroenterology (In Press).
Johnson,L.R., Aures,D. and Yuen,L., 1969.
Pentagastrin induced stimulation of the in vitro incorporation of ^{14}C-leucine into protein of the gastrointestinal tract.
Am. J. Physiol. 217:251.
Johnson,L.R., Steining,G.F., and Grossman,M.I., 1970.
The effect of sulfation on the gastrointestinal actions of caerulein.
Gastroenterology 58:208.
Lin,T.M., 1972.
Gastrointestinal actions of the C-terminal tripeptide of gastrin.
Gastroenterology 63:922.
Mainz,P.L., Black,O., and Webster,P.D., 1973.
Hormonal influences on pancreatic growth.
Gastroenterology 64:A83.
Mayston,P.D., and Barrowman,J.A., 1971.
The influence of chronic administration of pentagastrin on the rat pancreas.
J. Exp. Physiol. 56:113.
Meyer,J.H., and Grossman,M.I., 1970.
Pancreatic bicarbonate response to various acids in the duodenum of dogs.
Am. J. Physiol. 219:964.

Meyer,J.H., Spingola,L.F., and Grossman,M.I., 1971.
Endogenous cholecystokinin potentiates exogenous secretion on pancrease of dog.
Am. J. Physiol. 221:742.

Meyer,J.H., Way,L.W., and Grossman,M.I., 1970.
Pancreatic response to acidification of various lengths of proximal intestine in the dog.
Am. J. Physiol. 219:971.

Miller,L.R., Jacobson,E.D., and Johnson,L.R., 1973.
Effect of pentagastrin on gastric mucosal cells grown in tissue culture.
Gastroenterology 64:254.

Preshaw,R.M., Cooke,A.R., and Grossman,M.I., 1965.
Stimulation of pancreatic secretion by a humoral agent from the pyloric gland area of the stomach.
Gastroenterology 49:617.

Stanley,M.D., Coalson,R.E., Grossman,M.I., and Johnson, L.R., 1972.
Influence of secretin and pentagastrin on acid secretion and parietal cell number in rats.
Gastroenterology 63:264.

FACTORS INFLUENCING MESENTERIC BLOOD FLOW

David G. Reynolds, John C. Kerr and Kenneth G. Swan

INTRODUCTION

Perfusion of the splanchnic vasculature is regulated by central and peripheral mechanisms. Changes in cardiac output or aortic pressure will influence splanchnic blood flow. However, regional blood flow can change without alteration of central hemodynamics through neural and humoral influences on regional vascular resistances. In this manuscript we will consider the neural and humoral mechanisms that influence intestinal blood flow. Special emphasis will be placed upon the adrenergic mechanisms which function within this circulation.

BLOOD FLOW AND INTESTINAL MOTILITY

Effects of Nerve Stimulation

Kewenter (1965) investigated the effects of vagal nerve stimulation on intestinal blood flow and motility. His results demonstrated that stimulation of the vagal nerve trunks had little, if any, effect on mesenteric blood flow and altered only intestinal motility. Stimulation of these parasympathetic nerves caused an increase in jejunal motility that was of much greater magnitude than the ileal motor response. Similar studies were conducted following treatment of the animals with adrenergic blocking agents such as guanethidine and ergotamine. Under these conditions, nerve stimulation caused an equal increase in both jejunal and ileal motility. It was, therefore, concluded that the vagal influences were primarily on smooth muscle and distributed equally over the length of the small intestine.

Intestinal blood flow has been considered to be inversely related to intestinal motility. Jacobson (1970) demonstrated that superior mesenteric arterial blood flow was reduced by only intense contractions of the intestinal musculature. Zeigler et. al. (1973) investigated the relationship between mesenteric blood flow and intestinal contractility. They measured superior mesenteric arterial blood flow with an electromagnetic blood flowmeter and monitored intestinal contractions with a balloon and catheter situated in the intestinal lumen. A motility index, which equaled the product of frequency and amplitude of contraction, was calculated from this latter parameter. Methacholine, a cholinergic agonist with little peripheral vascular effects, was infused directly into the superior mesenteric artery and increased the motility index fourfold without significantly changing mesenteric blood flow. It would thus appear that, within reasonable limits of activity, intestinal motility and blood flow are independent variables.

The effects of splanchnic nerve stimulation long have been recognized to cause vasoconstriction of the splanchnic vasculature (Grim, 1963). Kewenter (1965) also studied the effects of splanchnic nerve stimulation on intestinal blood flow and motor activity. His results indicate that the vasomotor effects of the stimulus were distributed uniformly over the length of the small intestine. However, the adrenergic nerve distribution to intestinal smooth muscle was predominantly to the distal small intestine and was reduced in the jejunum. These observations were interpreted as evidence that the functional gradient of peristaltic activity is a result of the dominant inhibitory nerve supply to the distal intestine.

Forsyth (1972) used a radioactive microsphere technique to evaluate the effects of sympathetic nervous system activity on regional distribution of cardiac output in conscious rhesus monkeys. He stimulated a systemic increase in activity of the sympathetic nervous system by subjecting the animals to one of the following three experimental conditions: hemorrhage of 30 to 50 per cent of total blood volume, emotional stress, or direct electrical stimulation of the hypothalamus. Each of these experimental conditions caused a reduction in the proportion of cardiac output distributed to the splanchnic circulation in general, with exception of the hepatic arterial system, which received a greater percentage of cardiac output during hemorrhage and emotional stress and no change in the percentage of cardiac output received during hypothalamic stimulation.

The vasomotor effects resulting from sympathetic nerve activity are due to the interaction of the endogenous catecholamines, norepinephrine and epinephrine, on adrenergic receptors. In the splanchnic vasculature, as in other regional circulations, alpha adrenergic receptor stimulation causes vasoconstriction while stimulation of beta adrenergic receptors causes vasodilation. Our understanding of the pharmacologic action of these agents largely has been defined from canine and feline experimentation. In general, both agents are thought to be vasoconstrictors of the splanchnic vasculature; however, Ross (1967) has presented evidence that epinephrine dilates the cat intestinal vasculature.

Effects of Catecholamines

We have studied the effects of direct intra-arterial injection of the endogenous catecholamines upon mesenteric hemodynamics in anesthetized dogs. Figure 1 presents the results of these studies using a logarithmic dose range of 10^{-3} to 10^{0} ug kg^{-1}. This dose range was selected since central hemodynamic effects, of small magnitude, were elicited only at the highest concentration. Both norepinephrine and epinephrine caused dose dependent decreases in mesenteric blood flow and since central effects only occurred at the highest concentration, the responses indicate constriction of intestinal vasculature. At the two intermediate doses, norepinephrine caused significantly greater vasoconstriction than epinephrine. The effects of differential adrenergic blockade on these responses were described in a previous report (Swan and Reynolds, 1971a). In that study it was demonstrated that, subsequent to alpha adrenergic blockade with phenoxybenzamine, the responses to norepinephrine were attenuated significantly whereas the responses to epinephrine were reversed to vasodilation. Beta adrenergic blockade with propranolol did not significantly alter these responses. Apparently, norepinephrine exerts a pure alpha adrenergic influence on this regional circulation while epinephrine has an affinity for both alpha and beta adrenergic receptors.

AUTOREGULATORY ESCAPE

Return to Preinfusion Levels

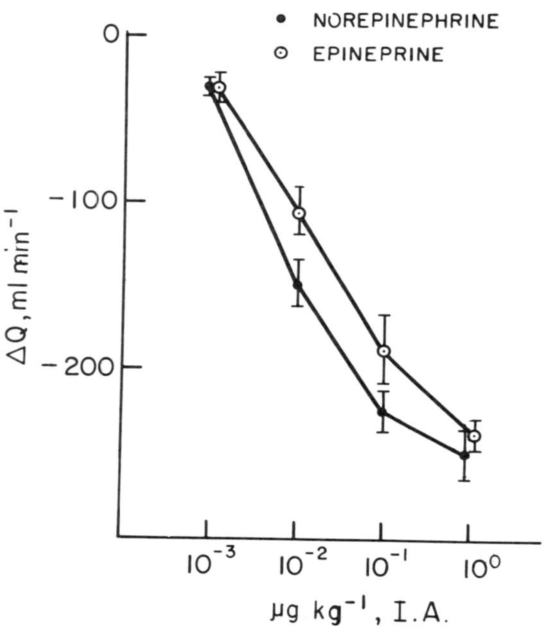

Fig. 1. Dose-response effects of epinephrine and norepinephrine injections into the superior mesenteric artery of dogs. Each point is the mean ± standard error of 5 experiments in 5 dogs. The ordinate is the change in mesenteric blood in ml min^{-1}. The abscissa is the logarithmic progression of dose in ug (base) kg^{-1}.

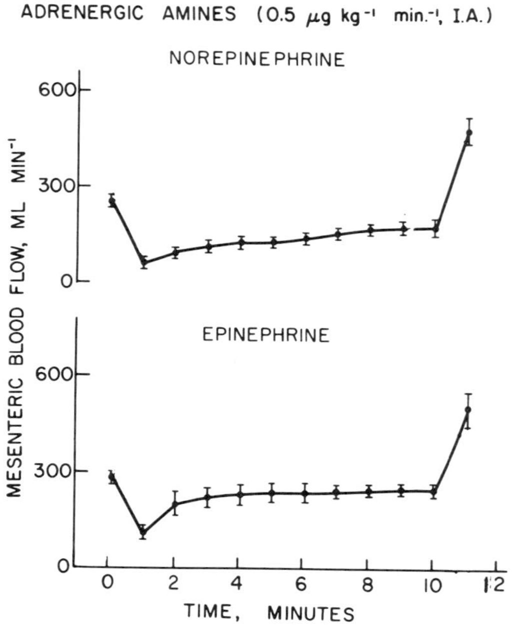

Fig. 2. Effects of 10 minute catecholamine infusion on canine mesenteric blood flow. Each point is the mean ± standard error of 5 experiments in 5 dogs.

Figure 2 illustrates the effects of epinephrine and norepinephrine when infused into the canine superior mesenteric artery for ten minutes. Both adrenergic amines caused a prompt, significant fall in mesenteric blood flow which then returned toward control over the duration of the infusion. During epinephrine infusion, blood flow returned to a value not significantly different from control within 3 to 4 minutes after the infusion started and remained at that level for the remainder of the infusion. The return of mesenteric flow during norepinephrine infusion occurred more gradually,and at the tenth minute of drug infusion the value was significantly below and above both control and peak constriction values. This phenomenon, a return of flow toward control during continued vasoconstrictor infusion, has been termed 'autoregulatory escape' (Folkow et al., 1964). Current evidence suggests that escape occurs as a result of relaxation of the same vascular elements that were constricted at the onset of drug infusion (Richardson and Johnson, 1969). However, Shanbour and Jacobson (1971) pointed out that the mechanism underlying escape has not been defined and suggested two possible mechanisms worth considering. First is the possibility that the adrenergic constrictor receptors may become refractory during continued exposure to adrenergic amines. Secondly, the possibility exists that unidentified dilator receptors may become activated during continued drug infusion or during continued nerve stimulation. Dopamine receptors may be involved since dopamine is a metabolic precursor of both epinephrine and norepinephrine. Stimulation of these receptors causes vasodilation of the intestinal vasculature.

Hyperemic Overshoot

Figure 2 demonstrates another characteristic of the effects of catecholamine infusion on the canine mesenteric circulation. Upon cessation of drug infusion, whether norepinephrine or epinephrine, mesenteric blood flow undergoes a hyperemic response in the form of an "overshoot" which increases flow significantly above control. The amplitude of the overshoot is remarkably consistent for both epinephrine and norepinephrine and also occurs following intra-arterial "bolus" type injections of these amines (Swan and Reynolds, 1971a). This response is probably not "reactive" hyperemia since it occurred following epinephrine infusion during which mesenteric flow had already returned to control. Shanbour and Jacobson (1971) suggested that the mechanism underlying autoregulatory escape also might be associated with the "overshoot" observed following cessation of vasoconstrictor infusion or splanchnic nerve stimulation. This possibility would be in agreement with a previous report in which we demonstrated that differential adrenergic blockade did not prevent autoregulatory escape or influence the magnitude of the "overshoot" that occurred following cessation of infusion of the adrenergic amines (Swan and Reynolds, 1971b).

The catecholamines have been incriminated in the irreversibility of shock by causing prolonged mesenteric ischemia (Lillehei et al., 1962). In this "adrenergic" theory of shock, experimental hypotention in the dog results in an increased plasma catecholamine concentration which induces mesenteric vasoconstriction, intestinal ischemia, and ultimately intestinal necrosis. The occurrence of autoregulatory escape, as demonstrated by the mesenteric vascular bed, argues against the validity of this concept. The data indicate that the intestine would not remain ischemic when perfused with blood containing elevated amounts of the endogenous catecholamines. Furthermore, independent studies in Jacobson's laboratory (Brobmann et al., 1970) and in our laboratory (Swan et al., 1971c) argue against the involvement of the splanchnic vasculature in the irreversibility of shock in subhuman primates. Unlike the canine intestine, the gut of both rhesus monkeys and baboons remains well perfused during the early phase of endotoxin shock due to a fall in mesenteric vascular resistance. It would, therefore, be important to compare the effects of the adrenergic amines on the intestinal vasculature of subhuman primates with those effects already presented for the canine gut.

Species Differences

The results of injections of the endogenous catecholamines into the superior mesenteric artery of baboons are shown in figure 3. When injected over the same dose range employed in the canine studies, norepinephrine caused dose dependent vasoconstrictor responses in the intestinal vasculature. Epinephrine, on the other hand, caused vasodilator responses when injected at the two lower doses and vasoconstrictor responses when injected at the two higher doses. The vasodilator responses to epinephrine injection were reversed to

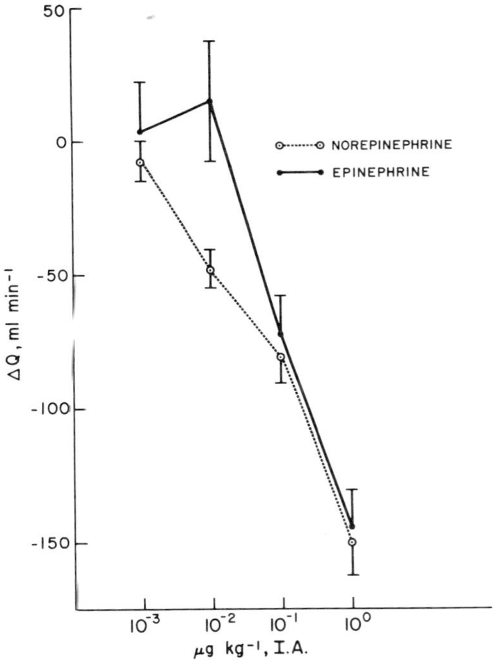

Fig. 3 Dose-response effects of epinephrine and norepinephrine injections into the superior mesenteric artery of baboons. Each point is the mean ± standard error of 5 experiments in 5 baboons.

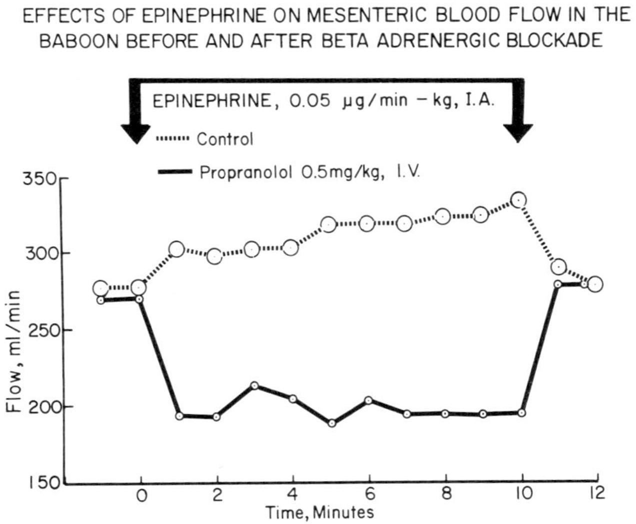

Fig. 4. Representative mesenteric vascular response to low dose epinephrine infusion into the superior mesenteric artery of a baboon.

vasoconstriction subsequent to treating the animal with the beta adrenergic antagonist, propranolol. Norepinephrine, when infused at the same rate used in the dog studies (0.5 ug kg^{-1} min^{-1}), elicited vasoconstrictor responses which were sustained throughout the ten minute infusion. There was neither evidence of autoregulatory escape nor the characteristic "overshoot" upon cessation of drug infusion. These observations suggest that autoregulatory escape does not occur within the mesenteric vasculature of the baboon. When infused at the same concentration, epinephrine brought about similar vasoconstrictor responses.

Plasma catecholamine levels were measured in our study of experimental endotoxemia in the baboon (Swan et al., 1971c). The combined plasma concentration of epinephrine and norepinephrine at the fourth hour of observation was slightly greater than 10 ug per liter of plasma and epinephrine accounted for over 75 per cent of the circulating catecholamines. On the basis of these measurements and knowing mesenteric arterial blood flow, an empiric calculation was made to determine the average rate of delivery of epinephrine to the small intestine. This amount (0.05 ug kg^{-1} min^{-1}) of the catecholamine was then infused into the superior mesenteric artery of anesthetized baboons and the results are shown in figure 4. Upon the onset of epinephrine infusion, there was a progressive increase in superior mesenteric arterial blood flow. Subsequent to beta adrenergic blockade with propranolol, this response was reversed to vasoconstriction that was sustained for the period of drug infusion. Mesenteric flow returned to control values following cessation of drug infusion and did not evidence an "overshoot". Thus, it would appear that the vasodilator influence of epinephrine at this concentration is a result of its interaction with beta adrenergic receptors. It is interesting, then, to consider the possibility that the progressive elevation of plasma epinephrine concentration during hypotension provides a mechanism that sustains the perfusion of the small intestine in subhuman primates subjected to experimental endotoxin shock.

CONCLUSIONS

The foregoing observations suggest the existence of specific differences between the splanchnic circulations of dog and monkey. Since man is phylogenetically closer to monkey than dog, one might expect the human gut to respond more like that of the monkey than the dog. One should be cautious, then, in extrapolating the results of canine experimentation directly to the human. In light of the observed differences in the mesenteric adrenergic mechanisms between these species, this caution might be extended to the current practice of vasoconstrictor therapy to control upper gastrointestinal bleeding. The vasomotor effects of each drug being considered for use in this manner should be verified in subhuman primates before being applied clinically to man. Such verification should evaluate both central and peripheral actions of the drug when delivered by the route, at the dose, and for the duration anticipated for therapeutic use.

REFERENCES

Brobmann,G.F., et al, 1970.
Mesenteric vascular responses to endotoxin in the monkey and dog.
Am. J. Physiol., 219:1464.

Folkow,B.D., et al, 1964.
The effect of the sympathetic vasoconstrictor fibers on the distribution of capillary blood flow in the intestine.
Acta Physiol. Scand., 61:458.

Forsyth,R.P., 1972.
Sympathetic nervous system control of distribution of cardiac output in unaesthetized monkeys.
Fed. Proc., 31:1240.

Grim,E., 1963.
The flow of blood in the mesenteric vessels, in Handbook of Physiology: Circulation, Sec. 2, Vol. II, P. 1439.
Am. Physiol. Soc., Washington, D.C.

Jacobson,E.D., 1970.
Intestinal motor activity and blooc flow.
Gastroenterology, 58:575.

Kewenter,J., 1965.
The vagal control of the jejunal and ileal motility and blood flow.
Acta Physiol. Scand., 65:(Suppl.)251.

Lillehei,R.C., Longerbeam,J.K., and Rosenberg,J.C., 1962.
The nature of irreversible shock: its relationship to intestinal changes, in Bock K.D., Shock: Pathogenesis and Therapy, p. 106.
Springer-Verlag, Berlin.

Richardson,D.R., and Johnson,P.C., 1969.
Comparison of autoregulatory escape and autoregulation in the intestinal vascular bed.
Am. J. Physiol., 217:586.

Ross,G., 1967.
Effects of epinephrine and norepinephrine on the mesenteric circulation of the cat.
Am. J. Physiol., 212:1037.

Shanbour,L.L., and Jacobson,E.D., 1971.
Autoregulatory escape in the gut.
Gastroenterology, 60:145.
Swan,K.G., and Reynolds,D.G., 1971a.
Adrenergic mechanisms in the canine mesenteric circulation.
Am. J. Physiol., 220:1779.
Swan,K.G., and Reynolds,D.G., 1971b.
Effects of intraarterial catecholamine infusions on blood flow in the canine gut.
Gastroenterology, 61:863.
Swan,K.G., Barton,R.W., and Reynolds,D.G., 1971c.
Mesenteric hemodynamics during endotoxemia in the baboon.
Gastroenterology, 61:872.
Seigler,M.G., and Swan,K.G., 1973.
Mesenteric blood flow and small intestinal motility in the dog.
Surgery, 73:649.

THE ROLE OF THE BRAIN IN THE CONTROL OF GASTRIC SECRETION

Frank P. Brooks

INTRODUCTION

The mammalian gastric mucosa is able to secrete acid in vitro (Carmona and Slangen, 1973). The ex vivo blood perfused canine stomach secretes acid when the vagi are stimulated electrically (Shaw and Urquhart, 1972). Nevertheless, the changes in gastric acid secretion in vivo after ablation or lesions in parts of the brain or stimulation of discrete areas in the brain (Brooks, 1967) suggest that under normal circumstances, the brain has a role in the control of gastric secretion.

EFFERENT PATHWAYS FROM BRAIN TO STOMACH

The vagal nuclei in the brain stem have long been assumed to be the main neuronal pool for efferent secretory fibers to the stomach. Recently, Kerr and Preshaw were able to block the acid secretory response to insulin hypoglycemia in a cat with a unilateral truncal vagotomy by destroying the contralateral dorsal motor nucleus of the vagus (Kerr and Preshaw, 1969). Norton and his associates stimulated acid secretion transiently in anesthetized dogs by inflating a balloon in the fourth ventricle and suggested that it was mediated by pressure on the vagal nuclei (Norton et al., 1972).

The hypothalamus is the next cephalad area of the brain identified with efferent connections to the stomach. In dogs (Davis et al., 1968) and rats (Brooks, 1967) lesions of the hypothalamus reduce the acid secretion in response to insulin hypoglycemia or 2-deoxy-d-glucose (2DG) (Ridley and Cirpili, 1969). In the rat the important control areas appear to be localized in a medial lateral plane while in the dog, anterior-posterior relationships are more significant. Kadekaro et al. found that intercollicular decerebration in cats prevented the acid-secretory response to 2DG, with similar results when lateral hypothalamic areas were destroyed (Kadekaro et al., 1972) (figure 1). Decortication was without effect. They concluded that the hypothalamus and median forebrain bundle system were the critical areas for responding to 2DG. Colin-Jones and Himsworth reached similar conclusions in the rat (Colin-Jones and Himsworth, 1969; Colin-Jones and Himsworth, 1970).

Stimulation of the hypothalamus can be used also to trace excitatory pathways. Hall and Smith found that electrical stimulation of the hypothalamus in monkeys over a 3 week period shifted the acid dose response to histamine to the left without changing the maximal response (Hall and Smith, 1969). This suggested that the oxyntic cells had become more sensitive to histamine. In rats, electrical stimulation of the posterior hypothalamus stimulated acid secretion if hypoglycemia resulted (Morrissey and Stephens, 1971). Drugs thought to inhibit activity in the higher centers of the visceral nervous system block acid secretion in response to 2DG (Pendleton et al., 1970). Intraventricular injection was effective at a lower dosage than intravenous administration (Ridley and Mann, 1973).

Injection of neurohumoral transmitters into the hypothalamus alters acid secretion. Carmona and Slangen found that the injection of norepinephrine into the lateral hypothalamic feeding area of rats stimulated acid output and the intake of food, while carbachol depressed food intake and acid output in the same rats (Carmona and Slangen, 1973) (figure 2). This implies that a different neurotransmitter in the same neuronal system can have opposite effects on the secretion of acid.

Lee and his associates found that acetylcholine was an excitant to acid secretion when injected into the amygdala of rats while serotonin was an inhibitor (Lee et al., 1969).

ACID RESPONSE TO HYPOGLYCEMIA AND GLUCOCYTOPENIA

The mechanism of the stimulus continues to evolve. Baron has

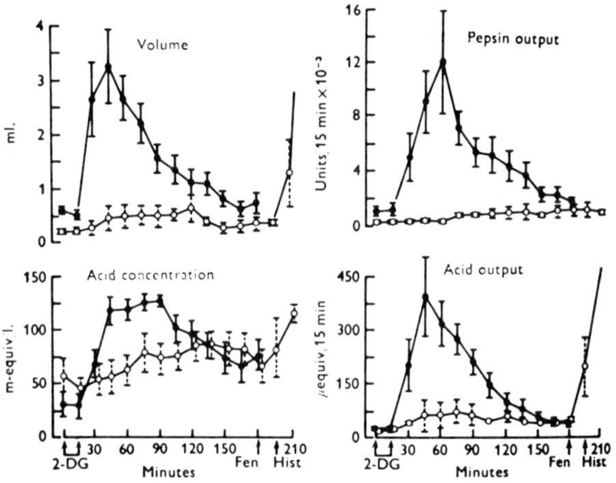

Fig. 1. Secretory response of eleven cats to 60 mg 2-deoxy-d-glucose/kg (●) and after (○) intercollicular transection of the brain stem. Mean values and standard error as a function of time (min) during and after injection of the drug. Arrows indicate administration of 2-DG (2-DG), promethazine hydrochloride (Fen) and histamine (Hist). (From Kadekaro, M. et al., J. Physiol. 221:6, 1972).

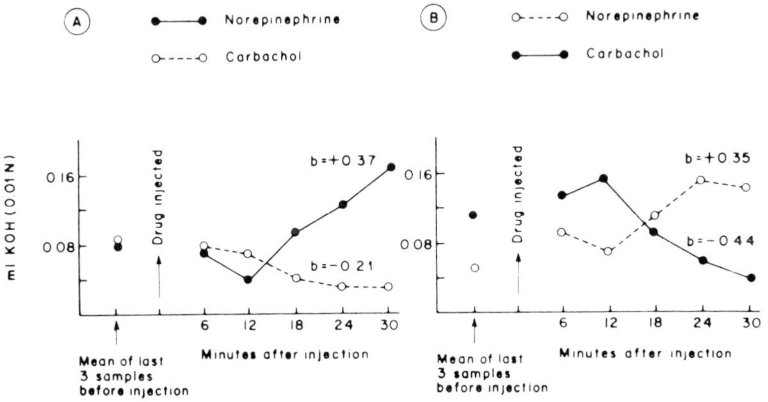

Fig. 2. Changes in acid output from rat stomachs in response to hypothalamic injections of norepinephrine and carbachol. b = slope of acid output. (From Carmona and Slangen, Physiology and Behavior 10:659, 1973).

demonstrated that the acid secretory response to insulin is dose-dependent (Baron, 1970). However the phenomenon is time-dependent as well. Cooke found no significant difference in the peak 15 minute acid output of dogs to doses of insulin ranging from 0.1 to 1.0 unit/kg, while the second and total 4 hour outputs differed markedly, with the response at 0.25 reaching less than one-half that at 0.5 U (Cooke, 1969) (table 1). Doses of insulin in the range of 0.03 to 0.06 U/kg stimulated acid secretion but the response was significantly less than that with 0.125 U (Stening and Isenberg, 1969). It has been shown that duration of hypoglycemia is a function of the dose of insulin (Brooks, 1967). That insulin may have complicating effects on acid secretion is indicated by Stadel and Rehfeld's observation that serum gastrin levels rose after insulin-hypoglycemia in man following truncal vagotomy (Stadel and Rehfeld, 1972).

Eisenberg et al. found no fatigue of the acid response in dogs during up to 24 hours of intravenous infusion of 2DG (Eisenberg et al., 1970).

These results indicate that over a wide range of doses of insulin, the initial acid secretory response is determined by a threshold of blood sugar in an all-or-none manner, but that after a short time period (over 15 minutes) the response becomes dose responsive with larger doses giving larger acid outputs up to a maximum.

BRAIN CONTROL OF GASTRIC SECRETIN

In a series of provocative if not convincing experiments Reigel and his colleagues have reported inhibition of basal and stimulated acid secretion in monkeys by transcranial or electrical stimulation of the amygdala (Reigel et al., 1969a; Reigel et al., 1969b; Reigel et al., 1970; Reigel et al., 1971). They claim to have isolated an inhibitory substance from jugular venous blood and from the gastric content of monkeys, and hypothesize that the inhibitor is released from the brain. The nature of the inhibitor is unknown but it is not gastrone.

Effects of Afferent Stimulation on Brain Mediated Acid Secretion

In a series of papers, Schapiro and his colleagues have presented observations indicating that the acid secretory response in dogs to insulin hypoglycemia is reduced by blinding, removal of the vestibular and auditory apparatus, and severing the olfactory tracts. The effects were shown to last for 4 months. Unfortunately dose response studies were not done (Schapiro et al., 1970a, 1970b, 1971, 1973).

Behavioral Effects on Acid Secretion

It seems reasonable to assume that the brain is involved in the mechanism of behaviorally induced-changes in gastric secretion although the action may be indirect e.g., on blood flow rather than on the oxyntic cells. Stacher et al. found that a hypnotically-induced catatonic state reduced acid secretion in humans (Stacher et. al., 1973). Badgley and his associates observed a decreased acid output during mental arithmetic (Badgley et al., 1969).

The effects of avoidance-conditioning and acute vs chronic stress on acid secretion continue to be controversial. Norman found no difference between the effect on acid secretion in humans, using a pH-sensitive telemetering capsule and in vivo neutralization with potassium bicarbonate, of the subjects being told that they could avoid shocks by lever pressing and being told that they could not influence the shocks. Both groups were shocked randomly (Norman, 1969). Pare found that shocks depressed volume but increased acid concentration in gastric fistula rats (Pare, 1972). Mikhail, using pylorus-ligated rats, found no effect of acute stress (electrical shocks for 14 hours) on acid secretion. Prolongation of the period of stress for 7 days resulted in a reduction of acid concentration (Mikhail, 1971).

Intracranial Injury and Stress-Effects on Acid Secretion

It is becoming apparent that intracranial injury may be relatively unique as a form of stress in its effect on gastric secretion. Norton et al. found that 12 hour night secretion exceeded 30 mEq in 12 of 19 patients with severe head trauma (Norton et al., 1970). Harrison and his associates on the other hand found a negative correlation between extent of burns and acid output over 12 hour collection periods (Harrison et al., 1972).

Stremple et al. found that acid secretion among 9 consecutive soldiers who suffered severe trauma in Vietnam and bled from acute gastric ulcers could be divided into three groups depending upon the nature of the trauma. Those with intracranial trauma had the highest acid outputs, those with spinal cord injuries came next and those with intraabdominal injury had the lowest 24 hour acid outputs (Stremple et al., 1972) (figure 3). In a similar group of patients, Bowen and his colleagues found higher serum gastrin levels in patients with CNS injury. There was no difference between patients without CNS injury whether they had stress ulcers or not (Bowen et al., 1973) (table 2). We have found that decerebration in dogs increased basal serum gastrin levels and, to an even greater degree, the levels after electrical stimulation of the vagi (Lanciault et al., 1973) (figure 4).

SUMMARY

The present state of the art defines the efferent pathway of behavioral and neurophysiological mechanisms acting via the brain to alter gastric acid secretion from the hypothalamus to the vagal nuclei. The response can be reduced by interrupting afferent input to the brain. Injury to the brain appears to stimulate interdigestive secretion of acid in many patients while other forms of stress may inhibit secretion.

Fig. 3. Daily changes in mean acid output of the nine bleeding patients separated by site of injury. Normal mean is 84 ± 36 mEq/24 hr. (From Strempel et al., Arch. Surg. 105: 179, 1972).

Fig. 4. Concentrations of serum gastrin and acid output following bilateral electrical stimulation of the vagus nerves in anesthetized decerebrated dogs. (From Lanciault et al., Am. J. Physiol. 225:548, 1973).

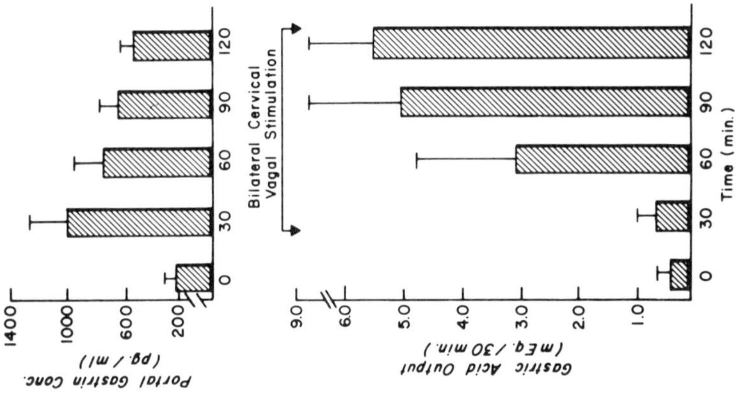

Figure 4

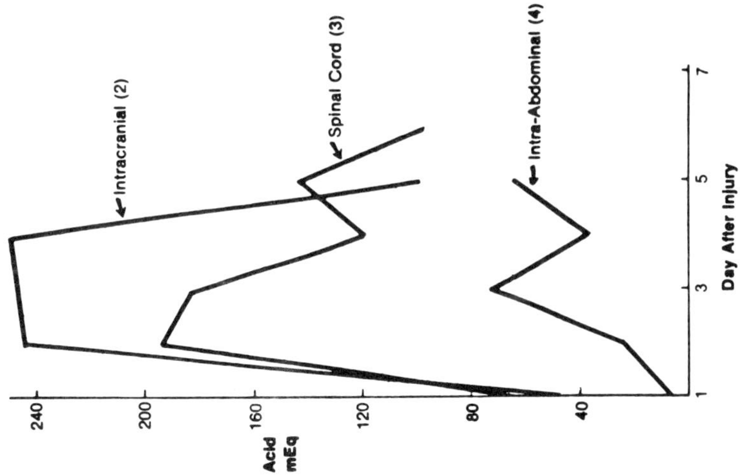

Figure 3

Table 1

Acid Output* in Response to Insulin and 2DG

Drug	Dose/kg	Highest 15 min. Acid Output	Acid Output 1st hr.	Acid Output 2nd hr.	Total 4 hr. Acid Output
Insulin	0.1 U	3.38 ± 1.38	5.18 ± 1.21	0.78 ± 0.22	6.00 ± 0.81
Insulin	0.25 U	4.27 ± 0.92	8.05 ± 0.80	2.67 ± 0.31	10.85 ± 0.72
Insulin	0.5 U	5.57 ± 0.88	12.03 ± 0.91	9.71 ± 0.71	22.03 ± 1.50
Insulin	1.0 U	5.67 ± 0.78	11.85 ± 0.82	15.16 ± 0.85	30.29 ± 2.62
2 DG	150 mg.	6.73 ± 1.12	18.69 ± 1.50	7.97 ± 0.89	30.06 ± 3.12

*Mean acid output in mEq ± Standard Error in mEq. (From Cooke, 1970)

Table 2

Serum Gastrin Levels in 39 Patients after CNS and Non-CNS Injury*

Patient Group	No. of Patients	Serum Gastrin (pg/ml)
(A) CNS injury	16	179 ± 40
(B) No CNS injury	23	77 ± 4
(C) CNS injury with stress ulcer	8	277 ± 67
(D) CNS injury without stress ulcer	8	131 ± 42
(E) No CNS injury with stress ulcer	10	82 ± 9
(F) No CNS injury without stress ulcer	13	73 ± 4

*Mean ± SEM for each group was calculated from the mean value for each patient within the group. A vs B, $P < .01$; C vs D, NS; E vs F, NS; C vs E, $P < .05$. (From Bowen et al., 1973).

REFERENCES

Badley,L.E., Spiro,H.M., and Senay,E.C., 1969.
Effect of mental arithmetic on gastric secretion.
Psychophysiology, 5:633.

Baron,J.H., 1970.
Dose response relationships of insulin hypoglycemia and gastric acid in man.
Gut, 11:826.

Brooks,F.P., 1967.
Central neural control of acid secretion, in handbook of physiology, Section 6: Alimentary Canal, Vol. II secretion., Edit. by C.F. Code.
Am. Physiol. Soc., Washington, C.C., p. 805.

Bowen,J.C., Fleming,W.H., and Thompson,J.C., 1973.
Elevated serum gastrin levels in Vietnam casualities with CNS injury.
Surg. Forum, 351.

Carmona,A., and Slanger,J.L., 1973.
Effects of chemical stimulation of the hypothalamus upon gastric secretion.
Physiol. and behavior, 10:657.

Colin-Jones,D.G., and Himsworth,R.L., 1969.
The secretion of gastric acid in response to a lack of metabolizable glucose.
J. Physiol., (London), 202:97.

Colin-Jones,D.G., and Himsworth,R.L., 1970.
The location of the chemoreceptor controlling gastric acid secretion during hypoglycemia.
J. Physiol., (London), 206:397.

Cooke,A.R., 1969.
Acid and pepsin secretion in response to endogenous and exogenous cholinergic stimulation and pentapeptide.
Aust. J. Exp. Biol. Med. Sci., 47:197.

Cummins,J.T., and Vaughan,B.E., 1964.
Acid secretion and the bioelectric potential in isolated rat stomach.
Intern. Congr. Biochem., New York, (Abstr.), 8:647.

Davis,R.A., Brooks,F.P., and Steckel,D.C., 1968.
Gastric secretory changes after anterior hypothalamic lesions.
Am. J. Physiol., 215:600.

Eisenberg,M.M., Chaiola,R.C., and Sugawars,K., 1970.
Sustained gastric secretion in response to 2 deoxy-d-glucose, indefatigability of the vagal mechanism.
Gastroenterology, 59:174.

Hall,W.H., and Smith,G.P., 1969.
Gastric secretory response to chronic hypothalmic stimulation in monkeys.
Gastroenterology, 57:491.

Harrison,A.M., Gaisford,J.C., and Wechsler,R.L., 1972.
Gastric secretion in the burned patient.
J. Trauma, 12:1041.

Kadekaro,M., Limo-Laria,C., Valle,L.E.R., and Velha, L.P.E., 1972.
The site of action of 2-deoxy-d-glucose mediating gastric secretion in the cat.
J. Physiol., (London), 221:1.

Kerr,F.W.L., and Preshaw,R.M., 1969.
Secretomotor function of the dorsal motor nucleus of the vagus.
J. Physiol., (London), 205:405.

Lanciault,G., Bonoma,C., and Brooks,F.P., 1973.
Vagal stimulation, gastrin release and acid secretion in anesthetized dogs.
Am. J. Physiol., 225:546.

Lee,Y.H., Thompson,J.H., and McNew,J.J., 1969.
Possible role of amygdala in regulation of gastric secretion in chronic fistula rats.
Am. J. Physiol., 217:505.

Mikhail,A.A., 1971.
Effects of acute and chronic stress situations on stomach acidity in rats.
J. Comp. Physiol. Psychol., 74:23.

Morrissey,S., and Stephens,D.N., 1971.
The role of the posterior hypothalamus in gastric acid secretion.
J. Physiol., (London), 221:14.

Norman,A., 1969.
Response contingency and human gastric acidity.
Psychophysiology, 5:673.
Norton,L., Fuchs,E., and Eisman,B., 1972.
Gastric secretory response to pressure on vagal nuclei.
Am. J. Surg., 123:13.
Pare,W.P., 1972.
Conditioning and avoidance responding effects on gastric secretion in the rat with chronic fistula.
J. Comp. Physiol. Psychol., 80:150.
Pendleton,R.G., Bartakovits,P., Miller,D.A., Mann,W.A., and Ridley,P.T., 1970.
Studies indicating a central antisecretory site of action for desmethylimipramine (DMI).
J. Pharmacol. Exp., 174:421.
Reigel,D.H., Barborcak,J.J., Larson,S.J., and Sances, A., Jr., 1969.
The effect of electroanesthesia on gastric acid secretion. Electrotherapeutic sleep and electro-anesthesia.
Proc. 2nd Internat. Sumposium Graz. Austria,8:296.
Reigel,D.H., Larson,S.J., and Sances,A., Jr., 1969.
Effect of limbic system stiumlation and electro-anesthesia upon gastric secretion.
Gastroenterology, 56:1192.
Reigel,D.H., Larson,S.J., and Sances,A., Jr., 1970.
Cerebral release of gastric acid inhibitor.
Surgery, 68:217.
Reigel,D.H., Larson,S.J., Sances,A., Hoffman,N.E., and Switala,K.J., 1971.
A gastric acid inhibitor of cerebral origin.
Surgery, 70:161.
Ridley,P.T., and Cirpili,E.O., 1969.
Suppression of 2-deoxy-d-glucose-augmented gastric secretion by hypothalamic lesions producing hyperphagia.
Am. J. Dig. Dis., 14:262.
Ridley,P.T., and Mann,W.A., 1973.
Central antisecretory action of desmethylimipramine in the rat.
Am. J. Dig. Dis., 18:493.

Schapiro,H., Wruble,L.D., Britt,L.G., and Bell,T.A., 1970.
Sensory deprivation on visceral activity. I. The effect of visual deprivation on canine gastric secretion.
Psychosom. Med., 32:379.
Schapiro,H., Gross,C.W., Nakamura,T., Wruble,L.D., and Britt,L.G., 1970.
Sensory deprivation on visceral activity. II. The effect of auditory and vestibular deprivation on canine gastric secretion.
Psychosom. Med., 32:515.
Schapiro,H., Britt,L.G., Gross,C.W., and Gaines,K.J., 1971.
Sensory deprivation on visceral activity. III. The effect of olfactory deprivation of canine gastric secretion.
Psychosom. Med., 33:429.
Schapiro,H., Britt,L.G., and Dohrn,R.H., 1973.
Sensory deprivation on visceral activity. IV. The effect of temporary visual deprivation on canine gastric secretion.
Am. J. Dig. Dis., 18:573.
Shaw,J.E., and Urquhart,J., 1972.
Parameters of the control of acid secretion in the isolated blood-perfused stomach.
J. Physiol., (London), 226:107P.
Smith,G.P., and Brooks,F.P., 1970.
Brain behavior and gastric secretion in progress in gastroenterology, Vol. II, (Edit. by G.B.J. Glass).
Grune and Stratton Inc., New York.
Stacher,L., Berner,P., and Naske,R., 1973.
Influence of suggestion of rest during hypnosis on gastric juice secretion.
Wien. Med. Wochenschr., 123:160.
Stadel,F., and Rehfeed,J.F., 1972.
Hypoglycemic release of gastrin in man.
Scand. J. Gastroenterology, 7:509.
Stening,G.F., and Isenberg,J.I., 1969.
Insulin-induced acid secretion after partial vagotomy in dogs and cats.
Am. J. Physiol., 217:962.

Stremple,J.F., Molot,M.D., McNamara,J., Moro,H., and Glass,G.B.J., 1972.
Post-traumatic gastric bleeding: Prospective gastric secretion composition.
Arch. Surg., 105:177.

PHARMACOLOGIC CONTROL OF GASTRIC SECRETION

David A. Brodie and Y. H. Lee

INTRODUCTION

The medical treatment of peptic ulcer disease has passed through various phases in its history, but the therapeutic dictum "no acid – no ulcer" remains as the accepted goal of anti-ulcer therapy. Even with the rapid advance of experimental test methods and significant drug discoveries in other fields of medicine, essentially the same therapeutic agents for ulcer treatment are in use today as compared to those of several decades ago. This does not mean that in the past 50 years no new agents have been introduced; however, it is reasonable to say that to date, no agents have been unequivocally successful in the clinic for increasing the rate of the ulcer healing process and preventing ulcer recurrence. It is only within the last 5 years that significant progress has been made toward better pharmacologic control of gastric secretion.

Since several reviews on drug-induced inhibition of gastric acid secretion have been published recently (Brodie, 1970; Thompson, 1972; Evers and Ridley, 1973), this presentation will deal with the highlights of the current research on drug inhibition of gastric secretion. Because gastrointestinal hormones and H_2 receptor antagonists will be discussed in detail by other speakers, these areas will not be included in this review.

Therapeutically useful drugs for the control of gastric secretion should be either inhibitors of acid and/or pepsin secretion or enhancers of mucus secretion. The mechanism of action could be by several routes –

1. Selective inhibition of vagal activity – either central or peripheral;

2. Alteration in mucosal blood flow;

3. Inhibition of enzymes controlling acid, pepsin or mucus production and/or release; or

4. Control of turnover of parietal and cheif cells.

The majority of drugs in use for therapy of peptic ulcer disease are anticholinergic agents which fall into the first group. There are no agents available at the present time which act by alteration of mucosal blood flow or control turnover of mucosal cell population. Most pharmacological research has been directed towards control of enzyme activity as the means of regulating gastric secretion. This review will deal mainly with this research after a brief mention of anticholinergic drugs.

ANTICHOLINERGICS

The belladonna alkaloids have been used in the treatment of peptic ulcer disease for over 30 years (Goodman and Gilman, 1941); their use was due to antimotility rather than antisecretory activity. In the mid-1950's the introduction of synthetic anticholinergics demonstrated that potent anticholinergic drugs could be used to reduce gastric acid secretion and that these drugs had a role in peptic ulcer therapy based on this action (Goodman and Gilman, 1955). The continuing popularity of these drugs – despite their disadvantages and contraindications – is indicated by the fact that in 1972, the prescription sales of this class of drugs was estimated to be 125 million dollars. One advantage of treatment with this type of agent is that the patient knows that the medicine is "doing something" when the side effects become apparent. The problem is whether the drugs are "doing something" to the gastric acid secretion as well as to the mouth, nose, urinary tract, intestine and eyes. Clinical trials of anticholinergics indicate that they provide relief of pain – possibly due to antimotility action – but the change in acid-pepsin secretion is moderate and of brief duration (Sun, 1962). There have not been any clinical studies indicating that therapy with these drugs speeds ulcer healing or reduces recurrence (Lennard-Jones, 1961; Friedlander, 1954; Melrose and Pinkerton, 1961). The short duration of acid inhibition combined with unacceptable side effects has spurred the search for new types of drugs to control gastric acid secretion.

GASTRIN ANTAGONISTS

Since gastrin is an important hormone in the regulation of gastric acid secretion, it is a logical therapeutic goal to seek a drug which inhibits its release or prevents it from stimulating parietal cell activity. The use of peptides with similar structures has not been successful in the search for an antagonist to the hormone, but compounds with thioacetamide structures have been shown experimentally to be potent gastrin antagonists (figure 1). SC-15396 (2-phenyl-2-(2-pyridyl)-thioacetamide) was the first compound to be claimed a "specific" gastrin antagonist (Cook and Bianchi, 1967; Lee and Bianchi, 1971). However, subsequent studies of this agent demonstrated that it inhibited histamine and insulin-induced gastric secretion in the rat (Lee and Thompson, 1968; Albinus and Sewing, 1969), the guinea pig (Albinus and Sewing, 1969), and the dog (Gillespie et al., 1968; Connell et al., 1968).

Furthermore, the drug did not block the extragastric effect of gastrin (Stening and Grossman, 1968), thus it appears that "antigastrin" is not the specific gastrin antagonist that it was hoped to be. But even if the compound is not a specific antigastrin substance, it still could be useful for the reduction of gastric secretion in the treatment of human peptic ulcer disease. Unfortunately, this compound was found to induce mammary adenocarcinoma in female rats (Lee, personal communication) and was not tested in the human.

Several analogs of SC-15396 have been synthesized and reported to be active: CMN-131 (pyridyl-2-thioacetamide hydrochloride) (Pascaud and Blouin, 1972); and SKF-59377 (N-methyl-2-(2-pyridyl) -d-methoxy-thioacetamide) (Groves et al., 1973) are among them. CMN-131 was found to be more potent than SC-15396 in inhibiting gastric secretion in the rat and Heidenhain pouch dog (Pascaud and Couline, 1972; Bleichner, 1973), and preventing experimental ulceration (Malen et al., 1971) while SKF-59377 was reported to be even more active than CMN-131 in the pylorus-ligated rat, gastric fistula rat and fistula squirrel monkey (Groves et al., 1973) as shown in figure 2.

Gastrin Antagonists

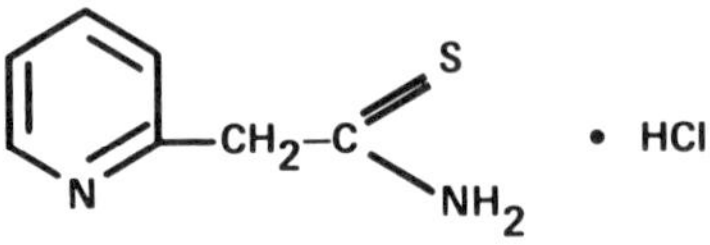

CMN 131
(Pyridyl-2-thioacetamide hydrochloride)

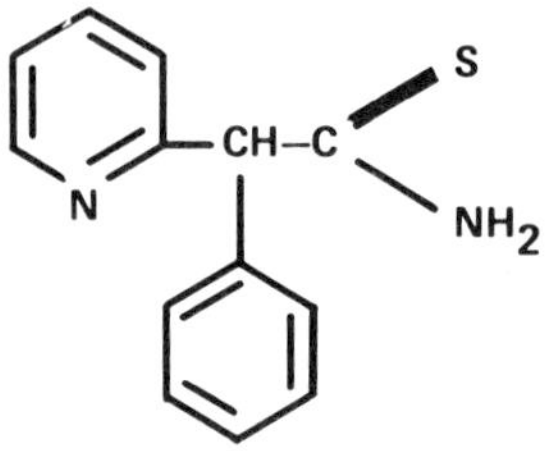

SC 15396
(2-phenyl-2(2-pyridyl)-
thioacetamide

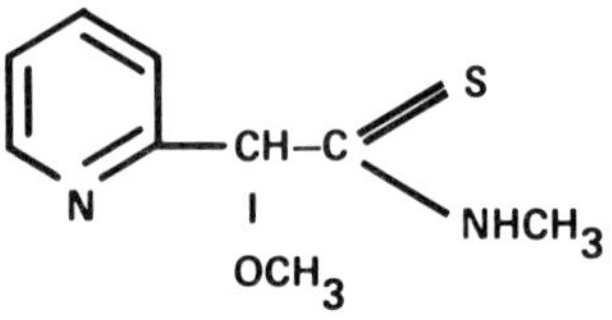

SK & F 59377
N-methyl-2-(2-pyridyl)-d-methoxy-
thioacetamide

Fig. 1. Chemical Structure of Gastric Antagonists.

COMPARATIVE ANTISECRETORY DATA

TEST	COMPOUND	ROUTE	ED_{50} mg/kg VOLUME	ED_{50} mg/kg TITRATABLE ACID CONCENTRATION	ED_{50} mg/kg ACID OUTPUT	ED_{Δ} 2.5 pH
PYLORUS	SK & F 59377	p.o.	3.8	1.3	1.0	2.3
LIGATED	SK & F 59377	i.v.	4.4	0.84	0.79	1.6
RAT	CMN 131	p.o.	4.5	4.1	2.6	4.2
	SC 15396	p.o.	NO DOSE RESPONSE	--	--	18.0
GASTRIC	SK & F 59377	p.o.	NO DOSE RESPONSE	3.1	1.3	
FISTULA	CMN 131	p.o.	NO DOSE RESPONSE	9.8	5.3	
RAT	SC 15396	p.o	87.0	60.0	36.0	
GASTRIC	SK & F 59377	p.o.	0.80	1.5	0.58	
FISTULA	CMN 131	p.o.	4.7	3.4	1.8	
MONKEY	SC 15396	p.o.	NO EFFECT	21.0	17.0	

(Data provided through the courtesy of Dr. William G. Groves, SK & F Lab)

Fig. 2. Comparative experimental antisecretory activity of 3 gastrin antagonists. ED 2.5 is the dose required to reduce pH from control values to 2.5. Test duration for all procedures was 2 hours; gastric juice was titrated to pH 7.4.

Since the thioamides have been found to be tumorigenic in rats, it will require lifetime studies of carcinogenicity in experimental animals before these compounds can be considered safe for therapeutic trial in man.

SYNTHETIC ANALOGS OF PROSTAGLANDINS

Natural prostaglandins, especially PGE_1 and PGE_2, have been demonstrated to be potent antisecretory and anti-ulcer agents in experimental animals (Ramwell and Shaw, 1968; Main, 1969; Robert et al., 1967, 1968; Robert and Phillips, 1968; Lee et al., 1973). However, because of a variety of pharmacological activities of prostaglandins, selective gastric activity remains a problem. As with the anticholinergics, the goal will be to synthesize analogs which avoid the undesirable effects but retain the potent antisecretory activity.

In the past few years, several synthetic analogs have been reported, such as SC-24665 (Lee and Bianchi, 1972) 15-methyl PGE_2 (Robert and Magerlein, 1973; Weeks et al., 1973; Karim et al., 1973) 16, 16-dimethyl PGE_2 methylester (Robert and Magerlein, 1973) and 9-oxoprostanoic acids (Lippmann, 1970; Lippmann, 1973, Lippmann and Seethaler, 1973) (figure 3).

SC-24665 was found to be orally active against pylorus ligation induced gastric ulcers in rats, histamine induced duodenal ulcers in guinea pigs, reserpine induced gastric ulcers in rats, pentagastrin induced duodenal ulcers in guinea pigs and cats, and exertion induced gastric ulcers in rats without producing significant hypotensive or uterine contractile activities (Lee and Bianchi, 1972). It also inhibited pentagastrin induced acid secretion in chronic fistula rats, cats and dogs (Lee and Bianchi, 1972). 15-Methyl PGE_2 and 16, 16-dimethyl PGE_2 exerted a systemic antisecretory effect against gastrin in Heidenhain pouch dogs both orally and parenterally and was even more potent than PGE_2 (Robert and Magerlein, 1973). In addition, in human studies, 15 (R) 15-methyl PGE_2 methyl ester was found to inhibit basal and pentagastrin stimulated acid secretion when administered orally or intravenously (Karim et al., 1973). However, no details of the experiment were given; nevertheless, diarrhea was observed along with antisecretory effects of SC-24665 (Lee and Bianchi, 1972), 15 methyl PGE_2 and 16, 16-dimethyl

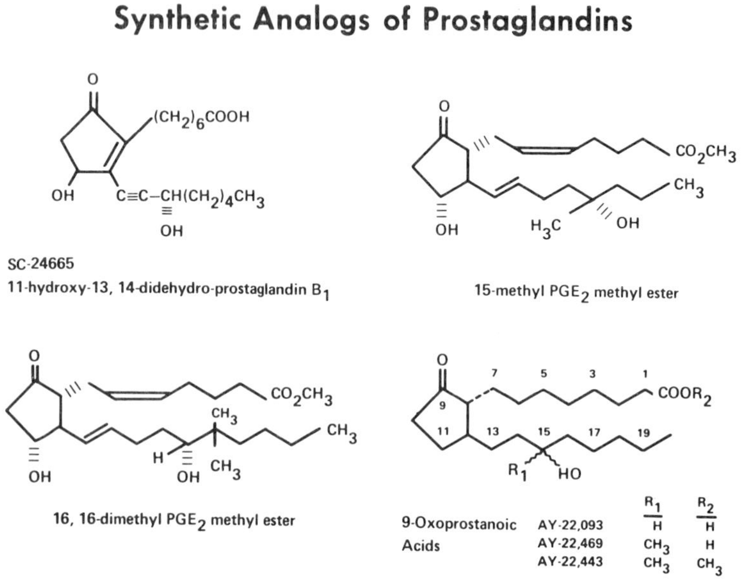

Fig. 3. Chemical structure of synthetic analogs of prostaglandins.

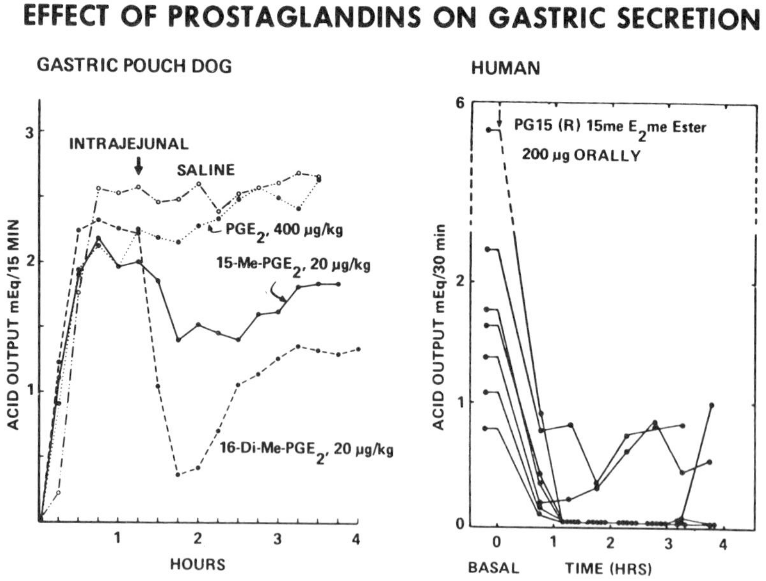

Fig. 4. Effect of prostaglandins on gastric secretion. The 15-methyl PGE_2 was active at 20 mg/kg in the dog and at 200 mg orally in humans on basal acid output.

PGE_2 (Robert and Magerlein, 1973). Thus, the problem of diarrhea will be one of the side effects that must be removed before the synthetic analogs of PG's are applied to the clinical treatment of peptic ulcer disease. These studies are summarized in figure 4.

MUCUS ENHANCERS

Carbenoxolone (biogastrone, duogastrone) is a glycrrhetinic acid derivative without anticholinergic or antisecretory activity (Robson and Sullivan, 1968; Baron and Sullivan, 1970; Jones and Sullivan, 1972). This drug (figure 5) has been reported to promote the healing of human chronic ulcer (Doll et al., 1962, Hill and Hutton, 1965, Horwich and Galloway, 1965, Watkinson, 1968) and there is some evidence that experimental ulcers, produced in rats by cautery, also heal faster under its influence (Kahn and Sullivan, 1968) (figure 5).

In addition, pretreatment with carbenoxolone can protect the gastric mucosa against stress erosions in the guinea pig (Lipkin and Ludwig, 1968) and against erosions produced in the rat by corticosteroids (Hoffmeister and Hoffmeister, 1971) and by compound 48/80 (Dean, 1968). In clinical studies, carbenoxolone was reported by British physicians to have a good effect on the acceleration of gastric ulcer healing based on the mean reduction in size of ulcer craters following 225 or 300 mg daily doses for one month or 50 to 100 mg t.i.d. for 5 weeks (Rosch and Ottenjahn, 1971; MacCaig, 1967 and 1970, Middleton et al., 1965; Ottenjahn and Rosch, 1970, Banks et al., 1967; Cocking and MacCaig, 1969; Perez, 1967; Doll et al., 1965; Doll et al., 1968; Geismer and Mosebech, 1970; Horwich and Galloway, 1965; Kunz, 1971; Lenz et al., 1971).

However, a similar undisputable beneficial effect was not observed in duodenal ulcer patients even with position released duogastrone (Heinkel, 1970; Watkinson, 1968; Perez, 1970; Amure, 1970; Craig et al., 1967; Cliff, 1968; Cliff-Jones and Lennard-Jones, 1968; Lawrence et al., 1968; Banforth, 1970). The mechanism of action is not known for certain, but probably involves increased mucus production. It has been suggested that carbenoxolone increases mucus turnover and discharge and even strengthens the gastric mucosal barrier (Cross and Hole, 1972; Dean, 1968; Lipkin, 1970; Goodier, 1968; Johnson, 1968; Menguy and Thompson, 1967; Gheorghia et al., 1972). Because of its sodium and water retention

Mucus Enhancers

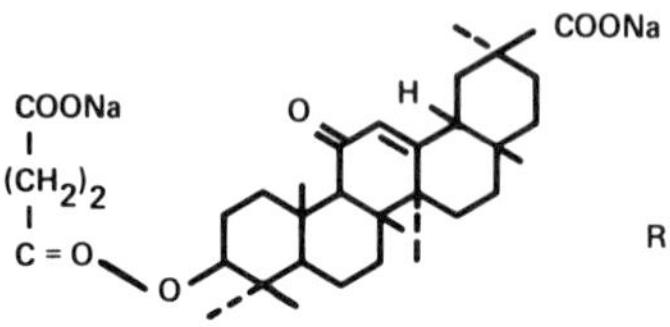

Carbenoxolone Sodium (Biogastrone, Duogastrone)

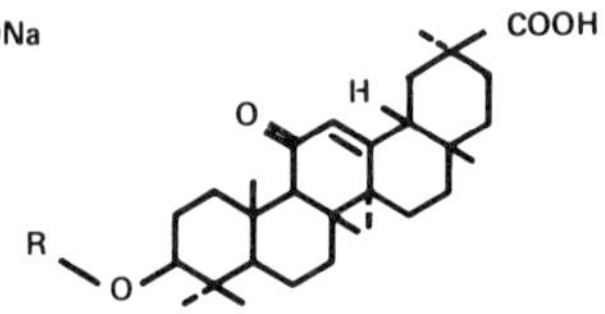

BX-24 (Lauroyl glycyrrhetinic acid)

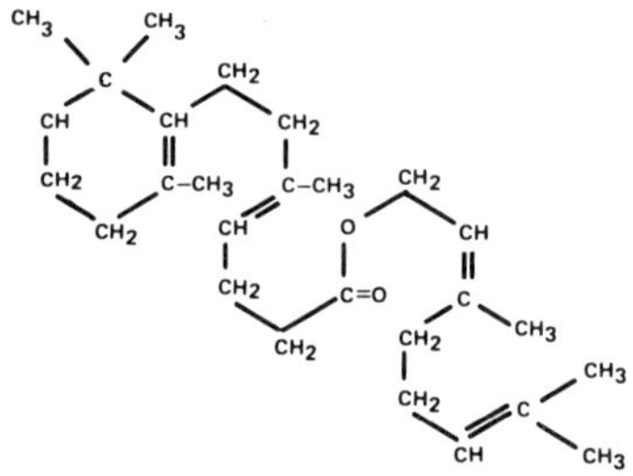

Geranyl farnesylacetate (Gefarnate, DA-688)

Fig. 5. Chemical structure of mucus enhancers.

property and hypopotassemia (Turpie and Thompson, 1965; Montgomery, 1967, 1970) several chemical modifications have been made, among them BX24, claimed to be free of undesirable side effects (Frasier et al., 1972).

Gefarnate (Geranyl farnesylacetate) (Adami et al., 1964; Murari, 1964) is a terpene which contains a number of isoprene units, the basic fragments from which pentacyclic ring structures like steroids can be snythesized and with which the triterpenoid, carbenoxolone, bears some structural resemblances. Experimental studies did not reveal an inhibitory effect on gastric secretion in rats (Adami et al., 1964). It has been claimed to promote gastric ulcer healing in clinical trials (Ponari, 1964; Ortone and Furno, 1968; Langman et al., 1973); while the mode of action is unknown it has been claimed to be a mucus enhancer (Takagi and Yano, 1972).

PEPSIN ANTAGONISTS

It has been postulated that acid alone is not responsible for ulcer disease but rather the presence of pepsin activated by acid which

Pepsin Antagonists

Depepsen (SN-263) Sulfated polysaccharide or Sodium amylosulfate (M. Wt. 60 x 10^6)

Pepstatins:

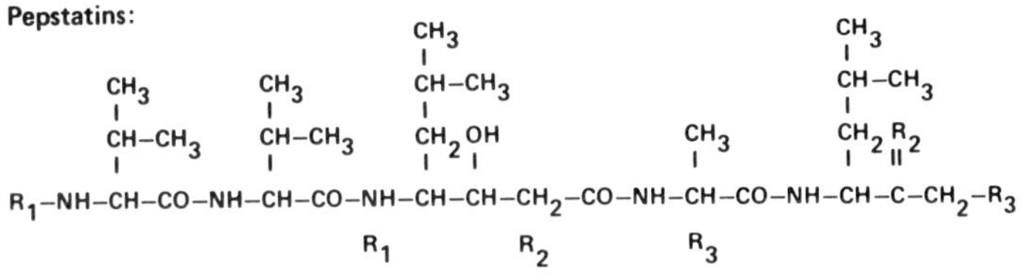

	R_1	R_2	R_3
Pepstatin A (Pepstatin)	*iso*-valeryl	< H, OH	–COOH
Pepstatin B	*n*-caproyl	< H, OH	–COOH
Pepstatin C	*iso*-caproyl	< H, OH	–COOH
Pepstanone A	*iso*-valeryl	=O	–H
S-PI	acetyl	< H, OH	–COOH

Example: Pepstatin A

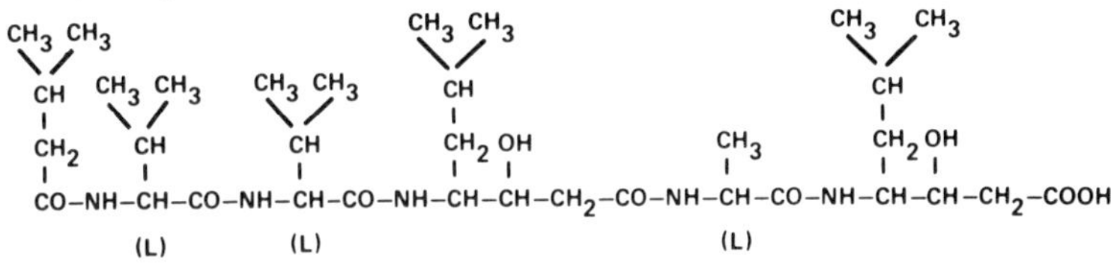

Fig. 6. Chemical structure of pepsin antagonists.

produces mucosal damage (Schiffrin and Kamarov, 1941, Schiffrin and Warren, 1942). If pepsin secretion is prevented or the released pepsin is bound and rendered inactive, acid secretion would not have to be depressed to achieve therapeutic results. Several agents have been reported as pepsin antagonists, such as depepsen and pepstatin, and have been studied in peptic ulcer disease (figure 6).

Depepsen (SN-263), a sulfated amylopectin polysaccharide, has been shown to reduce ulcer incidence in experimental animals (Bianchi and Cook, 1964; Lee and Bianchi, 1971), but there was no effect on gastric acid secretion (Cook and Drill, 1967). This agent has no anticholinergic activity and appears to act by (1) direct binding between free SN-263 and pepsin to form an enzyme inhibitor complex and (2) by binding of SN-263 to the substrate (Cammarata et al., 1971). In clinical trial, in addition to its antipeptic activity, Zimmon et al. (1969) reported that an oral dose of 0.5 gm hourly (9 a.m. to 8 p.m.) for 12 days increased the rate of healing of gastric ulcer (Sun, 1965, 1967; Cayer and Ruffin, 1967). However, the effectiveness of depepsen for duodenal ulcer therapy remains controversial (Sun and Ryan, 1970).

Pepstatin (Isovaleryl [L-valyl-L-valyl-4-amino-3-hydroxy-6-methylheptanoly-L-alanyl-4-amino-3-hydroxy-6-methylheptanoic acid]) (Morishima et al., 1970) was discovered in streptomyces culture filtrates and has been shown to be a specific inhibitor of acid proteases (Umezawa et al., 1970; Aoyagi et al., 1971). It has a strong protective effect against pylorus-ligated rat stomach ulcers (Umezawa et al., 1970). In human studies at the daily oral dose of 50 to 400 mg q.i.d., it reduced gastric juice protease activity and had a beneficial effect in human gastric ulcer on the rate of ulcer healing and reduction in the size of ulcer. There were no noticeable side effects but pain relief was not achieved (Ito et al., 1972; Harunii et al., 1972; Hara et al., 1972). The suggested mechanism of action was by pepsin binding (Kunimoto et al., 1972).

EVALUATION OF ANIMAL SPECIES USED FOR THE STUDY OF GASTRIC ANTISECRETORY DRUGS

The ideal experimental preparation for the study of antisecretory drugs would, of course, be one which mimics acid secretion in the peptic ulcer patient. The animal species would be inexpensive, tolerate surgery well, have a high basal acid secretion, tolerate drugs and produce a pharmacological profile predictive for the clinic. Since this ideal preparation does not exist, it is worthwhile examining the advantages and disadvantages of species available for the study of drug action on gastric secretion.

The most widely used animal is the rat, due principally to the use of the pylorus ligation operation which provides an animal with high values for gastric acidity, pepsin and volume. In general, data from the rat is well accepted for the study of potential antisecretory drugs, principally because anticholinergic agents are quite potent in this species. However, within the last few years, it has become clear that it is not possible to rely upon the rat to predict all types of drug action for the human. This has most recently been brought out in the study of the drug Burimimide, which has minimal antisecretory activity in the rat, possibly due to the insensitivity of this species to histamine, but has good activity in the dog.

Because of the swing away from the anticholinergic type of drug, other species have been examined as an alternative to the rat. At the present time there is no one species which will reliably mimic the human peptic ulcer patient. It is often overlooked that the cat was the animal used for the discovery of the hormone gastrin and this species has been used successfully in many laboratories for mechanism of action studies of acid secretion. There are also studies indicating that the squirrel monkey has a number of advantages as a test animal, such as low cost, small size, ease of handling and a high gastric acidity. However, the number of drug studies published in the species are small and those indicate that the squirrel monkey is not as reactive to known antisecretory agents as is the rat or the dog.

The species which appears to be most similar to man in the study of gastric secretion is the pig, and there have been several publications indicating that this species would have many advantages as a test animal (Huber and Wallin, 1965). The disadvantage of the pig is its size and cost; however, these can be overcome by the use of the miniature pig, whose weight and price approximate those of the dog. Although there have been several papers published indicating the utility of this animal, it has not achieved any measure of popularity and perhaps requires the discovery of particular pharmacological sensitivity before more work will be done with this animal.

At this time, the dog is the animal of choice for the study of drug action on gastric secretion. These animals are readily available and have the added advantage that at the current time they are used extensively for acute and chronic testing of new drugs. Major disadvantages in using the dog are that the animals do not secrete high acid levels spontaneously and so require administration of a secretory stimulant in order to test therapeutic agents. It is also known that dogs vomit rather easily which may cause loss of the drug and inhibition of gastric secretion due to nausea. Even with these disadvantages, the wide-spread use of the dog for gastrointestinal research has given the species an aura of acceptability, and it is unlikely at the present time that new drugs could be tested in the human without at least some idea of activity in the canine species.

As more data accumulate on pharmacological action of the antisecretory drugs in various animal species, it will be possible to achieve a better evaluation of which animal species best predicts clinical activity. In many instances, drugs which are highly active in the rat as antisecretory agents have little or no activity against gastric secretion in the dog. It is unlikely that drugs will be taken to the clinic for testing on the basis of rat data alone. This suggests that future testing of anti-acid secretion drugs will depend in large measure on activity demonstrated in the dog. The rat, however, may remain a useful animal for the study of drugs which act on mucus, pepsin or gastrointestinal motility. This may indicate a future dichotomy in which antisecretory agents will be tested entirely in the dog while anti-ulcer agents will be screened and evaluated primarily in the rat.

In the future there may be two types of drugs available for peptic ulcer therapy, one based on the "no acid – no ulcer" dictum with studies conducted in the dog, and the other based on stimulation of healing factors developed from rat ulcer models.

REFERENCES

Adami,E., Marazzi-Uberti,E., and Turba,C., 1964.
Pharmacological research on gefarnate, a new synthetic isoprenoid with an anti-ulcer action.
Arch. Int. Pharmacodyn., 147:113.

Albinus,M., and Sewing,K-Fr., 1969.
The effect of SC-15396, atropine and mepyramine ongastrin-, bethanechol-and histamine-stimulated gastric acid secretion in rats and guinea pigs.
J. Pharm. Pharmacol., 21:656.

Amure,B.O., 1970.
Clinical study of duogastrone in the treatment of duodenal ulcers.
Gut, 11:171.

Aoyagi,T., Kunimoto,S., Morishima,H., Takeuchi,T., and Umezaqa,H., 1971.
Effect of pepstatin on acid proteases.
J. Antibiot., 24:687.

Bachrach,W.H., 1958.
Anticholinergic drugs survey of the literature and some experimental observations.
Am. J. Dig. Dis., 3:743.

Bamforth,M., 1970.
An appraisal of duogastrone in general practice, in Baron,J.H., and Sullivan,F.M., Carbenoxdone Sodium.
Butterworths, (London), p. 153.

Bank,S., Marks,I.N., Palmer,P.E.S., Groll,A., and Van Eldik,E., 1967.
A trial of carbenoxolone sodium in the treatment of gastric ulceration.
S. Afr. Med. J., 41:297.

Baron,J.H., and Sullivan,F.M., 1970.
Carbenoxolone sodium.
Butterworths, (London), p. 171.

Bianchi,R.G., and Cook,D.L., 1964.
Antipeptic and antiulcerogenic properties of a synthetic sulfated polysaccharide (SN-263).
Gastroenterology, 47:409.

Bleichner,G., 1973.
Modeles Experimentaux Pour L'etude Des Inhibiteurs De La Secretion Gastrique Effets Compares d'un inhibiteur non anti-cholinergique et de l'Atropine (These).
Medicales et Universitaires, Paris, p. 118.

Brodie,D.A., 1970.
Induced inhibition of gastric secretion, in Glass, G.B.J., progress in gastroenterology, Vol. II.
Grune and Stratton Inc., New York.

Cammarata,P.S., Bianchi,R.G., and Fago,F.J., 1971.
Mechanism of the antipeptic action of amylopectin sulfate (SN-263), an antiulcer mucin-like agent.
Gastroenterology, 61:850.

Cayer,D., and Ruffin,J.M., 1967.
Effect of depepsen in the treatment of peptic ulcer.
Ann. N.Y. Acad. Sci., 140:744.

Cliff,J.M., 1968.
A trial of carbenoxolone capsules in royal navy, in Robson,J.M., and Sullivan,F.M., a symposium on carbenoxolone sodium.
Butterworths, (London), p. 239.

Cliff,J.M., and Mitton-Thompson,G.J., 1970.
A double-blind trial of carbenoxolone sodium capsules in the treatment of duodenal ulcer.
Gut, 11:167.

Cocking,J.B., and MacCaig,J.N., 1969.
Effect of low dosage of carbenoxolone sodium on gastric ulcer healing and acid secretion.
Gut, 10:219.

Collin-Jones,D.G., Lennard-Jones,J.E., Howel Jones,J., Misiewicz,J.J., and Langman,M.J.S., 1968.
Carbenoxolone capsules (Duogastrone) in duodenal ulcer: preliminary results of clinical and experimental studies, in Robson,J.M., and Sullivan, F.M., a symposium on carbenoxolone sodium.
Butterworths, (London), p. 209.

Connell,A.M., Hill,R.A., Macleod,I.B., Sircus,W., and Thomson,C.G., 1968.
Effects of SC-15396 on gastric secretion.
Gut, 9:641.

Cook,D.L., Eich,S., and Cammarata,P.S., 1963.
Comparative pharmacology and chemistry of synthetic sulfated polysaccharides.
Arch. Int. Pharmacodyn., 141:1.

Cook,D.L., and Bianchi,R.G., 1967.
SC-15396: a new antiulcer compound possessing anti-gastrio activity.
Life Sci., 6:1381.

Cook,D.L., and Drill,V.A., 1967.
Pharmacological properties of pepsin inhibitors.
Ann. N.Y. Acad. Sci., 140:724.

Craig,O., Hunt,T., Kimerling,J.J., and Parke,D.V., 1967.
Carbenoxolone in the treatment of duodenal ulcer.
Practitioner, 199:109.

Cross,S., Rhodes,J., and Hole,D., 1972.
Carbenoxolone: its protective action against bile damage to gastric mucosa in canine pouches.
Gastroenterology, 62:737.

Dean,A.C.B., 1968.
Protective effect of carbenoxolone in drug-induced lesions of the stomach, in Robson,J.M., and Sullivan,F.M., a symposium on carbenoxolone sodium.
Butterworths, (London), p. 33.

de Marcos Perez,V.M., 1967.
El Carbenoxolone Sodico en el Tratamiento de la Ulcera Peptica del Estomago.
Rev. Esp. Enferm. Apar. Dig., 26:3.

de Marcos Perez,V.M., 1970.
The treatment of duodenal ulcer with carbenoxolone sodium, in Baron,J.H., and Sullivan,F.M., carbenoxolone sodium.
Butterworths, (London), p. 131.

Doll,R., Hill,I.D., Hutton,C., and Underwood,D.J., 1962.
Clinical trial of a triterpenoid liquorice compound in gastric and duodenal ulcer.
Lancet, 2:793.

Doll,R., Hill,I.D., Hutton,C.F., 1965.
Treatment of gastric ulcer with carbenoxolone sodium and oestrogens.
Gut, 6:19.

Doll,R., Langman,M.J.S., and Shawdon,H.H., 1968.
Treatment of gastric ulcer with carbenoxolone:

antagonistic effect of spironolactone.
Gut, 9:42.

Evers,P.W., and Ridley,P.T., 1973.
Agents affecting gastrointestinal functions.
Ann. Reports in Medicinal Chemistry, 8:93.

Fraser,P.M., Doll,R., and Langman,M.J.S., 1972.
Clinical trial of a new carbenoxolone analogue (BX 24), zinc sulfate and vitamin A in the treatment of gastric ulcer.
Gut, 13:459.

Friedlander,P.H., 1954.
Ambulatory treatment of duodenal ulcers, effect of fruit juice, olive oil, hexamethonium and methantheline.
Lancet, 1:386.

Gheorghiu,T.H., Frotz,H., Klein,H.J., and Hubner,G., 1972.
Protective action of carbenoxolone sodium on gastroduodenal mucosa: a study of its effects on mucus secretion in human and in rats.
Gastroenterology, 64:732.

Geismar,P., and Mosbech,J., 1970.
Carbenoxolone sodium in the treatment of gastric ulcer, in Baron,J.H., and Sullivan,F.M., carbenoxolone sodium.
Butterworths, (London), p. 83.

Gillespir,G., McCusker,V.I., Bedi,B.S., Debas,H.T., and Gillespir,I.E., 1968.
Further experimental observations on the gastric acid secretion inhibitor SC 15396.
Gastroenterology, 55:81.

Goddie,T.E.W., 1968.
Histopathology of gastric ulcers treated with carbenoxolone, in Robson,J.M., and Sullivan,F.M., a aymposium on carbenoxolone sodium.
Butterworths, (London), p. 111.

Goodman,L., and Gilman,A., 1941.
The pharmacological basis of therapy 1st Ed.
MacMillan Company, New York, p. 476.

Goodman,L., and Gilman,A., 1955.
The pharmacological basis of therapy 2nd Ed.
MacMillan Company, New York, p. 559.

Groves,W.G., Schlosser,J.H., Brennan,F.T., and Ridley, P.T., 1973.
Some gastrointestinal effects of N_methyl-α (2-pyridyl)-α-methoxythioacetamide H Cl (SK&F 59377).
Pharmacologist, 15:238.
Hara,Y., Ogoshi,K., Tobida,Y., Tsuzuii,K., Zihara,S., Niha,M., and Zubada,K., 1972.
Clinical effect of pepstatin against pepticulcer.
Shindan to Chiryo (Japan), 60:1111.
Harunii,T., Ito,K., and Kinozumi,N., 1972.
Clinical studies on antipepsin agent (pepstatin)-double blind test.
Shinyaku to Rinsho, (Japan), 21:121.
Heinkel,K., 1970.
The treatment of duodenal ulcer with duogastrone, in BaronkJ.H., and Sullivan,F.M., Carbenoxolone sodium.
Butterworths, (London), p. 149.
Hoffmeister,H., and Hoffmeister,A.W., 1971.
Das Steroidulcus des Magens. Experimentelle Untersuchungen zu dessen Verhutung.
Z. Gesamti. Exp. Med., 156:195.
Horwich,L., and Galloway,R., 1965.
Treatment of gastric ulceration with carbenoxolone sodium: clinical and radiological evaluation.
Br. Med. J., 2:1274.
Huber,W.G., and Wallin,R.F., 1965.
Gastric secretion and ulcer formation in the pig, in Bustad,L.K., and McClellan,R.O., Swine in Biomedical Research, Battelle-Northwest.
Richland,Washington, p. 121.
Itob,K., Harunii,T., and Kinozumi,N., 1972.
The clinical study of antipepsin (Pepstatin) (II).
Shinryo to Shinyaku, (Japan), 9:111.
Johnson,F.R., 1968.
The cytological approach to the evaluation of drug action on gastric mucosa, in Robson,J.M., and Sullivan,F.,., a symposium on carbenoxolone sodium.
Butterworths, (London), p. 93.

Jones,F.A., and Sullivan,F.M., 1972.
Carbenoxolone in gastroenterology.
Butterworths, (London), p. 88.

Karim,S.M.M., Carter,D.C., Bhana,D., and Ganesan,P.A., 1973.
Effect of orally and intravenously administered prostaglandin 15 (R) 15-Methyl E_2 on gastric secretion in man.
Advances in the Biosciences, 9:255.

Khan,M.G., and Sullivan,F.M., 1968.
The pharmacology of carbenoxolone sodium, in Robson,J.M., and Sullivan,F.M., a symposium on carbenoxolone sodium.
Butterworths, (London), p. 5.

Kunimoto,S., Aoyagi,T., Morishima,H., Takeuchi,T., and Umezawa,H., 1972.
Mechanism of inhibition of pepsin by pepstatin.
J. Antibiotics, 25:251.

Kunz,O., 1971.
Erfahrungen mit carbenoxolon - natrium.
Med. Klin., 66:822.

Langman,M.J.S., Knapp,D.R., and Wakley,E.J., 1973.
Treatment of chronic gastric ulcer with carbenoxolone and gefarnate.
Br. Med. J., 3:84.

Lawrence,J.H., Manton,D.J., Mandl,K., and Montgomery, R.D., 1968.
A three-months assessment of duogastrone therapy in chronic duodenal ulcer, in Robson,J.M., and Sullivan,F.M., a symposium on carbenoxolone sodium.
Butterworths, (London), p. 217.

Lee,Y.H., and Thompson,J.H., 1968.
Inhibition of gastric secretion in the rat by SC-15396.
J. Pharmacol., 3:366.

Lee,Y.H., and Bianchi,R.G., 1971.
Use of experimental peptic ulcer modles for drug screening, in Pfeiffer,C.J., progress in peptic ulcer.
Munksgaard, Copenhagen, Denmark, p. 329.

Lee,Y.H., and Bianchi,R.G., 1972.
The antisecretory and antiulcer activity of a prostaglandin analog, SC-24665, in experimental animals.
Fifth International Congress of Pharmacology, San Francisco, (Abstr.), 816.

Lee,Y.H., Cheng,W.D., Bianchi,R.G., Mollison,K., and Hansen,J., 1973.
Effects of oral administration of PGE_2 on gastric secretion and experimental peptic ulcerations.
Prostaglandins, 3:29.

Lennard-Jones,J.E., 1961.
Experimental and clinical observations on poldine in treatment of duodenal ulcer.
Br. Med. J., 1:1071

Lenz,J., Hartel,W., and Schuster,G., 1971.
Behandlung florider gastroduodenalulzera mit carbenoxolon vor der Magenresektion.
Med. Klin., 66:553.

Lipkin,M., and Ludwig,W., 1968.
Carbenoxolone pretreatment and the production of restraint-stress induced erosions in guinea pigs, in Robson,J.M., and Sullivan,F.M., a symposium on carbenoxolone sodium.
Butterworths, (London), p. 41.

Lipkin,M., 1970.
Carbenoxolone sodium and the rate of extrusion of gastric epithelial cells, in Baron,J.H., and Sullivan,F.M., carbenoxolone sodium.
Butterworths, (London), p. 11.

Lippmann,W., 1970.
Inhibition of gastric acid secretion by a potent synthetic prostaglandin.
J. Pharm. Pharmacol., 22:65.

Lippmann,W., and Seethaler,K., 1973.
Oral anti-ulcer activity of a synthetic prostaglandin analogue (9-Oxoprostanoic acid: AY-22,469).
Experientia, 29:993.

Lippmann,W., 1973.
Oral antigastric acid secretory activity synthetic prostaglandin analogues (9-Oxoprostanoic acids).
Experientia, 29:990.

MacCaig,J.N., 1970.
Endoscopic control of carbenoxolone therapy, in Baron,J.H., and Sullivan,F.M., carbenoxolone sodium.
Butterworths, (London), p. 91.
Main,I.H.M., 1969.
Effects of prostaglandin E_2 (PGE_2) on the output of histamine and acid in rat gastric secretion induced by pentagastrin or histamine.
Br. J. Pharmacol., 36:214P.
Malen,C.E., Danvee,B.H., and Pascaud,X.B.L., 1971.
New thiocarboxamides derivatives with specific gastric antisecretory properties.
J. Med. Chem., 14:244.
Melrose,A.G., and Pinkerton,I.W., 1961.
Clinical evaluation of goldine methosulphate.
Br. Med. J., I:1096.
Menguy,R., and Thompson,A.E., 1967.
Regulation of secretion of mucus from the gastric antrum.
Ann. N.Y. Acad. Sci., 140:767.
Middleton,W.R.J., Cooke,A.R., Stephen,D., and Skyring, A.P., 1965.
Biogastrone in inpatient treatment of gastric ulcer
Lancet, 1:1031.
Montgomery,R.D., 1967.
Side effects of carbenoxolone sodium: a study of ambulant therapy of gastric ulcer.
Gut, 8:148.
Montgomery,R.D., 1970.
Long-term follow-up of gastric ulcer treated with carbenoxolone, with particular reference to malignant change, in Baron,J.H., and Sullivan,F.M., carbenoxolone sodium.
Butterworths, (London), p. 99.
Morishima,H., Takita,T., Aoyagi,T., Takeuchi,T., and Umezawa,H., 1970.
The structure of pepstatin.
J. Antibiot., 23:263.
Murari,F., 1964.
Pharmagological investigation on gefarnate, a new synthetic compound against gastric ulcer.
Med. Exp., 11:361.

Ortone,G., and Furno,F., 1968.
Il gefarnato nella terapia dell 'ulcera peptica.
Minerva Med., 59:5647.
Ottenjahn,R., and Rosen,W., 1970.
Therapie des ulcus ventriculi mit carbenoxolon-Natrium.
Med. Klin., 65:74.
Pascaud,X.B., and Blouin,M.M., 1972.
Gastric antisecretory properties of pyridly-2-thioacetamide (CMN 131) in the Heidenhain pouch dog.
In Fifth International Congress on Pharmacology, San Francisco, (Abstr.), 1057.
Ponari,O., 1964.
Design of planned clinical trials in the study of antiulcerative drugs.
Arzneimittel-Forsch., 14:207.
Ramwell,P.W., and Shaw,J.E., 1968.
Prostaglandin inhibition of gastric secretion.
J. Physiol., (London), 195:34P.
Robert,A., and Phillips,J.P., 1963.
Inhibition by prostaglandin E_1 of gastric secretion in the dog.
Gastroenterology, 54:1263.
Robert,A., Nezamis,J.E., and Phillips,J.P., 1967.
Inhibition of gastric secretion by prostaglandins.
Am. J. Dig. Dis., 12:1073.
Robert,A., Nezamis,J.E., and Phillips,J.P., 1968.
Effect of prostaglandin E_1 on gastric secretion and ulcer formation in the rat.
Gastroenterology, 55:481.
Robert,A., and Magerlein,B.J., 1973.
15-Methyl PGE_2 and 16, 16-dimenthyl PGE_2: potent inhibitors of gastric secretion.
Advances in the Biosciences, 9:247.
Robson,J.M., and Sullivan,F.M., 1968.
A symposium on carbenoxolone sodium.
Butterworths, (London), p. 263.
Rosch,W., and Ottenjahn,R., 1971.
Doppelblindstudie mit Carbenoxolon-Natrium bei Ulcus ventriculi.
Med. Klin., 66:383.

Schiffrin,M.J., and Komarov,S.A., 1941.
The inactivation of pepsin by compounds of aluminum and magnesium.
Am. J. Dig. Dis., 8:215.

Schiffrin,M.J., and Warren,A.A., 1942.
Some factors concerned in the production of experimental ulceration of the GI tract in cats.
Am. J. Dig. Dis., 9:205.

Stening,G.F., and Grossman,M.I., 1968.
The effect of SC-15396 on gastrin stimulated pancreatic secretion.
Proc. Soc. Exp. Biol. Med., 128:430.

Sun,D.C., 1962.
Comparative study on the effect of glycopyrrolate and propantheline on basal gastric secretion.
Ann. N.Y. Acad. Sci., 99:153.

Sun,D.C.H., 1965.
Antipeptic agents in the treatment of peptic ulcer.
Curr. Ther. Res., 7:790.

Sun,D.C., 1967.
Effect of a synthetic sulfated polysaccharide (SN-263) on gastric peptic activity in humans.
Ann. N.Y. Acad. Sci., 140:747.

Sun,D.C., and Ryan,M.L., 1970.
A controlled study of the use of propantheline and amylopectin sulfate (SN-263) for recurrences in duodenal ulcer.
Gastroenterology, 58:756.

Takagi,K., and Yano,S., 1972.
Effect of anti-ulcer drugs on gastric mucous heposamine in rats subjected to several ulcerogenic conditions.
Chem. Pharm. Bull., 20:1170.

Thompson,J.H., 1972.
Gastrointestinal disorders - peptic ulcer disease, in Rubin,A.A., Medicinal Research Series 6, Search for New Drugs.
Marcel Dekker, Inc., N.Y., p. 115.

Turpie,A.G.G., and Thompson,T.J., 1965.
Carbenoxolone sodium in the treatment of gastric ulcer with special reference to side-effects.
Gut, 5:591.

Umezawa,H., Aoyagi,T., Morishima,H., Matsuzaki,M., Hamada,M., and Takeuchi,T., 1970.
Pepstain, a new pepsin inhibitor produced by actinomycetes.
J. Antibiot., 23:259.

Watkinson,G., 1968.
Treating ulcer disease with carbenoxolone sodium.
Postgrad. Med., 44(5):92.

Weeks,J.R., DuCharme,D.W., Magee,W.E., and Miller,W.L., 1973.
The biological activity of 15 (S)-15-methyl analogues of prostaglandins E_2 and $F_2\alpha$.
J. Pharmacol. Exp. Ther., (In Press).

Zimmon,D.S., Miller,G., Cox,G., and Tesler,M.A., 1969.
Specific inhibition of gastric pepsin in the treatment of gastric ulcer.
Gastroenterology, 56:19.

SESSION III.

SECRETORY AND ABSORPTIVE ACTIVITIES OF INTESTINE AND BILIARY TRACT

ION TRANSPORT IN LARGE AND SMALL INTESTINE

Henry J. Binder

INTRODUCTION

The small and large intestine has digestive, absorptive and secretory functions. The attention of physiologists, biochemists and gastroenterologists has been directed almost exclusively towards the study of the absorptive and digestive functions. From 1940 to 1968 little mention of an intestinal secretory function was made but this neglect has been partially rectified during the past five years. This presentation of intestinal ion transport will summarize the characteristics of electrolyte absorption in jejunum, ileum and colon and then emphasize the ubiquity of net secretion. We will propose that active electrolyte secretion is frequently the driving force for net secretion, may be controlled by cyclic adenosine monophosphate (cyclic AMP) and may represent a neutral sodium anion secretory process.

ABSORPTION

The small intestine absorbs large quantities of water and electrolytes. Although average daily dietary intake is only 1.5 liters, the fluid contributed to the small intestine from salivary, gastric, biliary and pancreatic secretions results in a total load or input to the small bowel of approximately eight to nine liters daily. Since flow across the ileal cecal valve is approximately 1 liter, the small intestine absorbs 7 to 8 liters daily. In contrast to the small intestine, significantly less water (less than 1 liter daily) is absorbed by the large intestine. Similar types of calculations can be made for electrolytes.

Both similarities and differences exist in the characteristics of electrolyte absorption at various levels of the intestine. It is generally agreed that water movement is secondary to active solute transport. Curran's double membrane hypothesis, as modified by the standing osmotic gradient theory of Diamond, provides an adequate explanation of solute-stimulated water flow. The sodium concentration of an isosmolar solution from which net sodium and water absorption will occur varies along the gastrointestinal tract. Net sodium absorption will not occur from solutions with sodium concentrations less than approximately 130, 50 or 25 mEq/L in the jejunum, ileum and large intestine respectively.

Despite some disagreement regarding the responsible mechanism, glucose stimulates sodium and water absorption in the jejunum, possibly in the ileum but not in the colon. Similarly, amino acids will stimulate water and sodium absorption in the small intestine but not in the colon; it is important to remember that non-electrolytes are actively absorbed in the small intestine but are not actively absorbed in the large intestine. To explain glucose stimulation of water and sodium absorption Schultz and Curran (1970) have advocated glucose stimulation of active Na transport and that water absorption then follows active solute transport. Fordtran has proposed that glucose absorption results in increased water flow which then augments Na movement across the intact human jejunum by solvent drag (Fordtran, Rector, and Carter, 1968). It is possible that these varying hypotheses result from the different methods and species employed.

The mechanism of potassium secretion throughout the intestinal tract is probably passive, driven by the existing electrical chemical concentration gradients. The direction of bicarbonate and chloride movement also varies along the gastrointestinal tract. Bicarbonate is absorbed in the jejunum but secreted in the ileum and colon; chloride, on the other hand, is secreted in the jejunum and absorbed in the ileum and colon. Although bicarbonate movement most likely represents active secretion and bicarbonate movement often appears reciprocally linked to chloride transport, active chloride transport has not been consistently demonstrated. Turnberg et al., (1970) in studies of the intact human ileum, and Binder and Rawlins (1973) in the <u>in vitro</u> rat colon have proposed sodium-hydrogen and chloride-bicarbonate exchanges to explain many aspects of electrolyte transport in the ileum and colon respectively.

Mineralocorticosteroids exert varying effects on ion transport. Aldosterone increases sodium absorption and potassium secretion in the large intestine, has no effect on sodium movement in the jejunum and may have minimal action on electrolyte transport in the ileum.

SECRETION

After this brief summary of electrolyte absorption, I want to devote the remainder of my time to the fascinating problem of intestinal electrolyte secretion. Cholera has been, in large part, responsible for the renewed interest in intestinal secretion. Large volumes of fluid with a composition resembling a high bicarbonate isotonic ultrafiltrate of plasma is produced in both clinical and experimental cholera. Several possible mechanisms, diminished absorption, active ion secretion, altered mucosal permeability and increased hydrostatic pressure, have been proposed to account for the net secretion of fluid. Since cholera exterotoxin will stimulate adenylate cyclase and induce secretion in an in vitro preparation in the absence of electrical, chemical, osmotic and hydrostatic concentration gradients (Field, et al., 1972; Kimberg, et al., 1971), the available evidence is, therefore, most consistent with the concept that net fluid secretion is secondary to active electrolyte secretion which is mediated by cyclic AMP.

Accumulation of fluid and electrolytes within a segment of the intestine has now been demonstrated in a large variety of situations besides cholera, and these phenomena can be divided into several categories. Net secretion of fluid and electrolytes indicates a condition in which there is net movement of fluid across the intestinal mucosa into the luminal solution but does not imply the mechanism responsible for this fluid accumulation. Secretion has been observed under normal conditions, in experimental and clinical situations, and has been induced by both physiologic and pathologic stimuli; net secretion has been demonstrated both in vitro and in vivo. Table 1 catalogues several examples of intestinal secretion and illustrates the diversity of its occurrence.

What is the mechanism for net fluid secretion? Several mechanisms have been proposed to account for net fluid secretion (Table2). These include: 1) active electrolyte secretion; 2) increased luminal osmolarity; 3) diminished absorption; 4) altered motility; 5) increased hydrostatic pressure; 6) changes in mucosal permeability; and

Table 1

Several Phenomena in Which Net Secretion Has Been Observed

A. "Normal"
   1. Guinea pig small intestine (Powell, Malawer and Plotkin, 1969)
   2. Rabbit appendix (Blackwood, Bolinger and Lifson, 1973)
   3. Germ-free rat cecum (Donowitz and Binder, unpublished observations)
B. Physiologic Stimuli
   1. Cyclic AMP (Field, 1970)
   2. Theophylline (Pierce, et al., 1971)
   3. Prostaglandins (Pierce, et al., 1971)
   4. Cholecystokinin (Moritz, et al., 1973)
   5. Secretin (Moritz, et al., 1973)
   6. Galactose (Taylor, et al., 1968)
   7. Vasopressin (Soergel, et al., 1967)
C. Pathologic Stimuli
   1. Bacterial enterotoxins (cholerax, E. coli, etc.)(Banwell and Scherr, 1973)
   2. Bile salts (dihydroxy)(Mekjian, Phillips and Hofman, 1971)
   3. Hydroxy fatty acids (Bright-Asare and Binder, 1973)
   4. Systemic Na depletion (Clarke, et al., 1967)
   5. Bethnecol (intravenous)(Tidball, 1961)
   6. Phenol derivatives (intraluminal)(Tidball, 1961)
   7. Luminal distention (Herrin and Meek, 1933)
D. Clinical Diseases
   1. Cholera (Banwell, et al., 1970)
   2. Celiac Sprue (Fordtran, et al., 1967)
   3. Tropical sprue (Gorbach, et al., 1969)
   4. Lactase deficiency (Kern and Struthers, 1966)
   5. Ulcerative colitis (Harris and Shields, 1970)
   6. Intestinal obstruction (Wright, 1971)
   7. Regional enteritis (Atwell and Duthie, 1964)
E. Experimental
   1. X-irradiation (Curran, et al., 1960)
   2. Nematode infestation (Symonds, 1962)
   3. Salmonella enterocolitis (Powell, et al., 1971)

4. Intestinal obstruction (Shields, et al., 1965)
5. Colchicine enteropathy (Goulston and Skyring, 1966)
6. Niacin deficiency (Nelson, et al., 1966)

Table 2

Possible Mechanisms Responsible for Net Secretion

1. Active electrolyte secretion
2. Diminished absorption
3. Increased luminal osmolarity
4. Alterations in motility
5. Increased hydrostatic pressure
6. Altered mucosal permeability
7. Changes in mucosal vascular perfusion

7) changes in vascular perfusion. 1) In vitro studies have demonstrated that active electrolyte secretion is present in cholera (Field, et al., 1972) and recent experiments have demonstrated that active electrolyte secretion is also stimulated by E. coli enterotoxin, theophylline, prostaglandins, cyclic AMP and bile salts. Few examples of net fluid secretion secondary to mechanisms other than active ion secretion have been described. 2) Increased luminal osmolarity will account for the fluid secretion observed in lactase deficiency but few other situations exist in which net secretion is secondary to increased osmotic pressure. 3) Although both net fluid secretion and diminished absorption occur in celiac sprue, it is unlikely that diminished absorption alone can result in net secretion unless a secretory process is also present. 4) Although changes in motility are frequently mentioned as a cause of diarrhea, it is uncertain how net secretion can result from increased intestinal transit alone. 5) Increased hydrostatic pressure is an attractive though unproven possibility, to account for the net secretion observed in intestinal obstruction. Finally, changes in either 6) mucosal permeability or 7) blood flow could result in net secretion though no proven examples are available.

Active electrolyte secretion may frequently represent the driving force of net secretion. As already noted, evidence is available that indicates the cholera enterotoxin as well as E. coli enterotoxin stimulates adenylate cyclase. Thus, one could speculate that cyclic

AMP may be a common mediator of active ion secretion.

In order to understand the mechanisms responsible both for net secretion and for diarrhea, we have studied the problem of cholerheic enteropathy, another example of net secretion of water and electrolytes. Diarrhea often occurs following ileal resection. This diarrhea is probably mediated by bile salts since perfusion of dog, human and rodent colon induces water and sodium secretion and the administration of cholestyramine, a bile salt binding resin, frequently controls this diarrhea. Since the mechanism of bile salt induced diarrhea was not known, in vitro studies of the effect of bile salts on colonic electrolyte transport were initiated (Binder and Rawlins, 1973). These studies demonstrated that taurochenodeoxycholic acid (TCDC) a conjugated dihydroxy bile salt, increased electrical potential difference and short-circuit current (Isc)(fig. 1). Ion flux studies demonstrated decreased sodium absorption, decreased chloride absorption and stimulation of bicarbonate secretion. Theophylline produced similar effects in parallel studies. TCDC inhibited the effect of theophylline on short-circuit current and prior administration of theophylline inhibited the effect of TCDC on Isc. Additional preliminary results have indicated that TCDC increases colonic mucosal cyclic AMP content. These results with bile salts are similar to the effect of both cholera enterotoxin and theophylline in the rabbit ileum and are interpreted as evidence that bile salt stimulates adenylate cyclase and that the electrolyte secretion stimulated by bile salts is also mediated by cyclic AMP.

These studies provide the basis for our hypothesis that the common mediator of active ion secretion is cyclic AMP. I expect that additional examples of cyclic AMP mediated secretion will frequently be reported in the next few years.

A model to explain the active electrolyte secretion of cholera had not been delineated by the initial in vitro studies of cholera enterotoxin. In experiments performed with Drs. Powell and Curran in both guinea pig and rabbit ileum, a model of a neutral Na anion secretory process has been proposed. These studies will be briefly summarized.

The guinea pig small intestine secretes fluid and electrolytes (Powell, Malawer and Plotkin, 1969), and in vitro studies of this mucosal preparation offered the possibility of dissection of the secretory process. Our studies (Powell, Binder and Curran, 1972)

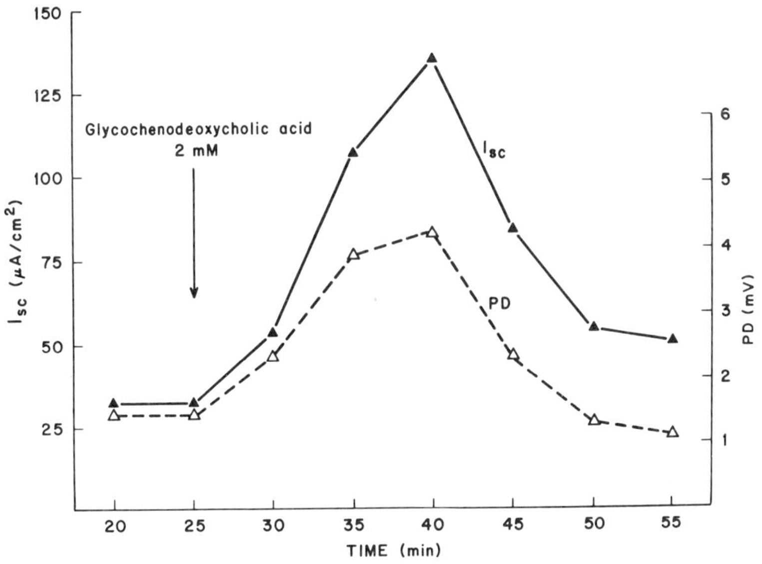

Fig. 1. Effect of 2 mM glycochenodeoxycholic acid (GCDC) on electrical potential difference (PD) and short-circuit current (Isc) across isolated rat colonic mucosa. The addition of GCDC to both mucosal and serosal solutions results in a prompt increase in both PD and Isc. The PD reflects serosal potential in respect to the mucosal side. Addition of theophylline produced similar effects. Additional studies indicated that these changes most likely secondary to active anion (HCO_3 and Cl) secretion (Binder and Rawlins, 1973).

demonstrated that both secretion and absorption were occurring simultaneously in the guinea pig ileum. Both the secretory and absorptive processes are active; the absorptive system is driven by an electrogenic sodium pump while the oppositely directed secretory mechanism is a neutral sodium-bicarbonate or sodium-chloride pump. The neutral pump has a greater affinity for HCO_3 than Cl. Theophylline stimulated the secretory process but not the absorptive one; ouabain inhibited the absorptive process but not the secretory process. Removal of bicarbonate and chloride from the in vitro media inhibited the neutral secretion but had no effect on sodium absorption and finally 3-0-methylglucose stimulated only sodium absorption but glucose increased both sodium absorption and secretion. Although studies of the effect of cycloheximide on cholera enterotoxin have suggested that the absorptive process is located in the villus and the secretory process in the crypt, our studies do not, in any way, provide information regarding the anatomical location of the absorptive and secretory processes.

Additional research on the effect of cholera enterotoxin on electrolyte transport in the rabbit ileum also suggests that neutral anion secretion may be common to many secretory processes (Powell, Binder and Curran, 1973). In these experiments, purified choleragen stimulated sodium, chloride and bicarbonate secretion with minimal augmentation of the short-circuit current. Removal of bicarbonate and chloride or sodium prevented the choleragen induced ion secretion. Therefore, similar neutral transport models have been proposed to explain electrolyte secretion both in the guinea pig ileum under "normal" conditions and electrolyte secretion in the rabbit ileum induced by cholera enterotoxin.

In conclusion, net secretion of water and electrolytes occurs under many conditions and is probably present in most diarrheal conditions. Although other possible mechanisms may, in part, be responsible for net fluid secretion in some situations, an active ion secretory process may be the driving force in most conditions. We postulate that cyclic AMP is the mediator of the secretory process and we propose that the secretory process may be best explained by a neutral Na anion mechanism.

REFERENCES

Atwell,J.D., and Duthie,H.L., 1964.
The absorption of water, sodium and potassium from the ileum of humans shwoing the effects of regional enteritis.
Gastroenterology 46:16.

Banwell,J.G., and Sherr,H., 1973.
Effect of bacterial enterotoxins on the gastrointestinal tract.
Gastroenterology 65:467.

Banwell,J.G., et al., 1970.
Intestinal fluid and electrolyte transport in human cholera.
J. Clin. Invest. 49:183.

Binder,H.J., and Rawlins,C.L., 1973.
Effect of conjugated dihydroxy bile salts on electrolyte transport in rat colon.
J. Clin. Invest. 52:1460.

Binder,H.J., and Rawlins,C.L., 1973.
Electrolyte transport across isolated large intestinal mucosa.
Am. J. Physiol. 225 (In Press).

Blackwood,W.D., Bolinger,R.A., and Lifson,N., 1973.
Some characteristics of the rabbit vermiform appendix as a secreting organ.
J. Clin. Invest. 52:143.

Bright-Asare,P., and Binder,H.J., 1973.
Stimulation of colonic secretion of water and electrolytes by hydroxy fatty acids.
Gastroenterology 64:81.

Clarke,A.M., Miller,M., and Shields,R., 1967.
Intestinal transport of sodium, potassium and water in the dog during sodium depletion.
Gastroenterology 52:846.

Curran,P.F., Wibster,E.W., and Hoyseplan,J.A., 1960.
The effect of x-irradiation on sodium and water transport in rat ileum.
Radiat. Res. 13:369.

Field,M., 1971.
Ion transport in rabbit ileal mucosa. II. Effect of cyclic 3', 5'-AMP.
Am. J. Physiol. 221:992.

Field,M., et al., 1972.
Effect of cholera enterotoxin on ion transport across isolated ileal mucosa.
J. Clin. Invest. 51:796.

Fordstran,J.S., et al., 1967.
Water and solute movement in the small intestine of patients with sprue.
J. Clin. Invest. 46:287.

Gorbach,S.L., et al., 1969.
Bacterial contamination of the upper small bowel in tropical sprue.
Lancet 1:74.

Goulston,K.J., and Skyringe,A., 1966.
The effect of colchicine on the absorption of water and electrolytes by rat jujunum.
Aust. J. Exp. Biol. Med. Sci. 44:93.

Harris,J., and Shields,R., 1970.
Absorption and secretion of water and electrolytes by the intact human colon in diffuse untreated protocolitis.
Gut 11:27.

Herrin,R.C., and Meek,W.J., 1933.
Distension as a factor in intestinal obstruction.
Arch. Int. Med. 51:152.

Kern,F., and Struthers,J.E., 1966.
Intestinal lactase deficiency and lactose intolerance in adults.
J. Am. Med. Assoc. 195:927.

Kimberg,D.V., et al., 1971.
Stimulation of intestinal mucosal adenyl cylase by cholera enterotoxin and prostaglandins.
J. Clin. Invest. 50:1218.

Mekhjian,H.S., Phillips,S.F., and Hofmann,A.F., 1971.
Colonic secretion of water and electrolytes induced by bile acids: Perfusion studies in man.
J. Clin. Invest. 50:1569.

Moritz,M., et al., 1973.
Effect of secretin and cholecystolinin on the transport of electrolyte and water in human jujunum.
Gastroenterology 64:76.
Nelson,R.A.,Code,C.F., and Brown,A.L., 1962.
Sorption of water and electrolytes, and mucosal structure, in niacin deficiency.
Gastroenterology 42:26.
Pierce,N.F., et al., 1971.
Effects of prostaglandins, theophylline and cholera enterotoxin upon transmural water and electrolyte movement in the canine jujunum.
Gastroenterology 60:22.
Powell,D.W., Malawer,S.J., and Plotkin,G.R., 1968.
Secretion of electrolytes and water by the guinea pig small intestine in vivo.
Am. J. Physiol. 215:1226.
Powell,C.W., et al., 1971.
Experimental diarrhea. I. Intestinal water and electrolyte transport in rat salmonella enterocolitis.
Gastroenterology 60:1053.
Powell,D.W., Binder,H.J., and Curran,P.F., 1972.
Electrolyte secretion by the guinea pig ileum in vitro.
Am. J. Physiol. 223:531.
Powell,D.W., Binder,H.J., and Curran,P.F., 1973.
Active electrolyte secretion stimulated by choletagen in rabbit ileum in vitro.
Am. J. Physiol. 225:781.
Schultz,S.G., and Curran,P.F., 1970.
Coupled transport of sodium and organic solutes.
Physiol. Rev. 50:637.
Shields,R., 1965.
The absorption and secretion of fluid and electrolytes by the obstructed bowel.
Br. J. Surg. 52:774.
Soergel,K.H., et al, 1968.
Effect of antidiuretic hormone of human small intestinal water and solute transport.
J. Clin. Invest. 47:1071.

Symons,L.E., 1960.
Pathology of infestation of the rat with nippostrongylus muris (Yokogawa) III. Jujunal fluxes in vivo of water, sodium and chloride.
Aust. J. Biol. Sci. 13:171.

Taylor,A.E., et al, 1968.
Effect of sugars on ion fluxes in intestine.
Am. J. Physiol. 214:836.

Tidball,C.S., 1961.
Active chloride transport during intestinal secretion.
Am. J. Physiol. 200:309.

Tidball,C.S., 1961.
Effect of substituted phenols on movement of water and protein across the intestine.
Am. J. Physiol. 200:305.

Turnberg,L.A., et al., 1970.
Interrelationships of chloride, bicarbonate, sodium, and hydrogen transport in the human ileum.
J. Clin. Invest. 49:557.

Wright,H.K., O'Brien,J.J., and Tilson,M.D., 1971.
Water absorption in experimental closed segment obstruction of the ileum in man.
Am. J. Surg. 121:96.

AMINO ACID HOMEOSTASIS IN THE SMALL GUT

E. S. Nasset

INTRODUCTION

In Cannon's original sense 'homeostasis' means maintenance of a steady state in the body fluid matrix, especially the blood. This concept can now be extended, in part, to include extra-corporeal fluid as represented by the contents of the small intestine. Evidence will be presented to demonstrate that amino acid homeostasis occurs early in the digestive process, and that both endogenous and exogenous proteins and amino acids are involved. The limits of homeostatic regulation of many constituents of blood are quite well-defined, but for gut contents the information is sparse and more work must be done to establish normal limits and how they may be altered by dietary or other means.

Most life scientists regard the small intestine simply as a reaction vessel in which foods are enzymatically hydrolyzed and from which the hydrolytic end products are transported to the circulating blood. This limited point of view excludes from consideration the uniquely active protein metabolism of the gut mucosa and other tissues as factors in digestion of protein and absorption of amino acids. When epithelial cells are shed from the free ends of villi into the lumen and cytolyzed, the cell contents are released and mixed with any ingesta that may be present. Apparently epithelial cell protein is digested and almost completely recovered from the lumen of the small bowel because little protein is lost in the feces. The mouth, pharynx, esophagus and stomach also contribute to the mixture of luminal endogenous protein that is always present. The digestive hydrolases constitute another source of endogenous protein in the gut lumen. Besides shed mucosal cells and digestive enzymes there are other sources of endogenous protein N in the gut lumen, such as mucoproteins, blood plasma and free amino acids in bile and succus entericus (table 1). The various possible sources of luminal endogenous protein N are generally known but they are not completely and individually quantified.

Table 1

Total Free Amino Acids (17) in Bile and Intestinal Juice

Rat, fasting, bile	3726 micromoles/liter, (N=3)
Rat, post cibal, bile	4061 micromoles/liter, (N=3)
Man, fasting, hepatic bile	769 micromoles/liter, (N=1)
Dog, fasting, hepatic bile	248 micromoles/liter, (N=1)
Dog, fasting, intestinal juice	993 micromoles/liter, (N=2)
Dog, post cibal, intestinal juice	1548 micromoles/liter, (N=2)

(Dog pancreatic juice contains little or no free amino acid)

The ingestion of any meal results in a mixture of proteins in the small intestine that usually includes more endogenous than exogenous protein N. This fact was established by analysis of gut contents after feeding single test meals to adequately nourished animals in which there was no possibility of complication from frank or incipient dietary deficiency (Nasset et al., 1955; Nasset and Ju, 1961).

AMINO ACID HOMEOSTASIS IN GUT LUMEN

Nasset, Schwartz and Weiss (1955) were the first to describe the relative constancy of the free amono acid pattern in the gut lumen. Some of their data are presented here as table 2 in a slightly modified form. Dogs were fed and 1½ hours later, under anesthesia, gastrointestinal contents were removed and analyzed for 15 free amino acids by microbiological assay. Owing to limitations of journal space, detailed analytical values for only 8 amino acids could be published.

Examination of free amino acid molar ratios in table 2 reveals extensive changes in the contents of the stomach when they pass into the small intestine and they are most marked after ingestion of the 2 protein-rich meals. The lesser changes after the non-protein meal are not unexpected, because only endogenous proteins and amino acids are present. The amino acid molar ratios of the 4 gut segments are not significantly different, regardless of the type of test meal. If labels are removed from table 2 it is difficult, if not impossible, to identify the data correctly.

Analysis of contents of the entire small gut after feeding ^{14}C-labeled casein to rats (Nasset and Ju, 1961) yielded results similar to those described above for the dog. In all our work, single test meals were given to fasting animals previously maintained with nutritionally adequate diets. The results obtained, therefore, represent responses of the digestive system to a single meal stimulus without benefit of previous experience or training of the animal. Bergen and Purser (1968) provided the most extensive corroboration of our results. They fed 3 diets containing 9% protein (casein, protozoal or bacterial protein) and a nitrogen-free diet for several days before removing contents from segments of jejunum and ileum for analysis. They hydrolyzed the contents completely in 6 N HCl and determined 16 amino acids present in the hydrolyzates. The distribution of amino acids was remarkably similar for all diets, and jejunal and ileal contents did not differ (Bergen and Purser, 1968, table V). It appears as if our determination of the free amino acids in gut contents, representing only partial hydrolysis of luminal proteins, was a representative sample of complete hydrolysis as carried out by Bergen and Purser. Their computed exogenous/endogenous amino acid ratios varied from 1:1 to 1:10 which is in the same range reported in earlier work of Nasset (1964).

Olmsted, Nasset and Kelley (1966) fed human subjects test meals of lean beef, gelatin, whole eggs or whole milk and determined free amino acids in gut contents. One and a half hours after meals, samples were collected at or slightly below the ligament of Treitz. Some of the data are presented in table 3. The mixture of free amino acids is very different from that obtainable by hydrolysis of the ingested proteins. Gelatin presents the most unusual mixture because its content of glycine, alanine and aspartic acid is much higher than the other 3 protein sources and the remaining 13 amino acids are all lower. Despite great variation in amino acid composition of the ingested proteins the amino acid pattern in the duodenum was greatly modified in the direction of more uniformity. The effect is not as pronounced in man, however, as it is in the dog and rat.

Experimental evidence demonstrates clearly that ingestion of any meal yields a mixture of free amino acids in the lumen of the small gut that is invariably significantly different from what is obtained by hydrolysis of the dietary protein in vitro. Data are available on the volumes and protein content of digestive secretions and on the amount of protein delivered to the gut lumen as a result of mucosal cell renewal (Nasset, 1965). Metabolic balance experiments indicate that most of the endogenous protein delivered to the alimentary canal must be hydrolyzed and recovered. Ingested protein may be diluted several-fold with endogenous protein, as demonstrated by feeding ^{14}C-labeled casein to rats and dogs (Nasset and Ju, 1961). Two facts are clearly evident: (a) large masses of endogenous protein are mixed with ingested protein in the small intestine of rat, dog and man, and (b) the hydrolysis of this mixture yields a pattern of free amino acids with relatively constant molar ratios.

RELATION TO AMINO ACID ABSORPTION

Proteins are usually hydrolyzed to amino acids and absorbed as such. If individual amino acids were normally absorbed at rates determined for them singly, one would expect certain changes in the luminal mixture of amino acids with time after feeding or in different segments of the bowel at the same time. The data in table 2 fail to demonstrate any consistent change in amino acid molar ratios in samples taken simultaneously from duodenum, jejunum and ileum. The contents of the whole small intestine of the rat at 1, 2, and 4 hours after feeding also fail to show consistent changes indicative of significant differences in the rates of absorption of various amino acids (Nasset and Ju, 1961). If such differences existed normally one would expect to find a corresponding disappearance of the rapidly absorbed amino acids and a relative accumulation of the slowly absorbed ones. Evidence of such differential absorption is not found in the experimental data cited above. The full significance of the data with respect to amino acid absorption during normal digestion is still unclear but the simplest interpretation is that free amino acids resulting from normal digestion disappear from the gut lumen at rates proportionate to their abundance.

Jejunal absorption of essential amino acids was investigated in human subjects by Adibi and Gray (1967). Equimolar solutions (1.2–20 mM) were introduced through one lumen of a double tube and the unabsorbed portions were recovered through the other lumen at some distance caudad. The results indicate a simple liner relationship between absorption and concentration for all amino acids tried at 1.2 and 3.0 mM but above 5.0 mM there was a wide divergence in rates of absorption. At the higher concentrations, methionine was absorbed most rapidly and threonine least rapidly. Olmsted et al. (1966) determined the concentration of free amino acids in human duodenum and upper jejunum 1½ hours after ingestion of beef muscle, gelatin, whole eggs or whole milk. The greatest concentrations were found after the beef meal, ranging from 0.17 mM leucine to 3.6 mM lysine. It is evident, therefore, that in the normal process of digestion in man the concentrations of free amino acids in the lumen are within the range in which all of them are absorbed equally well.

Digestibility of Endogenous Proteins

Endogenous proteins are almost completely digested and absorbed because there is no significant loss in the stool. Experimental evidence indicates that the mixture of enzymes present in the intestine is auto-digestible. Pancreatic juice instilled for 10 min into the duodenum of rats, previously freed of pancreatic enzymes by diversion of pancreatic juice, had its trypsin reduced 25–33%, its chymotrypsin 56–82% and its lipase 82–92% (Pelot and Grossman, 1962). The evidence indicates that digestive enzymes are readily inactivated and hydrolyzed under conditions that prevail in the lumen of the small intestine. Rats were fed meals containing equal quantities of ^{14}C-labeled casein and ^{75}Se-labeled pancreatic juice proteins (Nasset et al., 1973). The results indicate that $^{14}C/^{75}Se$ ratios of gut contents failed to show a progressive change from 1 to 4 hours post cibum, which suggests that both labeled proteins left the intestine at the same rate. The $^{14}C/^{75}Se$ ratios of plasma point to the same conclusion.

AMINO ACID METABOLISM OF INTESTINAL MUCOSA

The mucosa of the digestive tract, especially the small intestine, has a more active protein metabolism than any other tissue of the body. Most cells of the small gut mucosa are turned over in 1½ to 3 days and as a result about 70–90 g of intracellular protein may be released in the intestinal lumen of an adult man every day (Nasset, 1965). As the cells leave their site of origin in the crypts of Lieberkühn they mature and move toward the tips of the villi where they are shed into the lumen. During their migration and maturation the cells develop the capacity to synthesize a large assortment of enzymes. Nordström et al. (1968) found the greatest concentration of certain enzymes to be in the apical half of the villus. Presumably this is the locus also of greatest absorptive activity, which suggests that mucosal cells may have the capacity to remove amino acids for immediate synthetic processes directly from the stream of amino acids in transit through the cells during absorption. Absorption probably never ceases because villous tips are constantly shedding cells and secretion of digestive juices continues at low rates even in interdigestive intervals.

Examination of free amino acid concentrations on both sides of the mucous membrane provide relevant information on this point. Nasset et al. (1963) fed zein, egg albumin and non-protein meals to dogs and 2 hours later determined free amino acids in the contents of segments of gut and in the corresponding mesenteric vein. The results showed unmistakable evidence that the amino acid pattern in the gut was considerably altered in passing through the mucosa (fig. 1). Some amino acids were subtracted and others added.

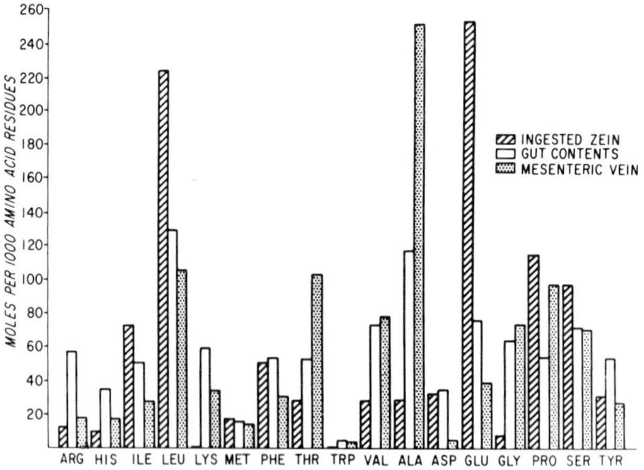

Fig. 1. Molar ratios of amino acids in ingested protein (zein), and simultaneous samples of contents in a segment of jejunum (2 h after ingestion of zein) and blood plasma in a mesenteric vein draining the same segment (from data of Nasset et. al., 81:343, 1963).

AMINO ACID HOMEOSTASIS IN HUMAN BLOOD PLASMA

Six healthy men were maintained on an adequate diet but every 4th day they ingested a variety of test meals, including isocaloric quantities (334 kcals) of corn oil (37.8 g) and cooked lean turkey meat (200 g). Blood samples for amino acid analysis were taken at 1, 2, 4 and 8 hours post cibum. The maximal increase in amino acid concentration occurred at 1 or 2 hours and the results at 1 hour are given in table 4 (Nasset et al., unpublished). The meal of corn oil evoked a rise in total amino acids 28% above the value in fasting and the meat meal caused a rise of 48%. Edible fat is known to be an adequate stimulus for the digestive system and the rise in plasma amino acids after such a meal is doubtless due to digestion and recovery of the endogenous protein and amino acids delivered to the gut. It is understandable that the meat meal caused a greater rise because both exogenous and endogenous amino acids were being absorbed.

The most significant aspect of these data is the constancy of molar ratios that is evident under all 3 conditions, i. e., fasting and ingestion of either a protein or a non-protein meal. These facts demonstrate that the body can and does tolerate large increases in total plasma amino acids but that the molar ratios do not change significantly. The evidence also indicates that the body's capacity to maintain a constant amino acid mixture in the blood is dependent in large part on the homeostatic mechanisms that function in the digestive system.

AMINO ACID HOMEOSTASIS AND PROTEIN METABOLISM

Starving prisoners of war recovered by the Allies in World War II, who could not tolerate intravenous protein hydrolyzates,were able to digest and absorb as much as 200–300 g of protein/day if taken by mouth (Burger et al., 1948). Obviously the digestive system of a starving man recovers its functional capacity in a very short period of re-alimentation and apparently other ill-defined nutritional advantages accrue from its recovery. Holm (1964) fed dogs a non-protein diet (80 kcal/kg/day) plus a supplement of 3 g of casein hydrolyzate by vein or by mouth. When hydrolyzate was given by mouth, plasma albumin and globulin remained normal. Hydrolyzate given by vein resulted in a drop of one-third in albumin and an increase of one-half in globulin. Hydrolyzate injected into the superior vena cava produced some pathological changes in the liver which were not present when intraportal injection was used. A mixture of 18 amino acids made to simulate casein is not nutritionally equivalent to casein, as judged by smaller weight gains and loss of appetite in rats (Ahrens et al., 1966). Intravenous injection of single amino acids or mixtures of a few of them in adult human subjects may evoke unfavorable signs and symptoms, such as hypotension, chills, fever, azotemia, hepatic dysfunction, nausea, vomiting, headache and disorientation (Floyd et al., 1966). Apparently the normal processes of digestion and absorption are essential for maximal utilization of dietary nitrogen.

AMINO ACID FORTIFICATION OF FOODS

Reference has been made to the adverse effects of intravenous injection of single amino acids or mixtures of a few of them as well as the inefficiency and possible toxicity of amino acid diets. Addition of a mixture containing all but one of the essential amino acids (imbalance) to a low protein but otherwise adequate diet leads to anorexia and if such a diet is force fed it can lead to pathological changes in pancreas and stomach (Nasset et al., 1967; Sidransky and Farber, 1958). Indications are that amino acids are not the innocuous compounds we have generally considered them to be, except in combinations as encountered in normal digestion and metabolism.

An important discovery, made in India, shows conclusively that a dietary deficiency disease can be induced by amino acid fortification of food. Pellagra was found to be prevalent in a population that rarely uses maize as food. The principal source (90%) of dietary protein is jowar (Sorghum vulgare), a kind of millet that has a very high leucine content. Suspecting that high leucine ingestion was related to the high incidence of pellagra, the Indian investigators produced black tongue in adult dogs and puppies by adding leucine to their low protein diets (Belavady and Gopalan, 1965; Belavady et al., 1967, 1968), and produced niacin deficiency in monkeys by feeding them diets containing jowar. Raghuramulu et. al., (1965) added 1.5% leucine to a 9% casein diet of rats and elicited increased urinary excretion of quinolinic acid and N′ methylnicotinamide. The authors suggested that excess dietary leucine interferes specifically with tryptophan-niacin metabolism. The investigations briefly described above emphasize again how important it is to maintain normal amino acid homeostasis and to proceed with caution before adopting a policy of amino acid fortification of foods for man.

SUMMARY

Ingestion of a meal gives rise to a mixture in the small gut lumen that usually contains more endogenous than exogenous protein. The molar ratios of amino acids resulting from the hydrolysis of this mixture are reasonably constant regardless of the composition of ingested protein. The free amino acid pattern in the lumen does not change significantly either with time or locus in the intestine. All amino acids seem to disappear from the lumen in proportion to their abundance in the mixture, which means that the great differences in rates of absorption of single amino acids demonstrated in vitro are not demonstrable under normal conditions in vivo.

Amino acid homeostasis in the gut lumen prevents wide fluctuations in the amino acid pattern of blood plasma and thus helps to preclude the development of anorexia and other deleterious effects of ingesting imbalanced amino acid mixtures or those devoid of one or more essential amino acids. The plasma amino acid molar ratios are not significantly altered by ingestion of either a protein or a nonprotein meal. In view of their rapid turnover, it is likely that the epithelial cells meet some of their immediate requirements by removal of amino acids directly from the stream of amino acids being absorbed.

Alimentation either by intravenous administration of amino acids or by ingestion of amino acid diets is nutritionally inferior to ingestion and normal digestion of foods and some ill defined nutritional advantages accrue to the animal from certain 'extra-digestive' functions of the alimentary system. The fortification of foods with amino acids may have unfavorable effects not yet suspected, especially in the rapidly growing infant. The normal mechanisms of amino acid homeostasis in the gut lumen are summarized in figure 2.

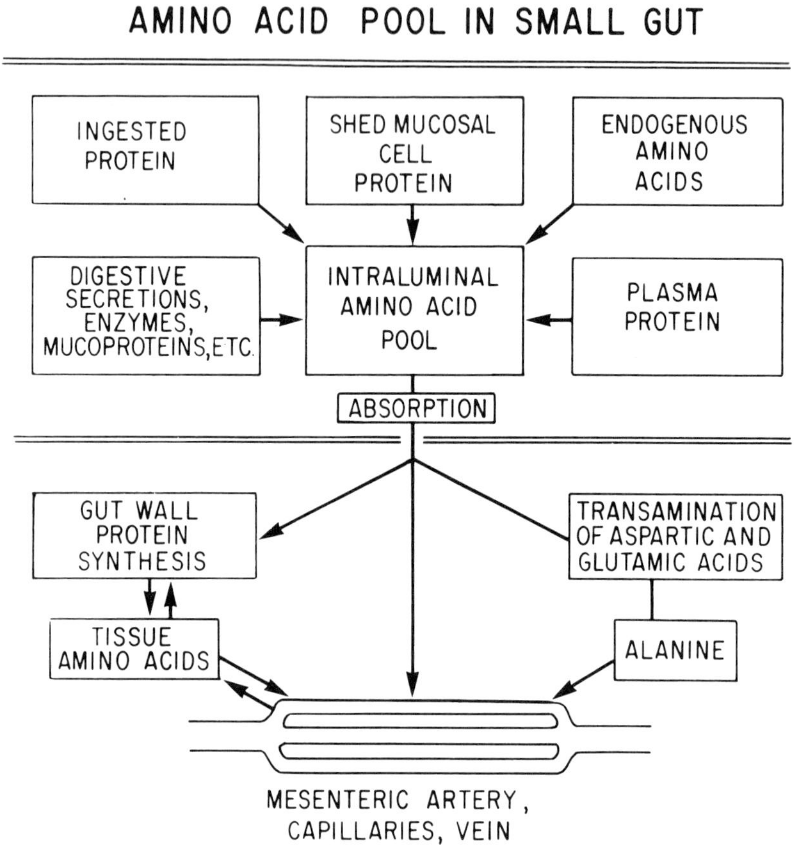

Fig. 2. Factors in amino acid homeostasis in the small gut.

REFERENCES

Adibi,S.A., and Gray,S.J., 1967.
Intestinal absorption of essential amino acids in man.
Gastroenterology 52:837.

Ahrens,R.A., Wilson,J.E.,Jr. and Womack,M., 1966.
Utilization of calories and nitrogen by rats fed diets containing purified casein versus a mixture, of amino acids simulating casein.
J. Nutri. 88:219.

Belavady,B., and Gopalan,C., 1965.
Production of black tongue in dogs by feeding diets containing jowar.
Lancet ii:1120.

Belavady,B., Madhaven,T.V., and Gopalan,C., 1968.
Production of nicotinic acid deficiency (black tongue) in pups fed diets supplemented with leucine.
Gastroenterology 53:749.

Belavady,B., Madhaven,T.V., and Gopalan,C., 1968.
Experimental production of niacin deficiency in adult monkeys by feeding jowar diets.
Lab. Invest. 18:97.

Bergen,W.G., and Purser,D.B., 1968.
Effect of feeding different protein sources on plasma and gut amino acids in the growing rat.
J. Nutr. 95:333.

Burger,G.C.E., Drummond,J.C. and Sandstead,H.R.,1948.
Malnutrition and starvation in western Netherlands, 1944-1945, Pt. 1, p. 91.
General State Printing Office, The Hague.

Floyd,J.C.,Jr., Fajans,S.S., Conn,J.W., Knopf,R.F., and Rull,J., 1966.
Stimulation of insulin secretion by amino acids.
J. Clin. Invest. 45:1487.

Holm,I., 1964.
Comparative studies of the plasma proteins on peroral, intravenous, intraportal and enteral administration of casein hydrolyzate.
Acta Chir. Scand. 325:108.

Nasset,E.S., Schwartz,P., and Weiss,H.V., 1955.
The digestion of proteins *in vivo*.
J. Nutr. 56:83.

Nasset,E.S., and Ju,J.S., 1961.
Mixture of endogenous and exogenous protein in the alimentary tract.
J. Nutr. 74:461.

Nasset,E.S., Ganapathy,S.N., and Goldsmith,D.P.J., 1963.
Amino acids in dog blood and gut contents after feeding zein.
J. Nutr. 81:343.

Nasset,E.S., 1964.
The nutritional significance of endogenous nitrogen secretion in non-ruminants, in Munro *The role of the gastrointestinal tract in protein metabolism.*
Blackwell, Oxford, pp. 83-96.

Nasset,E.S., 1965.
Role of the digestive system in protein metabolism.
Fed. Proc. 24:953.

Nasset,E.S., Ridley,P.T., and Schenk,E.A., 1967.
Hypothalamic lesions related to ingestion of an imbalanced amino acid diet.
Amer. J. Physiol. 213:645.

Nasset,E.S., Ju,J.S., and McConnel,K.P., 1973.
Comparative digestibility of casein and pancreatic juice proteins in the rat.
Nutr. Reports Internat. 7:643.

Nordstrom,C., Dahlqvist,A., and Josefsson,J., 1968.
Quantitative determination of enxymes in different parts of the villi and crypts of rat small intestine. Comparison of alkaline phosphatase, disaccharidases and dipeptidases.
J. Histochem. Cytochem. 15:713.

Olmsted,W.W., Nasset,E.S., and Kelly,M.L.,Jr., 1966.
Amino acids in postprandial gut contents of man.
J. Nutr. 90:291.

Pelot,D., and Grossman, M.I., 1962.
Distribution and fate of pancreatic enzymes in small intestine of the rat.
Amer. J. Physiol. 202:285.

Raghuramulu,N., Narasigna Rao,B.S., and Gopalan,C., 1965.
Amino acid imbalance and tryptophan-niacin metabolism. I. Effect of excess leucine on the urinary excretion of tryptophan-niacin metabolites in rats.
J. Nutr. 86:100.

Sidransky,H., and Farber,E., 1958.
Chemical pathology of acute amino acid deficiencies. I. Morphological changes in immature rats fed threonine-, methionine- or histidine-devoid diets.
Arch. Path. 66:119.

MECHANISM OF THE INTESTINAL ABSORPTION OF SUGARS AND AMINO ACIDS

Robert K. Crane

INTRODUCTION

The development of our current ideas on mechanism in this area of intestinal absorption has been so thoroughly covered by recent reviews (Schultz and Curren, 1970; Crane, 1968) that I have no wish to go over the same ground again. Instead I would like to try to clarify for you what are the issues and disputes as to mechanism and the bases for them.

As of today, most, I think, would concede that the absorption of glucose or amino acids from the lumen of the gut into the blood stream ultimately depends upon the activity of energy-coupled specific translocation processes located in the brush border pole of the epithelial cells of the gut mucosa.

Also as of today, many would concede that Na^+ is a requirement for the active cellular accumulation of sugars and amino acids and many would, as well, subscribe to some modification of the concept of co-transport of substrate and sodium ion (Crane et al., 1961) as the basis for this requirement and for energy-coupling.

As I have said, most and many; but by no means all. For example, Capraro's group (Esposito et al., 1973) is convinced that transport phenomena are more efficient "in vivo" than "in vitro". Consequently, they believe that because we work *in vitro* we see only the brush border process and are left unaware of a far more important active extrusion process in the baso-lateral membranes. They will not concede the brush border localization of active transport though they do agree that the process we have studied is linked in some way with sodium ion. There are others who will not do that. As perhaps best exemplified by Förster and Matthäus (1973), there are those who strongly argue that we are dead wrong and that Na^+ has nothing to do with the process.

With this degree of caveat let me tell you briefly where I think we are on (1) the question of Na^+-dependency and whether it is a constant of glucose and amino acid transport by the gut, (2) the meaning of Na^+-dependency for the events of translocation and (3) the meaning of Na^+-substrate co-transport for energy coupling.

THE Na^+-DEPENDENCY OF SUGAR AND AMINO ACID ABSORPTION

For reasons that I will try to make clear, it seems to me that there is little room for further doubt that the brush border membrane of the intestinal epithelial cell, as studied in vitro, has the property of being more permeable to glucose and related sugars and to some amino acids when Na^+ is present than when it is absent. Whatever else may be a matter of hypothesis requiring further proof, this permeability response to Na^+ is, I believe, established.

You may recall that Bihler, Hawkins and Crane (1962) first demonstrated an effect of Na^+ on membrane permeability independent of its effect on active transport. Using energy-depleted tissue incapable of active transport, we found that Na^+ enhanced the entry of those sugars which would have been actively transported under normal conditions, and only those sugars. This observation was fundamental to a discrimination among the various hypotheses which have been advanced for the mechanism of Na^+-dependent active transport. It suggested the presence of a simple carrier activated or enhanced in its activity by Na^+.

As so well reviewed by Schultz and Curran (1970), numerous other in vitro studies with intact tissue over the years by test methods more sensitive and more quantitative than those used by us have given results which are readily interpreted in the same way; that is, the presence of Na^+ enhances membrane glucose and amino acid permeability. Moreover this membrane property has finally been confirmed in a most clear way. Hopfer et al. (1973) have isolated rat brush borders and from them prepared highly purified membrane in vesicular form. The cores of the microvilli are gone, the cytoplasm is gone and these empty vesicles are out of contact with energy-yielding reactions. Nonetheless they display the phenomena anticipated from our deductions. D-glucose is taken up and released from the vesicles faster than L-glucose and the uptake of D-glucose is specifically enhanced by Na^+, among all ions tested. Inhibition by phlorizin and D-galactose and the phenomenon of countertransport were also seen.

In view of all this, is there a possibility of dispute about this particular aspect of Na^+-dependency of transport? One could say there is not, if the in vitro situation were specifically referred to. But dispute there is and dispute arises because this property of the brush border membrane so clear in vitro is not clearly expressed when sugar absorption is studied in vivo.

Early studies with in vivo loops of rat intestine seemed to confirm the anticipated Na^+-dependency of glucose absorption (Ponz and Lluch, 1964). However, peroral perfusion studies on man were less supportive. Olsen and Ingelfinger (1968), for example, found that sugar absorption is not as strictly dependent on luminal Na^+ as would be expected from in vitro studies. Also Saltzman et al. (1972), using the triple-lumen tube technique, find that glucose absorption is minimally or not at all reduced when the Na^+ concentration in the solutions perfused through the chosen segment of gut is reduced from high levels to concentrations which are known to be ineffective in supporting glucose permeability in vitro. They have extended these observations to the rat and the dog with the same general result. Meanwhile, the effect of Na^+ on glucose permeability and uptake by human intestine in vitro turns out to be readily demonstrated (Elsas et al., 1970). There is no possibility that the results, either way, are species dependent. The problem, however, remains; a prediction from the in vitro properties of the brush border membrane is not found in vivo. The question is why.

An answer to this question is not at hand. At the moment there are several possibilities. For example, the notion could be entertained that the effect of Na^+ on glucose entry is strictly an in vitro phenomenon; that the brush border membrane in the living cell is unaffected by Na^+ and that the appearance of Na^+-sensitivity is a phenomenon of functional degeneration following disruption of the normal supply of oxygen and nutrients from the circulation. Surely, to take this view would be to retreat to vitalism. I know of no studies on the properties of the brush border membrane of the absorbing cells of the gut, in vivo. Such studies as there are relate to the mucosal surface as a whole in which, for one example, secretory phenomena may well have been overlooked as a contributing factor to overall function. This is substantially the conclusion reached by Fleshler and Nelson (1970) from their studies of L-alanine absorption in dogs. They believe that the necessary Na^+ ions for absorption are contributed by the mucosal wall.

Semenza (1972) suggests that the difference between in vivo and in vitro is not at the level of the membrane but at the level of a barrier to diffusion, an unstirred layer, adjacent and external to the membrane. He suggests that the efflux of Na^+ noted by Fleshler and Nelson goes first into the unstirred layer before appearing in the lumen and is available at the location to activate the glucose permeability of the membrane and to be recycled inwardly by co-transport.

Some attention to this possibility is being paid in Fordtran's laboratory (Bieberdorf, personal communication) by using replacements for Na^+ other than mannitol. Mg^{++} has been used in an effort to displace Na^+ from a possibly negatively charged boundary at the mucosal surface. Despite these efforts, it is still found that 50 percent, at least, of active sugar transport by the ileum is independent of Na^+ added to the perfusion solution.

There is as yet no mutual ground for accommodation of these divergent results. Semenza (1972) has pointed out that the numerous methods for study of in vitro intestinal transport have been divised to provide an advantage for study of one or another portion of the overall process of intestinal absorption. Do our difficulties in resolving the Na^+ question suggest that some important component of the overall absorptive process has not yet been measured in vitro and another new and discriminating method needs to be devised?

THE MEANING OF Na^+-DEPENDENCE FOR TRANSLOCATION

We have so far considered the Na^+-dependence of glucose translocation across the brush border membrane in its simplest terms as merely an increase in the permeability of the membrane for glucose. Early on it was indeed possible to propose that Na^+ merely activated transport without participating in it. However, we (Crane et al., 1961) postulated co-transport of Na^+ and sugar because of the perceived need to couple energy with the carrier. These was supportive evidence for co-transport in the form of the effect of a reversed Na^+ gradient on sugar flux (Crane, 1964) and in the form of an effect of sugar on the in vitro transmural potential and short circuit (Schultz and Zalusky, 1964). However, more substantial proof of co-transport came from direct measurements of the simultaneous flux into rabbit ileum of Na^+ and amino acid (Curran et al., 1967) or Na^+ and sugar (Goldner et al., 1969). The interdependence of Na^+ and substrate movements which our hypothesis demanded was confirmed. And so it remains. In all studies where looked for, there has been found concommitant with an increase of sugar of amino acid permeability of the brush border membrane by presence of Na^+, an increase in Na^+ permeability of the brush border membrane by the presence of sugar or amino acid. It cannot be overemphasized that substrate dependent Na^+-transport should be viewed in the same way and as an expression of the same membrane events as Na^+-dependent substrate transport (Crane, 1967).

The failure of the in vitro studies on Na^+-dependent sugar transport to predict the in vivo consequences generally found has been discussed above as has the problem this failure creates. Turning the other side, however, there is no failure and no problem. There is no failure of in vitro studies on substrate-dependent Na^+ transport to predict the in vivo consequences. Substrate-dependent Na^+ transport occurs in vivo and it has been measured in the intact human intestine (Sachar et al., 1969). Is it not substrate-dependent Na^+ transport which is the basis of treating the devastating salt and water loss of cholera (Hirshhorn et al., 1968; Nalin et al., 1970) by giving saline with added glucose and amino acid to drink?

THE MEANING OF Na^+-SUGAR CO-TRANSPORT FOR ENERGY COUPLING

For the reasons I've set out above, I believe that the brush border plasma membrane contains carriers and that Na^+ and sugar or amino acid can be and are co-transported. Thus it is my view that there can be little doubt that the potential exists for energy to be coupled to the carrier by means of an imposed gradient or flux of Na^+ or the substrate. We have demonstrated such a coupling for sugar in the gut cell. Such a coupling has been demonstrated for amino acid in the pigeon red cell by Vidaver (1964) and in the Ehrlich cell by Eddy (1968). Coupling occurs. In fact, to go further afield you may recall that Peter Mitchell (1962) based the symport part of his chemiosmotic theory for bacteria on our view of Na^+ and sugar coupling in the gut. He proposed that a hydrogen ion gradient could drive galactoside transport in E. coli. The fact is that this coupling so closely related to Na^+substrate co-transport has now been demonstrated (Kashket and Wilson, 1973). It seems to me that the question can be no longer whether co-transport and consequent energy coupling can or does occur. The question is whether this kind of coupling, when it occurs, is the prime source of energy; that is, whether sufficient gradient of flux driving force is available to account for the observed active transport. This question has been approached at length and in various ways and there is yet no clear answer to it.

Recent work on this question has been mostly with cell types other than the gut and hence, of course, with amino acids. It can be summed up that, currently, both the view that cation gradients are not sufficient and the view that they are sufficient are supported. On the one hand, calculations of energy input vs. energy need indicate that only about half the needed energy can be provided by cation gradients (Schafer and Heinz, 1971). On the other hand, when cation gradients are specifically and selectively abolished by gramicidin (Terry and Vidaver, 1972) so also is amino acid active transport.

Some work has been done with the intestine and, as made quite clear by Smyth (1971), the question of energy coupling is still an open one. Overall, it may be said, the intestinal epithelial cell is probably a more favorable cell for coupling to occur than some others. The reason for this is that the necessary events seem to be clearly separated. Studies on tissue (Tomasini and Dobbins, 1970; Stirling, 1972) and isolated membranes (Hopfer, personal communication) agree with the proposition that Na^+ and sugar enter together at the brush border membrane and Na^+ is ejected from the cell at the lateral membrane. There is thus the possibility for the brush border→lateral membrane flux of Na^+ to drive sugar accumulation without the need to establish large, overall lumen-cell Na^+ gradients.

Lately, the concept of co-transport has been challenged by Kimmich (1970) with a proposal of a more direct coupling of ATP energy to sugar and amino acid transport. In this initial proposal border co-transport of Na^+ was left out. In a more current version (Kimmich, 1973) co-transport of Na^+ is back in with, additionally, the recognition that if the events of Na^+ and sugar co-transport, on the one hand, and Na^+ pumping, on the other, are physically separated, as they seem to be, this scheme cannot work.

The search for final answer to the role of Na^+ goes on.

REFERENCES

Bihler,I., Hawkins, K.A. and Crane, R.K., 1962.
Studies on the mechanism of intestinal absorption of sugars. VI. The specificity and other properties of Na^+-dependent entrance of sugars into intestinal tissue under anaerobic conditions, *in vitro*.
Biochem. Biophys. Acta. 59:94.

Crane, R.K., Miller, D. and Bihler, I., 1961.
The Restrictions on the possible mechanisms of intestinal active transport of sugars, in *Membrane Transport and Metabolism*.
Edit by A. Kleinzeller and A. Kotyk, New York. Acad. Press, pg. 439.

Crane, R.K., 1964.
Uphill outflow of sugar from intestinal epithelial cells induced by reversal of the Na^+ gradient. Its significance for the mechanism of Na^+-dependent active transport.
Biochem. Biophys. Res. Comm. 17:481.

Crane, R.K., 1967.
Gradient Coupling and the membrane transport of water soluble compounds: A general mechanism? Vol. in *Colloquia on the Protides of the Biological Fluids*, edit. by H. Peeters.
Elsevier, Amsterdam, Vol. XV, p. 227.

Crane, R.K., 1968.
Absorption of Sugars, in "*Alimentary Canal*", edit by C.F. Code.
Handbook of Physiology, Vol. III.
Am. Physiol. Society, Washington, pg. 1323.

Curran, P.F., Schultz, S.G., Chez, R.A. and Fuisz, R.E., 1967.
Kinetic relations of the Na-aminoacid interaction at the mucosal border of the intestine.
J. Gen. Physiol. 50:1261.

Eddy, A.A., 1968.
The effects of varying the cellular and extra-cellular concentrations of sodium and potassium ions on the uptake of glycine by mouse ascites-tumor cells in the presence and absence of sodium cyanide.
Biochem. J. 108:489.

Elsas, L.J., Hillman, R.E., Patterson, J.H. and Rosenberg, L.E., 1970.
Renal and intestinal hexose transport in familial glucose-galactose malabsorption.
J. Clin. Invest. 49:576.

Esposito, G., Faelli, A. and Capraro, V., 1973.
Sugar and Electrolyte Absorption in the Rat
Pflugers Arch. 340:335.

Fleshler, B. and Nelson, R.A., 1970.
Sodium dependency of L-alanine absorption in canine Thiry-Vella loops.
Gut 11:240.

Forster, H. and Matthaus, M., 1973.
Some comments on the Coupling between Intestinal Absorption of Glucose and Sodium.
FEBS letters, 31:75.

Goldner, A.M., Schultz, S.G. and Curran, P.F., 1969.
Sodium and sugar fluxes across the mucosal border of rabbit ileum.
J. Gen. Physiol. 53:362.

Hirschorn, N., Kinzie, J.L., Sachar, D.B., Northrop, R.S., Taylor, J.O., Ahmad, S.Z. and Phillips, R.A., 1968.
Decrease in net stool output in cholera during intestinal perfusion with glucose-containing solutions.
N. Eng. J. Med. 279:176.

Hopfer, U., Nelson, K., Perrotto, J.L. and Isselbacher, K.J., 1973.
Glucose transport by isolated brush border membranes of rat small intestine.
J. Biol. Chem. in press.

Kashket, E.R. and Wilson, T.H., 1973.
Proton-coupled Accumulation of Galactoside in Streptococcus lactis 7962.

Proc. Nat. Acad. Sci. USA, 70:2866.
Kimmich, G.A., 1970.
Active Sugar Accumulation by isolated Epithelial Cells. A new model for sodium-dependent metabolite transport.
Biochemistry 9:3669.
Kimmich, G.A., 1973.
Coupling Between Na^+ and Sugar Transport in Small Intestine.
Biochem. Biophys. Acta. 300:31.
Mitchell, P., 1962.
Molecule, Group and Electron Translocation through Natural Membranes.
Biochem. Soc. Symp. 22:142.
Nalin, D.R., Cash, R.A., Rahman, M. and Yumus, M.D., 1970.
Effect of glycine and glucose on sodium and water absorption in patients with cholera.
Gut 11:768.
Olsen, W.A. and Ingelfinger, F.J., 1968.
The role of sodium in intestinal glucose absorption in man.
J. Clin. Invest. 47:1133.
Ponz, F. and Lluch, M., 1964.
Influence of the Na^+ concentration on the *in vivo* intestinal absorption of sugars.
Rev. Espan. Fisiol. 20:179.
Sachar, D.B., Taylor, J.O., Saha, J.R. and Phillips, R.A., 1969.
Intestinal transmural electric potential and its response to glucose in acute and convalescent cholera.
Gastroenterology 56:512.
Saltzman, D.A., Rector, F.C., Jr. and Fordtran, J.S., 1972.
The role of intraluminal sodium in glucose absorption *in vivo*.
J. Clin. Invest. 51:876.
Schafer, J.A. and Heinz, E., 1971.
The effect of reversal of Na^+ and K^+ electrochemical potential gradients on the active transport of amino acids in Ehrlich ascites tumor

cells.
Biochem. Biophys. Acta 249:15.
Schultz, S.G. and Zalusky, R., 1964.
The interaction between active sodium and active sugar transport.
J. Gen. Physiol. 47:1043.
Schultz, S.G. and Curran, P.F., 1970.
Coupled transport of sodium and organic solutes.
Physiol. Rev. 50:637.
Semenza, G., 1972.
Some aspects of intestinal sugar transport, in "Transport Across the Intestine", edit by W.L. Burland and P.D. Samuel, Churchill Livingstone. A. Glaxo Symposium, Edinburgh and London, p. 78.
Smyth, D.H., 1971.
Sodium-hexose interactions.
Philas. Trans. R. Soc. Lond. Biol. Sci. 262:121.
Stirling, C.E., 1972.
Radioautographic localization of sodium pump sites in rabbit intestine.
J. Cell Biol. 53:704.
Terry, P.M. and Vidaver, G.A., 1972.
The effect of gramicidin on the Na^+-dependent accumulation of glycine by pigeon red blood cells.
Biochem. Biophys. Res. Comm. 47:539.
Tomasini, J.T. and Dobbins, W.O., 1970.
Intestinal Mucosal Morphology During Water and Electrolyte Absorption: A light and electron microscopic study.
Am. J. Dig. Dis. 15:226.
Vidaver, G.A., 1964.
Glycine transport by hemolyzed and restored pigeon red cells.
Biochemistry 3:795.

FAT ABSORPTION

Peter R. Holt and Susanne Bennett Clark

INTRODUCTION

The purpose of this presentation is to summarize the present status of our knowledge of normal fat absorption, with particular emphasis upon recent advances, and to present the implications of mainly unpublished areas of investigation from our laboratory.

The intestinal absorption of non-lipid substances such as carbohydrates and proteins is dependent upon a digestive phase in which high molecular weight substrates are hydrolized into low molecular weight products that are able to penetrate into the mucosal cell. In considering the absorption of non-lipid substances most emphasis is placed upon their transfer into and out of the mucosal cell rather than on the intraluminal or intracellular reactions. The diffusion of compounds through the lipoidal portion of the membrane of the cell is extremely slow, and diffusion through the hypothetical water-filled pores probably is limited in quantity. Specific protein receptors are, however, present in the membrane of the cell which permit rapid transmembrane passage of water-soluble substances into the aqueous cell interior. In contrast, lipid molecules such as long chain free fatty acids which traverse the membrane face different problems during absorption.

FATTY ACID TRANSPORT

The Cell Membrane

The transport of lipids and long chain free fatty acids across the

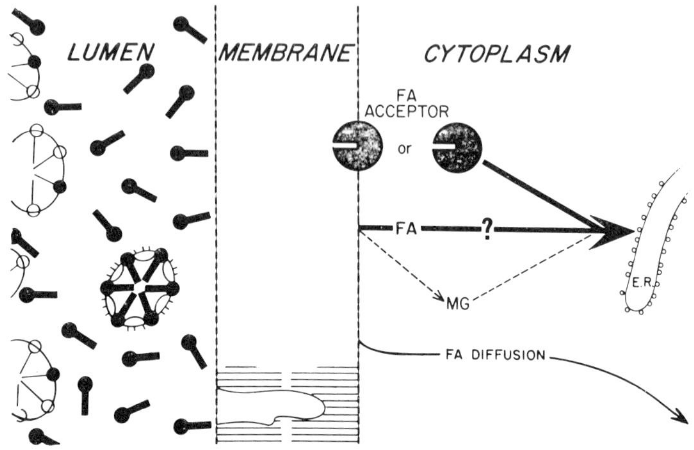

Fig. 1. Diagrammatic Representation of Fatty Acid Uptake and Release from the Microvillus Membrane of the Intestinal Mucosal Cell. The concentration of fatty acid monomers in the unstirred water layer surrounding the microvillus determines membrane uptake rate. Transport to the endoplasmic reticulum probably involves a protein carrier.

same predominantly lipid membrane is rapid since dissolution occurs readily. However, on each side of the membrane fatty acids must move in an aqueous environment. On the luminal side is an unstirred water layer and on the mucosal side the cytoplasm is also predominantly comprised of water. The recent work of Dietschy and coworkers have emphasized that the rate of transfer of free fatty acid through the unstirred water layer is slow (Wilson et al., 1971), and that in slice and everted sac experiments this step appears to be rate-limiting for fatty acid uptake by the cell (Sallee and Dietschy, 1973). On the other hand, calculations derived from studies of maximal triolein absorption in the rat (Bennett et al., 1973) and studies by Weiss and Holt (Weiss and Holt, 1971) in man indicate that overall fatty acid absorption is directly related to the micellar concentration of fatty acid in the lumen, which is in turn determined by the concentration of luminal bile salts within the normal range. It seems likely then that the concentration of fatty acid monomers in the unstirred water layer adjacent to the mucosal cell is well maintained by the micellar concentration of free fatty acid normally present in the lumen and that this barrier is unlikely to be rate-limiting for overall fat absorption in vivo. Data showing that in the total absence of bile in the lumen absorption of dietary triglyceride is well maintained (Morgan, 1964) support the concept that monomolecular diffusion is sufficiently rapid to maintain reasonable fat absorption.

After leaving the membrane absorbed fatty acid must reach the endoplasmic reticulum, site of formation of fatty acid CoA and subsequent reesterification of fatty acid to triglyceride. The endoplasmic reticulum is situated some distance from the base of the microvillus, so that absorbed fatty acid must be detached from the membrane and then be transported to the site of subsequent esterification. Although no direct experimental data are available, it would seem likely that the diffusion of fatty acid through the aqueous cytoplasm would be as slow as that calculated for diffusion through the unstirred water layer on the outer side of the membrane. The recent work of Ockner (Ockner et al., 1972) and of Kessler (Kessler and Mishkin, 1973) suggests that a mucosal fatty acid binding protein is present in the cell that may be of great importance in the transfer of fatty acid from the membrane to the endoplasmic reticulum. This protein may be associated with the membrane itself (Kessler and Mishkin, 1973) or be present as an acceptor molecule in the cytoplasm on the inner side of the membrane. By reducing the concentration of free fatty acid on the inner side of the membrane, such a binding protein mechanism would enhance the diffusion gradient of free fatty acid through the membrane and thus increase overall absorption into the cell. In vitro work from our laboratories also suggests that an excess of monoglyceride in the cell may sequester absorbed fatty acid in a separate pool where rapid esterification does not occur, and under these circumstances fatty acid diffusion into the cell is also enhanced (Marubbio et al., 1974). Within the endoplasmic reticulum two separate and independent pathways by which fatty acid CoA can be esterified to triglyceride are known (Senior, 1964). Two studies in vivo, one in the rat (Mattson and Volpenhein, 1964), and one in man (Kayder et al., 1967) indicate that the monoglyceride pathway normally predominates. However, it appears likely that the α-glycerophosphate pathway for triglyceride synthesis may substitute effectively if the monoglyceride esterification pathway is inhibited (Kern and Borgstrom, 1963). Controlling mechanisms for these two pathways have not been elucidated to date, nor have the associated consequences of fatty acid esterification through one versus another pathway been studied.

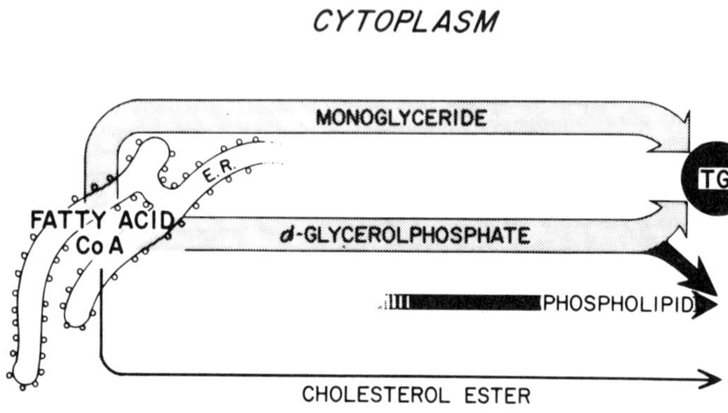

Fig. 2. Diagrammatic Representation of the Pathways Controlling Mucosal Triglyceride Synthesis. Note that the quantitative significance of phospholipid synthesis via the α-glycerophosphate pathway is unknown.

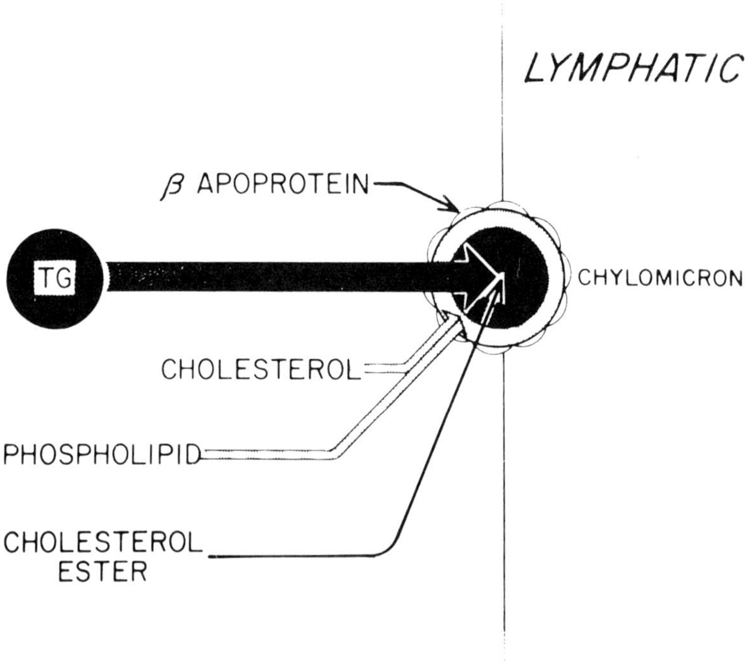

Fig. 3. Diagrammatic Representation of the Incorporation of Components into the Chylomicron. Triglyceride, cholesterol and fat soluble vitamins enter the core whereas free cholesterol, β-apoprotein and phospholipid are incorporated into the chylomicron coat.

Although phospholipid synthesis in the cell can occur by diversion of fatty acid from diglyceride in the α-glycerophosphate pathway, the quantitative significance of this CD-Pcholine pathway to normal phospholipid synthesis is unknown and the source of phospholipid for chylomicron formation and for replacement of phospholipid in cell and subcellular membranes is poorly understood.

Formation of Chylomicron

Chylomicron formation is also unclear. The chylomicron is the carrier complex for the large amount of absorbed triglyceride that must be transported through the aqueous environments of lymph and blood stream. Nonpolar lipids such as triglyceride, cholesterol esters and fat soluble vitamins occupy the center of the chylomicron particle; the coat contains a specific protein (β- apoprotein), phospholipid and free cholesterol (Frederickson et al., 1967). The assembly of this particle appears to occur above and around the Golgi apparatus of the cell (Jersild and Clayton, 1971) and the "pre-chylomicron" thus formed passes readily by unknown mechanisms out of the cell and into the lymphatics of the intestinal villus. Although some differences in the composition of the pre-chylomicron released from mucosal cells and the chylomicron harvested from mesenteric lymphatics have been described (Redgrave, 1971) it is likely that chylomicron synthesis is almost entirely a mucosal cellular event. At present there is little information available about chylomicron formation in vivo and this is an area in which we are working actively at present. Some aspects of our work will be discussed below. We consider it a reasonable working hypothesis that chylomicron formation or release may require the presence of all the three components that are found in the chylomicron coat.

Although many studies in the past decade have concentrated on aspects of the digestion and solubilization of dietary triglyceride, there are still important gaps in our overall knowledge. Detailed studies of fat absorption have almost universally been performed with liquid triglyceride (usually triolein or olive oil). One can envisage that triglyceride oil after ingestion is present in the aqueous environment of the gastrointestinal tract as large oil globules. Before the triglyceride digestion products, monoglyceride and fatty acids, can be formed three steps must occur. Triglycerides are hydrolyzed at the oil-water interface by the action of pancreatic lipase with the

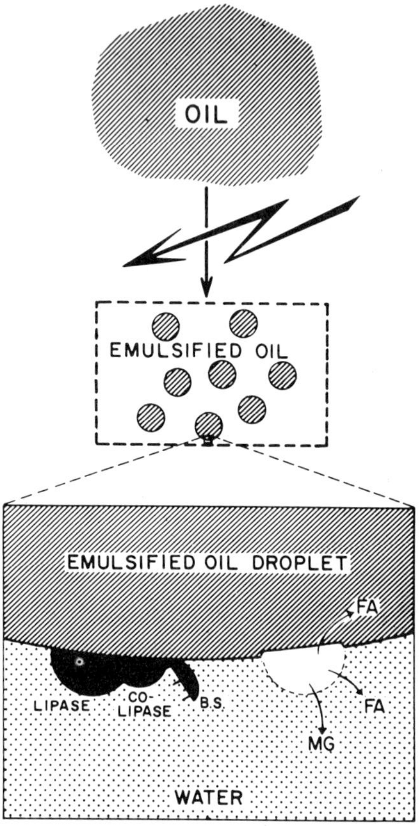

Fig. 4. Diagrammatic Representation of the Requirements for Normal Triglyceride Lipolysis. Emulsion formation requires mechanical energy and stabilizers. Enzyme activity involves lipase and colipase. Continued lipolysis demands removal of the products, free fatty acid and monoglyceride from the site of enzyme action by solubilization by amphipathic compounds.

formation of free fatty acid and β-monoglyceride. The classical experiments of Desnuelle and his group showed that the rate of lipolysis was related to the surface area of oil available to the enzyme (Desnuelle and Savary, 1963). Normally pancreatic lipase is present in the intestinal lumen in great excess and malabsorption occurs only with severe reduction of pancreatic enzyme secretion into the gut. The action of lipase involves a small protein molecule secreted in pancreatic juice termed co-lipase. Recent information suggests that its function is to protect the enzyme lipase from denaturation by bile salt (Borgstrom, 1967). Emulsification is the process whereby large lipid droplets are converted to small lipid droplets and then are stabilized, preventing coalescence of droplets. This process of emulsification greatly increases the surface area of triglyceride available for lipolysis. Emulsification requires mechanical energy (which is most efficiently produced by a shearing force) and the presence of the stabilizers, which are usually physiologic amphipaths. Bile salts and other amphipathic molecules also function to strip the triglyceride lipolytic products, free fatty acids and monoglycerides from the site of enzyme action by micellar solubilization thereby allowing enzyme action on the triglyceride substrate to continue. Thus, emulsification, lipase action and the presence of amphipathic solubilizers are all essential for normal triglyceride lipolysis; however, the quantitative importance of these mechanisms in maintaining normal fat digestion is not entirely clear.

Role of Bile Salt

Many recent reviews have described the solubilizing activity of bile salts and the other natural amphipaths in the small intestinal lumen (Dietschy, 1972; Hofmann and Kern, 1971). Within the normal range of concentration of bile salts in the lumen the concentration of free fatty acid in the aqueous phase is directly related to the bile salt concentration (up to about 20 mMolar bile salts). In addition, the partition of free fatty acid between the oil and aqueous phases in the intestinal lumen (which may be experimentally separated by ultracentrifugation (Hofmann and Borgstrom, 1964)) is dependent upon pH, since un-ionized fatty acid will distribute in part into the oil phase. Furthermore, free fatty acid partition is also related to the volume of the oil phase present (Borgstrom, 1967). Thus, an expanded oil phase and low pH will reduce the concentration of free fatty acid in the micellar or aqueous phase independent of bile salt concentration.

ABSORPTION SITES

Differences between Bowel Segments

For many years we have used a method of intraduodenal infusion of a test triglyceride, emulsified triolein, in the awake restrained rat

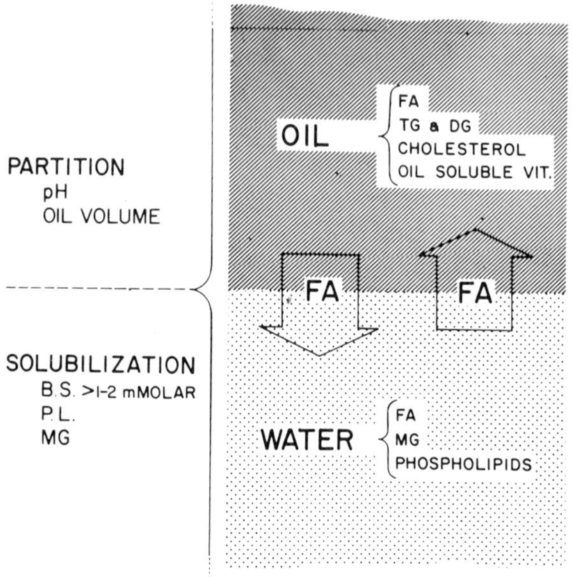

Fig. 5. Diagrammatic Representation of the Distribution of Lipids between Oil and Water Phases in the Intestinal Lumen. The partition of free fatty acids is dependent upon both the intraluminal pH and the volume of the oil phase.

in order to study the rate-determining steps governing intestinal fat absorption. The test lipid can be perfused for prolonged period at a steady rate and controlled steady state conditions for digestion and absorption can be established. This model has been used to compare the absorption rate and characteristics of triglycerides of varying compositions (Bennett and Holt, 1968) and also the interaction of differing triglycerides during the absorptive process (Bennett and Holt, 1969). Recently, one of us (SBC) made the intriguing observation that if the whole length of the intestine was stressed to absorb large amounts of fat the distal intestine (segments 6, 7, & 8 when the small intestine is divided into ten equal segments) accumulated fat during prolonged perfusion whereas the fat concentration in the proximal intestine (segments 2–5) failed to rise (Bennett et al., 1973). The total mucosal uptake and tissue lipid accumulation during maximal perfusion of triolein for varying times (one to six hours) suggested that accumulation was not due to significant regional differences in the mucosal uptake of test fat from the intestinal lumen, but was due to a failure to release fat from the distal small intestine. The absorbed test fat was present in the mucosa almost entirely as triglyceride so that the accumulation did not result from a defect in mucosal triglyceride synthesis in the distal intestine. This observation has been pursued and to date we can state that distal intestinal accumulation occurs also one month following resection of the proximal intestine and reanastomosis or surgical transposition of proximal and distal intestine.

Very recent studies of the direct perfusion of lipids into either the jejunum or the ileum have directly demonstrated impaired lymphatic transport of triglyceride following absorption from the distal intestine. It appears, therefore, that the distal intestine is intrinsically different from the proximal bowel in its handling of absorbed fat. It is intriguing to speculate, although not yet proven, that chylomicron formation might be deficient in this part of the intestine. However, two alternative possibilities, that in this area of the bowel prechylomicrons are normally formed but cannot as readily pass into the submucosa, or that lymphatic drainage is impaired, cannot be ruled out. Direct demonstration of differences in intracellular prechylomicron formation between proximal and distal intestine is needed to prove altered chylomicron synthesis.

Electron Microscopy Studies

Electron microscopic observations on proximal and distal intestinal segments following maximal duodenal perfusion in collaboration with Dr. Seymour Sabesin of the University of Tennessee School of Medicine, has demonstrated the massive accumulation of very large lipid droplets in segments 6 to 8 at the end of three or four hours of perfusion whereas such large droplets are rarely found in the upper intestine. The lipid droplets in the wall of the distal intestine varied in size from 1,000 to 11,000 millimicrons and in the proximal intestine were rarely greater than 2,000 to 3,000 millimicrons in diameter. Lipid vesicles demonstrated in the submucosa in all regions of the intestine were at all times 500 to 700 millimicrons in diameter. Following cessation of the intestinal perfusion, large lipid droplets continued to be evident in electron micrographs from distal intestine for as long as six to nine hours whereas the jejunum was practically empty of fat already after three hours.

This electron microscopic appearance of the distal intestine in our normal rats closely resembles the picture of human α-β-lipoprotenemia (Dobbins,1968) and also resembles the appearance following the experimental administration of protein synthesis inhibitors followed by fat feeding in animals (Sabesin and Isselbacher, 1965). To expand upon this observation further we previously studied an animal model in which similar intestinal accumulation of triglyceride was found in the proximal intestine as well. This model was the essential fatty acid deficient rat, which showed mild fat malabsorption and in whom the only significant defect in the absorptive process that was detected was the failure to release absorbed triglyceride into the lymph (Bennett et al., 1973). Since the major effect of essential fatty acid efficiency is a compositional alteration in phospholipid it is tempting to speculate that a change in the phospholipid of the chylomicrons was responsible for a defect in fat release into the lymph. Rather similar electron micrographs of small intestine have been seen in inosotol-deficient gerbils (Hegsted et al., 1973) and in marmosets on high fat, high cholesterol diets (Driezen et al., 1971). O'Doherty, Kakis and Kuksis (O'Doherty et al., 1973) working with choline-deficient animals have implied that fat accumulation occurred within intestinal mucosal cells also under these conditions and suggested that a cellular phospholipid deficiency might be responsible for impaired chylomicron formation. At present it is uncertain whether any effect of phospholipid upon chylomicron formation or release exists, whether due to unavailability of phospholipid itself for chylomicron synthesis or whether mediated through a requirement for phospholipid for normal protein synthesis in the endoplasmic reticulum or Golgi. In any case, these preliminary observations suggest that many intracellular actors may contribute to control the formation and/or release of chylomicrons from intestinal mucosal cells. Our further understanding of this process in normal and disease states requires that these variables be clarified.

Emulsion Formation

Finally, we should like to discuss recent unpublished work from our laboratory that is concerned with an early step in fat digestion in the upper gastrointestinal tract following triglyceride feeding, the process of emulsion formation. The only important information on emulsion formation following fat feeding is derived from a study by Sir Alistair Frazer and his associates in Birmingham reported in 1944

(Frazer et al., 1944). This study, incidentally, resulted in Frazer's proposal of the "partition theory" for fat absorption (Frazer, 1944). Frazer's group used unphysiologic amounts of natural amphipaths, which undoubtedly were chemically very impure, in an attempt to form spontaneous emulsions in the test tube, and suggested that bile salts, monoglyc rides, and fatty acid soaps were the stabilizers for emulsion droplet formed in the intestine. Furthermore, they also suggested that small intestinal emulsion particles were about 0.5 microns in diameter. We have recently been restudying this problem using pure amphipathic compounds in physiologic amounts and confirm that bile salts and fatty acid soaps, together with phospholipid and monoglyceride are excellent stabilizers for emulsion droplets once formed. However, significant concentrations of emulsified triglycerides cannot be found in the stomach and it appears from our preliminary experiments that the pylorus also does not create sufficient mechanical shearing force to make small emulsions particles. Studies in normal human volunteers suggest that appreciable amounts of unemulsified test corn oil can be recovered from the duodenum. However, a significant emulsion phase is probably necessary for normal digestion since the rate of pancreatic lipolysis appears to be directly related to the surface area available for enzyme action. It seems important to pursue these studies in order to determine where the force responsible for creating small emulsion particles in the upper intestine of man is generated. It also seems likely that in some disease states emulsion formation might be impaired and that this might lead to fat malabsorption.

In summary, despite considerable advances in our understanding of the physiology of intestinal fat digestion and absorption, significant gaps in our knowledge still exist. In particular, it appears essential to test one by one the events leading to normal triglyceride absorption in intact animals and in man, in order to understand better the final product of triglyceride absorption, the formation of chylomicrons. We hope that such understanding might allow for future experimental manipulation of this normal process in order to create chylomicrons that might be less atherogenic.

REFERENCES

Bennett Clark,S., et al, 1973.
Fat absorption in essential fatty acid deficiency: a model experimental approach to studies of the mechanism of fat malabsorption of unknown etiology.
J. Lipid Res., 14:581.

Bennett Clark,S., and Holt,P.R., 1968.
Rate limiting steps in steady state intestinal absorption of trioctanoin-1-^{14}C. Effect of biliary and pancreatic flow diversion.
J. Clin. Invest., 47:612.

Bennett Clark,S., and Holt,P.R., 1969.
Inhibition of steady-state intestinal absorption of long-chain triglyceride by medium-chain triglyceride.
J. Clin. Invest., 48:2235.

Bennett Clark,S., Lawergren,B., and Martin,J., 1973.
Regional intestinal absorptive capacities for triolein: an alternative to markers.
Am. J. Physiol., 225:574.

Borgstrom,B., 1967.
Partition of lipids between emulsified oil and micellar phases of glyceride-bile salt dispersions.
J. Lipid Res., 8:598.

Borgstrom,B., and Erlanson,C., 1971.
Pancreatic juice co-lipase: physiological importance.
Biochim. Biophys. Acta, 242:509.

Desnuelle,P., and Savary,P., 1963.
Specificities of lipases.
J. Lipid Res., 4:369.

Dietschy,J.M., (Edit.), 1972.
Symposium on bile acids.
Arch. Int. Med., 130:473.

Dobbins,W.O., 1966.
An ultrastructural study of the intestinal mucosa in congenital B apoprotein deficiency with particular emphasis upon the intestinal absorptive cell.
Gastroenterology, 50:195.

Driezen,S.B., Levy,M., and Bernick,S., 1971.
Diet induced jejunal lipodystrophy in the cotton-top marmoset.
Proc. Soc. Exp. Biol. Med., 138:7.
Frazer,A.C., 1944.
The absorption of triglyceride fat from the intestine.
Physiol. Rev., 24:103.
Frazer,A.C., Schulman,J.H., and Stewart,H.C., 1944.
Emulsification of fat in the intestine of the rat and its relationship to absorption.
J. Physiol., 103:306.
Frederickson,D.S., Levy,R.I., and Lees,R.S., 1967.
Fat transport in lipoproteins: an integrated approach to mechanisms and disorders.
N. Engl. J. Med., 276:34.
Hegsted,D.M., et al, 1973.
Inisotol deficiency: an intestinal lipodystrophy in the gerbil.
J. Nutr., 103:302.
Hofmann,A.F., and Borgstrom,B., 1964.
The intraluminal phase of fat digestion in man: the lipid content of the micellar and oil phases of intestinal content obtained during fat digestion and absorption.
J. Clin. Invest., 43:247.
Hofmann,A.F., and Kern,F., Jr., 1971.
The significance of bile acids in gastrointestinal and hepatic disease.
Disease-a-Month.
Jersild,R.A., Jr., and Clayton,R.T., 1971.
A comparison of the morphology of lipid absorption in the jejunum and ileum of the adult.
Rat. Am. J. Anta., 131:481.
Kayden,H.J., Senior,J.R., and Mattson,F.H., 1967.
The monoglyceride pathway of fat absorption in man.
J. Clin. Invest., 46:1695.
Kern,F., Jr., and Borgstrom,B., 1965.
Quantitative study of the pathways of triglyceride synthesis by hamster intestinal mucosa.
Biochim. Biophys. Acta, 98:520.

Kessler,J.I., and Mishkin,S., 1973.
Demonstration of fatty acid-binding proteins associated with the brush borders of hamster intestinal epithelium.
J. Clin. Invest., 52:47a.

Marubbio,A.T., Jr., et al, 1974.
Monoglyceride modification of rat jejunal absorption of fatty acid.
J. Lipid Res., (In Press).

Mattson,F.H., and Volpenhein,R.A., 1964.
The digestion and absorption of triglycerides.
J. Biol. Chem., 239:2772.

Morgan,R.G.H., 1964.
The effect of bile salts on the lymphatic absorption by the unanesthetized rat of intraduodenally infused lipids.
Quart. J. Exp. Phys., 49:457.

Ockner,R.K., et al, 1972.
A binding protein for fatty acids in cytosol of intestinal mucosa, liver, myocardium, and other tissues.
Science, 177:56.

O'Doherty,P.J.A., Kakis,G., and Kuksis,A., 1973.
Role of luminal lecithin in intestinal fat absorption.
Lipids, 8:249.

Redgrave,R.G., 1971.
Association of Golgi membranes with lipid droplets (Pre-Chylomicrons) from within intestinal epithelial cells during absorption of fat.
Aust. J. Exptl. Biol. Med. Sci., 49:209.

Sabesin,S.M., and Isselbacher,K.J., 1965.
Protein synthesis inhibition: mechanism for the production of impaired fat absorption.
Science, 147:1149.

Sallee,V.L., and Dietschy,J.M., 1973.
Determinants of intestinal mucosal uptake of short-and medium-chain fatty acids and alcohols.
J. Lipid Res., 14:475.

Senior,J.R., 1964.
Intestinal absorption of fats.
J. Lipid Res., 5:495.

Weiss,J.B., and Holt,P.R., 1971.
Controlling factors during intestinal fat absorption in man.
J. Clin. Invest., 50:97a.

Wilson,F.A. Sallee,V.L., and Dietschy,J.M., 1971.
Unstirred water layers in intestine: rate determinant of fatty acid absorption from micellar solutions.
Science, 174:1031.

ENTEROHEPATIC CIRCULATION OF BILE ACIDS

Gershon W. Hepner

INTRODUCTION

In man the two primary bile acids, cholic and chenodeoxycholic acid, as well as their bacterial metabolites, deoxycholic and lithocholic acid, are excreted by the liver as conjugates of glycine and taurine (Sjoval, 1960; Garbutt et al., 1971), stored in the gallbladder between meals and released from the gallbladder when it contracts under stimulus of cholecystokinin-pancreoxymin, an intestinal hormone liberated from the duodenal mucosa by products of food digestion such as fat and amino acids (Go et al., 1970; Ertan et al., 1971). In the bile, bile acids help to maintain cholesterol in micellar solution, preventing its precipitation and the formation of cholesterol gallstones: within the intestinal lumen bile acids participate in the absorption of fat (Hofmann and Small, 1967). They are largely reabsorbed in the ileum (Bergstrom et al., 1963; Dietschy, 1968; Tyor et al., 1972) but some reabsorption also occurs in the colon (Samuel et al., 1968); jejunal reabsorption, if it occurs at all, is minimal (Wingate et al., 1973). Reabsorption of bile acids, their return to the liver and their resecretion into the bile and intestinal lumen gives rise to their enterohepatic circulation.

NORMAL BILE ACID METABOLISM

Bile Acid Alterations and Absorption Modes

During enterohepatic circulation bile acids may be entirely unaltered, or they may undergo two modifications: a) bacterial biotransformation, b) hepatic modification. The bacterial biotransformations to which bile acids are susceptible are caused by fastidiously anerobic bacteria which in health are found only in the ileum and colon (Gorbach, 1971; Mallory et al., 1973). These bacterial biotransformations are:

1. deconjugation of glycine- or taurine-conjugated bile acids with liberation of the free steroid (bile acid) and the free amino acid (glycine or taurine) moieties.

2. 7-dehydroxylation of the steroid moiety with formation of lithocholic acid from chenodeoxycholic acid (Hellstrom and Sjovall, 1961) and deoxycholic acid from cholic acid (Hellstrom and Sjovall, 1961; Lindstedt et al., 1957). Lithocholic acid, being poorly soluble, is poorly reabsorbed (Low-Beer et al., 1969) but nevertheless does have a small enterohepatic circulation (Norman and Palmer, 1964). Deoxycholic acid is as soluble as its precursor and at least as well reabsorbed, if not better (Hepner et al., 1971): it therefore has a considerable enterohepatic circulation.

There are two hepatic modifications of bile acids in man: 1) reconjugation of reabsorbed free bile acids with amino acids (glycine or taurine) prior to resecretion into the bile, 2) sufation of the glycine or taurine conjugates of lithocholic acid (Palmer, 1967; Palmer and Bolt, 1971). In man neither lithocholic nor deoxycholic acid are rehydroxylated (Norman and Palmer, 1964; Hepner et al., 1972; Hanson and Williams, 1971).

The theoretical modes whereby bile acids may be reabsorbed and recirculate enterohepatically may be summarized thus:

1. reabsorption of the unchanged conjugated bile acid
2. reabsorption of the dehydroxylated conjugated bile acid
3. reabsorption of the unaltered steroid moiety of the deconjugated bile acid, which is reconjugated in the liver prior to recycling
4. reabsorption of the dehydroxylated steroid moiety of the deconjugated bile acid which is reconjugated in the liver prior to recycling
5. reabsorption of the amino acid moiety of the deconjugated bile acid

The last is only a theoretical possibility since, following deconjugation, liberated glycine and taurine are oxidised by intestinal bacteria and not reabsorbed as such (Hepner et al.,1972a; Hepner et al.,1972b;

Hepner et al., 1973).

Bile Acid Pool and Turnover

Using a simple algebraic model for the enterohepatic circulation, in which an assumption is made of steady state and constant pool size, with bile acid loss replaced by concomitant hepatic synthesis, it is possible to calculate bile acid deconjugation and efficiency of intestinal reabsorption by determining the fractional turnover rate of other amino acid moiety and steroid moiety of conjugated bile acids (Hepner et al.,1972a; Hepner et al.,1972b; Hepner et al., 1973). The pool P is secreted C times daily into the duodenum. The fraction of the pool which is absorbed as the conjugated bile acid or the free steroid moiety (f_{abs} . pool) is increased by the synthesis of P ($1\text{-}f_{abs}$) per cycle or C.P ($1\text{-}f_{abs}$) daily. If some bile acid is deconjugated by bacterial enzymes within the intestinal lumen before returning to the liver, bile acid conjugation equals the sum of bile acid synthesis plus the amount of unconjugated bile acid returning to the liver. The mole fraction of the pool reabsorbed in conjugated form, N_{conj}. does not require conjugation; the unconjugated fraction absorbed per cycle equals P.f_{abs} ($1\text{-}N_{conj}$). Bile acid conjugation therefore equals C.P ($1\text{-}f_{abs} + f_{abs}$ ($1\text{-}N_{conj}$)) which can be reduced to C.P ($1\text{-}f_{abs}\cdot N_{conj}$). For conjugated bile acids conjugation, and hence deconjugation, equals the daily synthesis of the amino acid moiety of the conjugated bile acids, and it is thus possible to calculate the percentage of the conjugated bile acid deconjugated per cycle per day.

Using doubly-labeled bile acids, the pool size, daily fractional turnover rate and synthesis rate of the steroid and amino acid moieties of cholylglycine, chenodeoxycholylglycine, deoxycholylglycine and cholyltaurine have been determined (table 1) (Hepner et al., 1972a; Hepner et al., 1972b; Hepner et al., 1973). The efficiency of intestinal absorption of the steroid moiety of these bile acids was approximately 95%, assuming 6 daily enterohepatic cycles (a figure which accords well with recent studies (Brunner et al., 1972) showing that in health the bile acid pool recirculates 4—8 times per day). In four subjects in whom the metabolism of cholyltaurine was compared with that of chenodeoxycholyltaurine, the daily fractional turnover rate of the former was smaller in every case (figure 1). Chenodeoxycholic acid therefore seems to be more efficiently conserved than cholic acid, in accordance with similar studies by Vlahcevic et al.

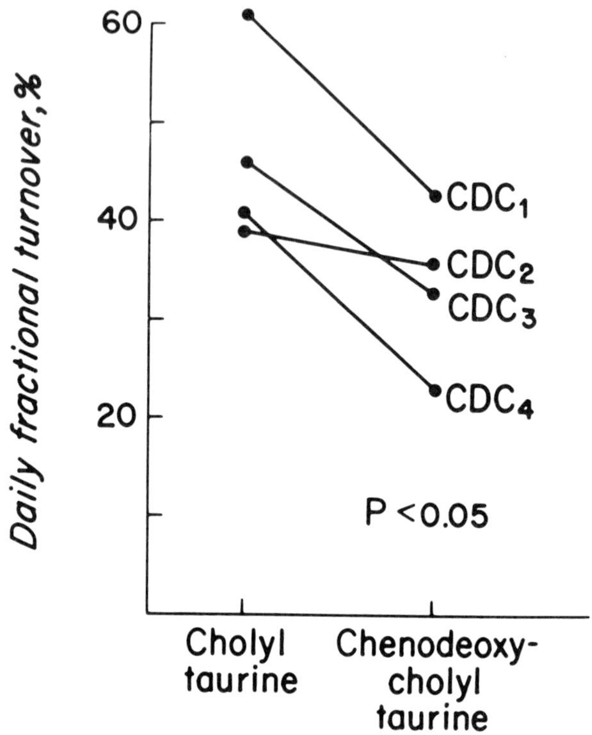

Fig. 1. Daily fractional turnover of cholyl moiety of cholyltaurine and chenodeoxycholyltaurine.

(Vlahcevic et al., 1971).

The daily fractional turnover rate of the glycine moiety of the glycine conjugated bile acids is about 120%, approximately three times that of the steroid moiety (table 1). This means that, assuming 6 enterohepatic cycles per day, about 20% of these bile acids are deconjugated per enterohepatic cycle. By contrast, only about 7% of cholyltaurine is deconjugated per cycle, and the same holds true for chenodeoxycholyltaurine (Hepner, Sturman, Thomas and Hofmann, unpublished data). Thus there is less deconjugation of taurine-conjugated than of glycine-conjugated bile acids during enterohepatic recirculation, due either to the greater resistance of taurine conjugated bile acids to bacterial deconjugated enzymes (Aries and Hill, 1970; Nair et al., 1967) or to greater efficiency of reabsorption of taurine-conjugated bile acids, with more proximal absorption and less

Table 1

Pool Size, Daily Fractional Turnover Rate and Synthesis Rate of Steroid and Amino Acid Moieties of Conjugated Bile Acid

	cholylglycine					chenodeoxycholylglycine				
		dft[1]		Synthesis			dft		Synthesis	
	pool	ch[2]	gly[3]	ch	gly	pool	CDC[4]	gly	CDC	gly
	mmoles	%		mmoles/day		mmoles	%		mmoles/day	
mean	3.00	38	106	1.05	3.18	1.61	29.9	125	0.47	1.98
SE	0.37	7	17	0.18	0.62	0.17	3.0	15	0.07	0.30

	deoxycholyglycine					cholyltaurine				
		dft		Synthesis			dft		Synthesis	
	pool	DC[5]	gly	DC	gly	pool	ch	taur[6]	ch	taur
	mmoles	%		mmoles/day		mmoles	%		mmoles/day	
mean	0.89	30.7	124	0.29	1.00	0.98	43.2	40.3	0.42	0.39
SE	0.10	4.0	9	0.05	0.15	0.10	3.7	4.4	0.05	0.04

1. Daily fractional turnover; 2. cholyl; 3. glycine; 4. chenodeoxycholy; 5. deoxycholyl
6. taurine

exposure to deconjugating bacteria. The greater fraction of bile acids is conjugated with glycine rather than taurine (Sjovall, 1960; Garbutt et al., 1971). This is probably due to the relative lack of the latter. When deconjugation is minimal, as in the neonate, most biliary bile acids are taurine conjugates (Enerantz and Sjovall, 1959; Poley et al., 1964); the fraction of taurine conjugates in the bile can be increased by feeding taurine (Hepner et al., 1973; Sjovall, 1959). Both these observations accord with the view that availability of taurine is the factor that limits its use for bile acid conjugation.

Absorption Sites

From the data, it is possible to infer the role of the terminal ileum and colon in the reabsorption of conjugated bile acids. Assuming 6 enterohepatic cycles per day and a glycine-conjugated bile acid pool of 5 mmoles, 30 mmoles of glycine-conjugated bile acids are secreted daily into the small intestine. Fecal loss, which in the steady state must equal daily synthesis, is 1.8 mmoles, or 0.3 mmole per cycle. Bile acid absorbed from the intestine as the free steroid moiety and as glycine-conjugated bile acid, is 28.2 mmoles. For glycine-conjugated bile acids 6 mmoles of glycine are used for bile acid conjugation, 1.8 for newly synthesized bile acid and 4.2 mmoles for reconjugation of bile acid absorbed in unconjugated form from the intestine. Thus 4.2/28.2, or about 15% of glycine-conjugated bile acids are absorbed in unconjugated form. This reabsorption presumably occurs in the distal ileum or colon, since it is there that anerobic deconjugating bacteria are found in greatest concentrations (Gorbach, 1971; Mallory et al., 1973; Gorbach and Tabaqchali, 1969), and free bile acids are found (Northfield and McColl, 1973; Mallory et al., 1973). For taurine-conjugated bile acids the daily fractional turnover rate of the steroid and taurine moieties is similar. The rate of deconjugation is about one third that of glycine-conjugated bile acids and therefore only about 5% of taurine-conjugated bile acids are absorbed in the terminal ileum and colon after deconjugation.

7-dehydroxylation is, like deconjugation, a bacterial biotransformation which occurs in the lumen of the distal small intestine and large intestine, and performed exclusively by fastidiously anerobic bacteria (Aries et al., 1971). Indeed, the organisms performing 7-dehydroxylation may be more fastidiously anerobic than those which deconjugate, since in vitro deconjugation, but not 7-dehydroxylation, has been performed using cell-free extracts from aerobic bacteria (Hepner et al., in press). In studies in which cholyl [^{14}C] glycine was administered to healthy control subjects, ^{14}C appeared in deoxycholyltaurine during the course of the study in only 4 of the 8 subjects who were studied (Hepner et al., 1972). The percentage of administered ^{14}C label that appeared in deoxycholylglycine was small in all cases, and it was concluded that although 7-dehydroxylation of cholylglycine can occur in vivo without prior deconjugation, 7-dehydroxylation mainly occurs following deconjugation of cholylglycine. (In vitro 7-dehydroxylation, in contrast to that occurring in vivo, can only occur when the substrate is the free bile acid (Aries et al., 1971)). In studies with cholyl [^{35}S] taurine no ^{35}S appeared in deoxycholyltaurine in the bile of any of 8 healthy controls who were studied (Hepner et al., 1973); for cholyltaurine, therefore, 7-dehydroxylation of the steroid moiety occurs only following deconjugation. In another study, the percentage of ^{3}H in deoxycholylglycine following the administration of [2-4-^{3}H] cholylglycine was studied in samples of duodenal bile taken from 12 healthy control subjects 24 hours following the administration of the labeled bile acid (Hepner et al., in press). In these subjects about 20% of cholylglycine was deconjugated per enterohepatic cycle, whereas about 2% of cholylglycine was 7-dehydroxylated at the same time. Since most of the 7-dehydroxylation occurs after deconjugation, these data indicate that in health not more than 10% of cholic acid liberated from cholylglycine is 7-dehydroxylated. The rate of deconjugation thus appears to exceed the rate of 7-dehydroxylation perhaps because deconjugating bacteria may be found more proximally than dehydroxylating bacteria (Percy-Robb et al., 1971).

ABNORMAL INTESTINAL AND BILIARY STATES

Ileal Disease

Abnormal metabolism of the steroid and amino moieties of conjugated bile acids have been described in patients with ileal disease, intestinal stagnant loops, gallbladder disease, biliary obstruction and celiac disease.

With ileal disease the conservation of the steroid moiety is impaired and its fractional turnover rate is increased (Austad et al., 1967; Stanley and Nemchausky, 1967; Heaton et al., 1968; Meihoff and Kern, 1968; Abaurre et al., 1969; Woodbury and Kern, 1971).

An increased percentage of the bile acid pool is exposed to the colon during each enterohepatic cycle, and while some reabsorption may occur there (Wingate et al., 1973), watery diarrhea termed "cholerrheic enteropathy" (more properly "cholanorrheic enteropathy") may ensue (Hofmann, 1967). Malabsorption of cholesterol due to ileal dysfunction could lead to decrease in bile acid pool size if the cholesterol pool were to decrease, since bile acids are metabolites of cholesterol. However, the malabsorption of cholesterol in fact leads to increased endogenous synthesis of cholesterol both in the liver and the intestine (Moutafis et al., 1968; Grundy et al., 1971) and to increased conversion of cholesterol into bile acids (Grundy et al., 1971). Thus the liver and intestine compensate for the increased loss of cholesterol, while the liver itself compensates for the increased loss of bile acids (Woodbury and Kern, 1971; Grundy et al., 1971; Dowling et al., 1970; Moore et al., 1969; Hofmann and Poley, 1972). Synthesis of bile acids may increase from 3 to 20 times normal, and the increased synthesis appears to correlate with the length of ileum resected (Woodbury and Kern, 1971; Hofmann and Poley, 1972).

Bile acid pool size diminishes, however, when malabsorption is so severe that increased hepatic bile acid synthesis cannot compensate for increased intestinal losses (Abaurre et al., 1969). Fat malabsorption may occur due to decreased jejunal bile acid concentration with decreased micellar solubilisation of lipids (Van Deest et al., 1968) and bile may become lithogenic (Dowling et al., 1972), leading to the observed increase in the incidence of cholesterol cholelithiasis in patients with ileal disease (Heaton and Read, 1969; Cohen et al., 1971). Increased deconjugation occurs and may be detected clinically by the "breath test" (Hepner et al., in press; Fromm and Hofmann, 1971; Sherr et al., 1971; Fromm et al., 1973) which will be described below. Increased deconjugation causes an increased requirement of amino acid for bile acid conjugation; the limited availability of taurine causes the percentage of taurine-conjugated bile acids to decrease with a reciprocal increase in the percentage of glycine conjugates (Garbutt et al., 1971; Austad et al., 1967; Abaurre et al., 1969). Deoxycholic acid may increase in the bile, due the increased exposure of bile acids to colonic anerobes following ileal malabsorption, but sometimes, however, deoxycholic acid disappears from the bile (Mitchell and Eastwood, 1972; Kern, 1971). This could be due to a) malabsorption of deoxycholic acid (but this is unlikely since it is not found in the stools of some of these patients), b) inhibition of 7-dehydroxylase by cholic acid, which is synthesized in increased amounts and thus may be found in the colon in increased concentrations (Floch et al., 1971; Percy-Robb and Collee, 1972), c) decrease in 7-dehydroxylating bacteria (Mallory et al., 1973), d) inhibition of 7-dehydroxylase by hydroxy fatty acids that are produced in the colon in excess because of the malabsorption of fat (James et al., 1961; Kinn and Spritz, 1968), and e) intestinal hurry, decreasing the time for the substrate, cholic acid, to react with 7-dehydroxylating enzymes (Percy-Robb et al., 1971; Garbutt et al.). There is little evidence to support any but the fifth mechanism.

Elegant experimental studies on the effect of ileal resection on the enterohepatic circulation of bile acids have been performed using rhesus monkeys (Dowling et al., 1965; Dowling et al., 1971; Small et al., 1972; Redinger and Small, 1972). These studies have facilitated a quantitative evaluation of bile acid loss following ileal resection, and of increased hepatic bile acid synthesis which occurs in response to the interruption of the return of bile acids to the liver. These studies have only limited relevance to human physiology since bile acid composition in the rhesus monkey differs significantly from that in the human (Redinger and Small, 1972). The rhesus monkey studies suggest that following ileal resection in the rhesus monkey a greater conservation of bile acids, presumably in the colon and possibly in the jejunum as well, occurs than has been described in humans with ileal resection. Certainly, the 20-fold increase in hepatic bile acid synthesis seen in some patients with ileal resection (Hofmann and Poley, 1972) was far greater than that seen in any of the rhesus monkey studies.

Intestinal stagnant loops

The intestinal stagnant loop syndrome is characterized by stagnation of intestinal content, secondary bacterial proliferation, and malabsorption of both fat and vitamin B_{12} (Booth et al., 1968). The pathogenesis of steatorrhea in this syndrome is imperfectly understood. Mucosal cell abnormalities have been seen by electron microscopy (Ament et al., 1972) but their cause is unknown. The bacterial proliferation is thought to be the cause of the bile acid abnormalities that characteristically occur when the stagnant loop is in the proximal part of the small intestine. Anerobic bacteria in the loops (Gorbach, 1971; Mallory et al., 1973; Gorbach and Tabaqchali, 1969; Mallory et al., 1973; Goldstein et al., 1961; Hill and Drasar, 1968; Mitvedt and Norman, 1967; Drasar and Shiner, 1969; Egger and Kessler, 1973) are capable of causing both 7-dehydroxylation and deconjugation (Aries and Hill, 1970; Nair et al., 1967; Aries et al., 1971; Egger and Kessler, 1973; Kim et al., 1966; Tabaqchali et al., 1968; Goldstein, 1971). When the loop is proximal, the secondary and free bile acids so formed accumulate (Northfield et al., 1973) since little, if any, jejunal absorption of bile acids occurs in man (Wingate et al., 1973). The increased deconjugation, with the increased requirements of amino acids for reconjugation, leads to a decrease in the percentage of taurine conjugated bile acids (Tabaqchali et al., 1968), as in patients with ileal resection (Austad et al., 1967; Abaurre et al., 1969). The increased concentrations of secondary, free and glycine-conjugated bile acids may contribute to the pathophysiology of the steatorrhea, but further studies on the interrelationship between intestinal flora, bile acids and mucosal structure and function clearly remain to be done.

Cholesterol Cholelithiasis and Cholecystectomy

The bile acid pool size of patients with cholesterol cholelithiasis is decreased (Hepner et al., in press; Vlahcevic et al., 1970; Bell et al., 1972). Conservation of the steroid moiety, as determined by its daily fractional turnover rate, appears to be normal and since bile acid synthesis equals the product of the pool size and the fractional turnover rate, bile acid synthesis is reduced. Enterohepatic cycling may be increased evidence of bacterial degradation of bile acids in these patients exists and suggests that enterohepatic cycling may be increased. This evidence includes a) increased deoxycholic acid concentrations in the bile, with concomitant increase in dihydroxy; trihydroxy ratio (Van der Linden, 1971; Heller and Bouchier, 1973), b) increased bacterial 7-dehydroxylation of [2-4-^{3}H] cholylglycine (Hepner et al., in press), and c) the presence of abnormal ketohydroxy bile acids (Hepner et al., in press). Such abnormal enterohepatic recycling may be secondary to disease of the gallbladder, or it may play a primary role in the pathogenesis of cholesterol cholelithiasis. Of especial interest is the observation that deoxycholic acid inhibits the synthesis of chenodeoxycholic acid (Low-Beer and Pomare, 1973); since the pool size of the latter is decreased in patients with cholesterol cholelithiasis it is tempting to speculate that this decrease may be related to the increase in bacterial degredation of cholic acid to deoxycholic acid, with a relative increase of the latter.

Following cholecystectomy, patients with cholesterol cholelithiasis have greatly increased bacterial degredation of their bile acid pool, with increased deoxycholic acid and abnormal keto-hydroxy bile acids in the bile as well as increased bacterial deconjugation of bile acids (Hepner et al., in press; Simmons et al., 1972; Pomare and Heaton, 1972).

Sprue

Patients with untreated adult celiac disease (non-tropical sprue), a disease in which there is subtotal villous atrophy of the proximal small intestinal but not usually of the ileal mucosa (Stewart et al., 1967), have been reported to have an increased bile acid pool size (Low-Beer et al., 1973). This is thought to be due to decreased enterohepatic recirculation of bile acids, explained as follows. The defective duodenal and jejunal mucosa leads to impaired release of cholecystokinin-pancreozymin (DiMagno et al., 1972), so that bile acids accumulate in the gallbladder rather than being released at mealtimes. Since bile acids remain in the gallbladder,bile acid feedback of hepatic bile acid synthesis is obviated and the bile acid pool size is able to increase (Low-Beer et al., 1973). Preliminary studies (Hepner, unpublished observations) have failed to show an increase in bile acid pool size in healthy volunteers who reduced the frequency of their enterohepatic cycles by abstaining from fat and proteins, and in the rhesus monkey fasting causes a decrease in bile acid pool size (Redinger et al., 1973). The observation in celiac patients therefore clearly needs more elucidation.

Tropical sprue differs from celiac disease anatomically in that the ileal as well as jejunal villous atrophy occur commonly (Lindenbaton, 1973). Bile acid pool size has not been measured in a group of these patients, but clearly it would be interesting to see the effect of the interaction of decreased enterohepatic cycling that might occur on account of the jejunal abnormality and the decreased ileal absorption due to ileal dysfunction. The former abnormality would predispose to an enlargement of the bile acid pool, the latter to a decrease. There are some data available on bile acid metabolism in a group of Bengali patients with this disease (Cassels et al., 1970; Nair et al., 1970). Free bile acids are found in the jejunum, but this is unlikely to be due to increased deconjugation per se since the ratio of taurine-conjugated to glycine-conjugated bile acids is increased rather than decreased. Biliary lithocholic acid decreases, while both chenodeoxycholic and deoxycholic acids decrease. Clearly further biliary studies are required to elucidate the abnormal bile acid metabolism that may occur in patients with this intriguing disease.

Hepato-Biliary Disease

The bile acid pool is not entirely confined to the enterohepatic circulation even in health. Bile acids can be assayed in the serum by either gas-liquid chromatography or radioimmunoassay (Sandberg et al., 1965; Roovers and Vanderhaege, 1968; Makino et al., 1969; Pellizari et al., 1973; Simmonds et al., 1974), and using either technique post-prandial rises in serum bile acids have been described (Roovers and Vanderhaege, 1968; Simmonds et al., 1974). In patients with hepato-biliary disease a variety of changes in bile acid metabolism have been described.

In cirrhosis, the bile acid pool size is decreased (Vlahcevic et al., 1971), as might be expected, since bile acids are synthesized in the liver. Deoxycholic acid concentration in the bile decreases. This may be due to more efficient reabsorption of the diminished cholic acid pool, with less exposure before reabsorption to 7-dehydroxylating bacterial enzymes. In keeping with this hypothesis, we have found (Hepner, unpublished observations) that deconjugation (like 7-dehydroxylation a bacterial biotransformation caused only by intestinal anerobes) is reduced in patients with cirrhosis in whom the bile acid pool size is diminished. Furthermore, we found that the percentage of taurine-conjugated bile acids rose in the bile, as was found in a previous study on serum bile acids in a group of cirrhotics (Neale et al., 1971); this finding, too, accords with decreased deconjugation, and hence relatively increased availability of taurine. There is an increased incidence of gallstones in cirrhotic patients (Bouchier, 1969; Nicholas et al., 1972), but this may not be related directly to the decreased bile acid pool size, since the stones in these patients have pigment rather than cholesterol nuclei (Nicholas et al., 1972; Vlahcevic et al., 1972). Serum bile acids are raised in patients with cirrhosis, and unconjugated bile acids, not found in the serum in health, but sometimes seen with cholestasis (Sandberg et al., 1965). have been reported.

Abnormal bile acids are found in serum and urine of patients with cholestasis (Makino et al., 1971; Williams et al., 1972; Murphy et al., 1972; Makino, 1973; Back, 1973; Yousef and Fisher, 1973; Javitt, 1968) and arginine conjugates have been found in the bile (Yousef and Fisher, 1973). Unusual bile acids in such patients could be of primary significance, and play a role in promoting cholestasis as has been experimentally produced with lithocholic acid (Javitt, 1968). On the other hand, unusual bile acids may be due to diminished exposure to intestinal bacterial or an increased exposure of bile acids to hepatocytes. An increased hepatic bile acid concentration has been described in patients with cholestasis (Murphy et al., 1972), but the significance of this finding has yet to be elucidated.

"Breath Test"

The enterohepatic circulation of cholylglycine acids may be conveniently assessed following the administration of cholyl [^{14}C] glycine by the "breath test" (Hepner et al., in press; Fromm and Hofmann, 1971; Sherr et al., 1971; Fromm et al., 1973) and that of cholyltaurine may be similarly studied by measuring the urinary excretion of ^{35}S following the administration of cholyl [^{35}S] taurine (Hanson and Williams, 1971). In health, the output of $^{14}CO_2$ 24 hours following the administration of cholyl [^{14}C] glycine correlates well with the rate of deconjugation of this bile acid (Hepner et al., 1972a; Hepner et al., 1972b; Hepner et al., 1973); this correlation also obtains when the rate of deconjugation is increased, as in patients with cholecystectomy (Hepner et al., in press). It is poor, however, in patients with greatly increased deconjugation due to ileal disease or ileal resection. In a group of patients with ileal resection studied by Fromm et al.(Fromm et al., 1973) the "breath test" was positive in only 18. In a similary study of 19 patients with regional ileitis or ileal resection, we found that the test was positive in only 12 patients (Hepner, unpublished observations). However, when we determined the percentage of $^{14}CO_2$ excreted in 24 hours which was excreted in the first 12 hours, we found that the technique clearly discriminated between healthy controls and patients with ileal dysfunction (figure 2). Modified thus, the breath test is an excellent non-invasive method of screening patients in whom the presence of an abnormal rate of bacterial deconjugation of conjugated bile acids is suspected.

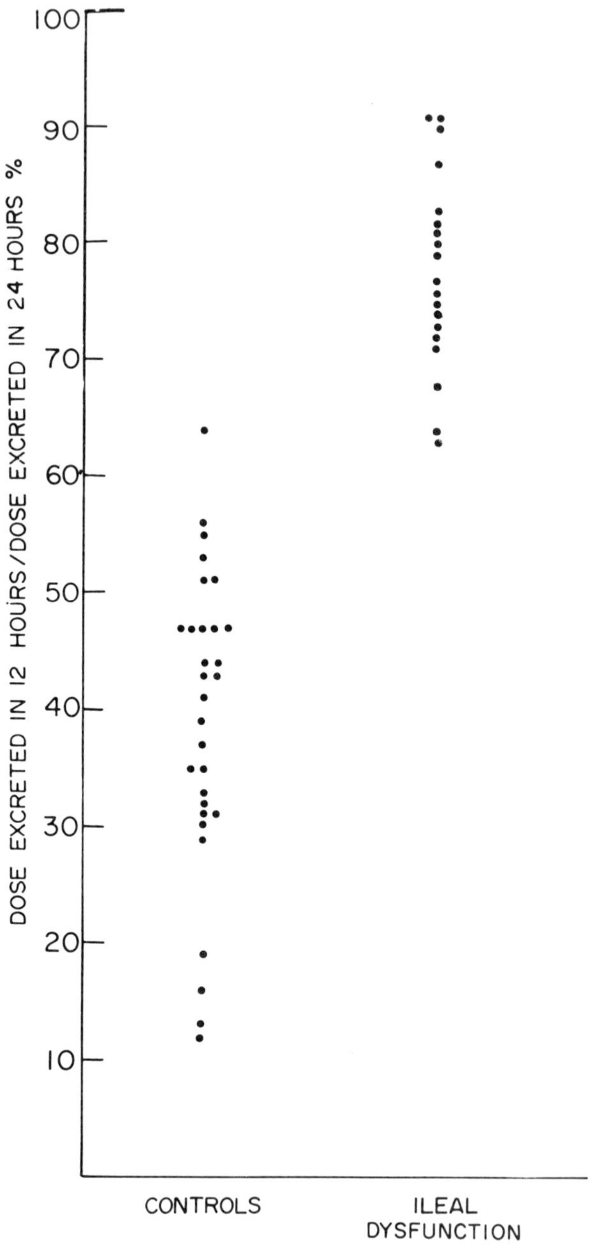

Fig. 2. Percentage of administered dose of cholyl [^{14}C] glycine excreted in $^{14}CO_2$ in 24 hours which was excreted in 12 hours.

REFERENCES

Abaurre,R., Gordon,S.G., Mann,J.G., and Kern,F., 1969.
Fasting bile salt pool size and composition after ileal resection.
Gastroenterology, 57:679.

Ament,M.E., Shimoda,S.S., Saunders,D.R., and Rubin,C.E., 1972.
Pathogenesis of steatorrhea in three cases of small intestinal stasis syndrome.
Gastroenterology, 63:728.

Aries,V.C., Goddard,P., and Hill,M.J., 1971.
Degredation of steroids by intestinal bacteria. III. 3oxo-5β-steroid Δ^{1}-dehydrogenase and 3-oxo-5β-Δ steroid ^{4}-dehydrogenase.
Biochim. Biophys. Acta., 248:482.

Aries,V., and Hill,M.J., 1970.
Degredation of steroids by intestinal bacteria. I. Deconjugation of bile salts.
Biochim. Biophys. Acta., 202:526.

Austad,W.I., Lack,L., and Tyor,M.P., 1967.
Importance of bile acids and of an intact distal small intestine for fat absorption.
Gastroenterology, 52:638.

Back,P., 1973.
Identification and quantitation determination of urinary bile acids excreted in cholestasis.
Clin. Chim. Acta, 44:199.

Bell,C.C., McCormick,W.C., Gregory,D.H., Law,D.H., Vlahcevic,Z.R., and Swell,L., 1972.
Relationship of bile acid pool size to the formation of lithogenous bile in male Indians of the Southwest.
Surg. Gynecol. Obstet., 134:473.

Bergstrom,V., Lundh,G., and Hofmann,A.F., 1963.
The site of absorption of conjugated bile salts in man.
Gastroenterology, 45:229.

Booth,C.C., Tabaqchali,S., and Mollin,D.L., 1968.
Comparison of stagnantloop syndrome with tropical sprue.
J. Clin. Nutr., 21:1047.

Bouchier,I.A.D., 1969.
Postmortem study of the frequency of gallstones in patients with cirrhosis of the liver.
Gut, 10:705.

Brunner,H., Hofmann,A.F., and Summerskill,W.H.J., 1972.
Daily secretion of bile acids and cholesterol measured in health.
Gastroenterology, 62:188, (Abstr.).

Cassels,J.S., Banwell,J.G., Gorbach,S.L. Mitra,R., and Mazumder,D.N.G., 1970.
Tropical sprue and malnutrition in West Bengal. IV. Bile salt deconjugation in tropical sprue.
Am. J. Clin. Nutr., 23:1579.

Cohen,S., Kaplan,M., Gottlieb,L., and Patterson,J., 1971.
Liver disease and gallstones in regional enteritis.
Gastroenterology, 60:237.

Dietschy,J.M., 1968.
Mechanisms for the intestinal absorption of bile acids.
J. Lipid Res., 9:197.

DiMagno,E.P., Go,V.L.W., and Summerskill,W.H.J., 1972.
Impaired cholecystokinin-pancreozymin secretion, intraluminal dilution, and maldigestion of fat in sprue.
Gastroenterology, 63:25.

Dowling,R.H., Bell,G.D., and White,J., 1972.
Lithogenic bile in patients with ileal dysfunction.
Gut, 13:415.

Dowling,R.H., Mack,E., and Small,D.M., 1970.
Effect of controlled interruption of the enterohepatic circulation of bile salts by biliary diversion and by ileal resection on bile salt secretion, synthesis and pool size in the rhesus monkey.
J. Clin. Invest., 49:232.

Dowling,R.H., Mack,E., and Small,D.M., 1971.
Primate biliary physiology. IV. Biliary lipid secretion and bile composition after acute and chronic interruption of the enterohepatic circulation in the Rhesus monkey.
J. Clin. Invest., 50:1917.

Drasar,B.S., and Shiner,M., 1969.
Studies on the intestinal flora. II. Bacterial flora of the small intestine in patients with gastrointestinal disorders.
Gut, 10:812.

Egger,G., and Kessler,J.I., 1973.
Clinical experience with a simple test for the detection of bacterial deconjugation of bile salts and the site and extent of bacterial overgrowth in the small intestine.
Gastroenterology, 64:545.

Enerantz,J.C., and Sjovall,J., 1959.
On the bile acids in duodenal contents of infants and children. Bile acids and steroids, 72.
Clin. Chim. Acta, 4:793.

Ertan,A., Brooks,F.P., Ostrow,J.D., Arvan,D.A., Williams,N., and Cerda,J.J., 1971.
Effect of jejunal amino acid perfusion and exogenous cholecystokinin on the pancreatic exocrine pancreatic and biliary secretions in man.
Gastroenterology, 61:686.

Floch,M.H., Gershengoren,W., Elliot,S., and Spiro,H.M., 1971.
Bile acid inhibition of the intestinal microflora--a function for simple bile acids?
Gastroenterology, 61:228.

Fromm,H., and Hofmann,A.F., 1971.
Breath test for altered bile-acid metabolism.
Lancet, 2:621.

Fromm,H., Thomas,P.J., and Hofmann,S.F., 1973.
Sensitivity and specificity in tests of distal ileal function: prospective comparison of bile acid and Vitamin B_{12} absorption in ileal resection patients.
Gastroenterology, 64:1077.

Garbutt,J.T., Lack,L., and Tyar,M.P., 1971.
Physiological basis of alterations in the relative conjugation of bile acids with glycine and taurine.
Am. J. Clin. Nutr., 24:218.

Garbutt,J.T., Wilkins,R.M., Lack,L., and Tyor,M.P.,
Bacterial modification of taurocholate during enterohepatic recirculation in normal man and patients with small intestinal disease.
Gastroenterology, 59:553.

Go,V.L.W., Hofmann,A.F., and Summerskill,W.H.J., 1970.
Pancreozymin assay in man based on pancreatic enzyme secretion potency of specific amino acids and other digestive products.
J. Clin. Invest., 49:1558.

Goldstein,F., 1971.
Mechanisms of malabsorption and malnutrition in the blind loop syndrome.
Gastroenterology, 61:780.

Goldstein,F., Wirts,C.W., and Dramer,S., 1961.
The relationship of afferent limb stasis and bacterial flora to the production of postgastrectomy steatorrhea.
Gastroenterology, 40:47.

Gorbach,S.L., 1971.
Intestinal microflora.
Gastroenterology, 60:1110.

Gorbach,S.L., and Tabaqchali,S., 1969.
Bacteria, bile and the small bowel.
Gut, 10:963.

Greim,H., Trulzsch,D., Czygan,P., Rudick,J., Hutterer, F., Schaffner,F., and Popper,H., 1972.
Mechanism of cholestasis. 6. Bile acids in human livers with or without biliary obstruction.
Gastroenterology, 63:846.

Grundy,S.M., Ahrens,E.H., and Salen,G., 1971.
Interruption of the enterohepatic circulation of bile acids in man: comparative effects of cholestyramine and ileal exclusion on cholesterol metabolism.
J. Lab. Clin. Med., 78:94.

Hanson,R.F., and Williams,G., 1971.
Metabolism of deoxycholic acid in bile fistula patients.
J. Lipid Res., 12:688.

Heaton,K.W., Austad,W.I., Lack,L., and Tyor,M.P., 1968.
Enterohepatic circulation of C^{14}-labeled bile salts in disorders of the distal small bowel.
Gastroenterology, 55:5.

Heaton,K.W., and Read,A.E., 1969.
Gallstones in patients with disorders of the terminal ileum and disturbed bile salt metabolism.
Brit. Med. J., 3:494.

Heller,F., and Bouchier,I.A.D., 1973.
Cholesterol and bile salt studies on the bile of patients with cholesterol gallstones.
Gut, 14:83.

Hellstrom,K., and Sjovall,J., 1961.
On the origin of lithocholic and ursodeoxycholic acids in man.
Acta Physiol. Scand., 51:218.

Hepner,G.W., Hofmann,A.F., Malagelada,J.R., Szczepanik, P.A., and Klein,P.D.
Increased bacterial degredation of bile acids in cholecystectomised subjects.
Gastroenterology, (In Press).

Hepner,G.W., Hofmann,A.F., and Thomas,P.J., 1972.
Metabolism of steroid and amino acid moieties of conjugated bile acids in man. I. Cholylglycine.
J. Clin. Invest., 51:1889.

Hepner,G.W., Hofmann,A.F., and Thomas,P.J., 1972.
Metabolism of steroid and amino acid moieties of conjugated bile acids in man. II. Glycineconjugated dihydroxy bile acids.
J. Clin. Invest., 51:1898.

Hepner,G.W., Sturman,J., Hofmann,A.F., and Thomas,P.J., 1973.
Metabolism of steroid and amino acid moieties of conjugated bile acids in man. III. Cholyltaurine.
J. Clin. Invest., 52:433.

Lindenbaton,J., 1973.
Tropical enteropathy.
Gastroenterology, 64:637.

Lindstedt,S., 1957.
The formation of deoxycholic acid from cholic acid in man. Bile acids and steroids 52.
Arkiv for Kemi, 11:145.

Low-Beer, T. S., and Pomare, E. W., 1973.
Regulation of bile salt pool size in man.
Brit. Med. J., 2: 338-340

Low-Beer,T.S., and Pomare,E.W., 1973.
Vholate pool size: its dependence on enterohepatic cycling frequency.
Gastroenterology, 64:763, (Abstr.).

Low-Beer, T. S., Pomare, E. W., Heaton, K. W., and Read, A. E., 1973
The effect of coeliac disease upon bile salts.
Gut, 14: 204-8

Low-Beer,T.S., Tyor,M., and Lack,L., 1969.
Effects of sulfation of taurolithocholic and glycolithocholic acids on their intestinal transport.
Gastroenterology, 56:721.

Makino,I., 1973.
Sulfated bile acid in urine of patients with hepatobiliary diseases.
Lipid, 8:47.

Makino,I., Nakagawa,S., and Mashimo,K., 1969.
Conjugated and unconjugated serum bile acid levels in patients with hepatobiliary disease.
Gastroenterology, 56:1033.

Makino,I., Sjovall,J., Norman,A., and Strandvik,B., 1971.
Excretion of 3β-hydroxy-4-cholenoic and 3β-hydroxy-5α-cholanoic acids in urine of infants with biliary atresia.
FEBS Letters, 15:161.

Mallory,A., Kern,F., Smith,J., and Savage,D., 1973.
Patterns of bile acids and microflora in the human small intestine.
Gastroenterology, 64:26.

Hill,M.J., and Drasar,B.S., 1968.
Degredation of bile salts by human intestinal bacteria.
Gut, 9:22.
Hofmann,A.F., 1967.
The syndrome of ileal disease and the broken enterohepatic circulation: cholerheic enteropathy.
Gastroenterology, 52:752.
Hofmann,A.F., and Poley,J.R., 1972.
Role of bile acid malabsorption in pathogenesis of diarrhea and steatorrhea in patients with ileal resection. I. Response to cholestyramine or replacement of dietary long-chain triglycerides with medium chain triglycerides.
Gastroenterology, 62:918.
Hofmann,A.F., and Small,D.M., 1967.
Detergent properties of bile salts: correlation with physiological function.
Ann. Rev. Med., 18:333.
James,A.T., Webb,J.P.W., and Kellock,T.D., 1961.
The occurrence of unusual fatty acids in fecal lipids from human beings with normal and abnormal fat absorption.
Biochem. J., 78:333.
Javitt,N., Ennerman,S., 1968.
Effect of sodium taurolithocholate on bile flow and bile acid excretion.
J. Clin. Invest., 47:1002.
Kern,F., 1973.
Disappearance of deoxycholic acid after ileal resection.
Gastroenterology, 64:123.
Kim,Y.S., Spritz,N., Blum,M., Terz,J., and Sherlock,P., 1966.
The role of altered bile acid metabolism in the steatorrhea of experimental blind-loop.
J. Clin. Invest., 45:956.
Kinn,Y.S., and Spritz,N., 1968.
Hydroxy acid excretion in steatorrhea of pancreatic and non-pancreatic origin.
N. Engl. J. Med., 179:1424.

Mallory,A., Savage,D., Kern,F., and Smith,J.G., 1973.
Patterns of bile acids and microflora in the human small intestine. II. Microflora.
Gastroenterology, 64:34.

Meihoff,W.E., and Kern,F., 1968.
Bile salt malabsorption in regional ileitis, ileal resection and mannitol-induced diarrhea.
J. Clin. Invest., 47:261.

Mitchell,W.D., and Eastwood,M.A., 1972.
Faecal bile acids and neutrol steroids in patients with ileal dysfunction.
Scand. J. Gastroenterology, 7:29.

Mitvedt,T., and Norman,A., 1967.
Bile acid transformations by microbial strains belonging to genera found in intestinal contents.
Acta Pathol. Microbiol. Scand., 71:629.

Moore,R.S., Frantz,I.D., and Buchwald,H., 1969.
Change in cholesterol pool size, turnover rate and fecal bile acids and sterol excretion after partial ileal bypass in hypercholesterolemic patients.
Surgery, 65:98.

Moutafis,D.C., Myant,N.B., and Tabaqchali,S., 1968.
The metabolism of cholesterol after resection of bypass of the lower small intestine.
Clin. Sci., 35:537.

Murphy,G.M., Jansen,F.H., and Billing,B.H., 1972.
Unsaturated monohydroxy bile acids in cholestatic liver disease.
Biochem. J., 129:491.

Nair,P.P., Banwell,J.G., Gorbach,S.L., Lilis,C., and Alcaraz,A., 1970.
Tropical sprue and malnutrition in West Bengal. III. Biochemical characteristics of bile salts in the small intestine.
Am. J. Clin. Nutr., 23:1569.

Nair,P.P., Gordon,M., and Reback,J., 1967.
The enzymatic cleavage of the carbon-nitrogen bond in 3α, 7α, 12α -trihydroxy-β-cholan-24-oylglycine.
J. Biol. Chem., 242:7.

Neale,G., Lewis,B., Weaver,V., and Panveliwalla,D., 1971.
Serum bile acids in liver disease.
Gut, 12:145.
Nicholas,P., Rinauso,P.A., and Conn,H.O., 1972.
Increased incidence of cholelithiasis in Laenac's cirrhosis.
Gastroenterology, 63:112.
Norman,A., and Palmer,R.H., 1964.
Metabolites of lithocholic acid-24-C^{14} in human bile and feces.
J. Lab. Clin. Med., 63:986.
Northfield,T.C., Drasar,B.S., and Wright,J.T., 1973.
Value of small intestinal bile analysis in the diagnosis of the stagnant loop syndrome.
Gut, 14:341.
Northfield,T.C., and McColl,I., 1973.
Postprandial concentrations of free and conjugated bile acids down the length of the normal human small intestine.
Gut, 14:513.
Palmer,R.H., 1967.
The formation of bile acid sulfates: a new pathway of bile acid metabolism in humans.
Proc. Nat. Acad. Sci., 58:1047.
Palmer,R.H., and Bolt,M.G., 1971.
Bile acid sulfates. I. Synthesis of lithocholic acid sulfates and their identification in human bile.
J. Lipid Res., 12:671.
Pellizari,E.D., O'Neil,F.S., Farmer,R.W., and Fabre, L.F., 1973.
Identification of lithocholic acid and measurement of other bile acids in serum of healthy humans.
Clin. Chem., 19:248.
Percy-Robb,I.W., Brunton,W.A.T., Gould,J.C., Kalan,K.N., McManus,J.P.A., and Sircus,W., 1971.
Composition and bile salt transforming capacity of the bacterial flora of ileal effluent in patients with ileostomies.
Scand. J. Gastroenterology, 6:625.

Percy-Robb,I.W., and Collee,J.G., 1972.
Bile acids: a pH dependent antibacterial system in the gut?
Brit. Med. J., 3:813.
Percy-Robb,I.W., Jalan,K.N., McManus,J.P.A., and Sircus, W., 1971.
Effect of ileal resection on bile salt metabolism in patients with ileostomh following proctocolectomy.
Clin. Sci., 41:371.
Poley,J.R., Dower,J.C., Owens,C.A., and Shickler,G.B., 1964.
Bile acids in infants and children.
J. Lab. Clin. Med., 63:838.
Pomare,E.W., and Heaton,K.W., 1972.
Increased bacterial degredation of bile salts in cholecystectomised subjects, in bile acids in human diseases, (Edit. by Back,P., and Gerok,W.).
F.K. Schattauer Verlag, Stuttgart, p. 209.
Redinger,R.N., Hermann,A.H., and Small,D.M., 1973.
Primate biliary physiology. X. Effects of diet and fasting on biliary lipid secretion and relative composition and bile salt metabolism in the rhesus monkey.
Gastroenterology, 64:610.
Redinger,R.N., and Small,D.M., 1972.
Bile composition, bile salt metabolism and gallstones.
Arch. Intern. Med., 130:618.
Roovers,J., Evrard,E., and Vanderhaege,H., 1968.
An improved method for measuring human blood bile acids.
Clin. Chim. Acta, 19:449.
Samuel,P., Saypol,G.M., Meilman,E., Mosbach,E., and Chafizadeh,M., 1968.
Absorption of bile acids from the large bowel in man.
J. Clin. Invest., 47:2070.
Sandberg,D.H., Sjovall,J., Sjovall,K., and Turner,D.A., 1965.
Measurement of human serum bile acids by gas-liquid chromatography.
J. Lipid Res., 6:182.

Sherr,H.P., Sasaki,Y., Newman,A., Banwell,J.G., Wagner, H.N., and Mendrix,T.R., 1971.
Detection of bacterial deconjugation of bile salts by a convenient breath-analysis technique.
N. Engl. J. Med., 285:656.

Simmonds,W.J., Korman,M.G., Go,V.L.W., and Hofmann, A.F., 1974.
Radioimmunoassay of conjugated bile acids in serum.
Gastroenterology, (In Press).

Simmons,F., Ross,A.P.J., and Bouchier,I.A.D., 1972.
Alterations in hepatic bile composition after cholecystectomy.
Gastroenterology, 63:466.

Sjovall,J., 1959.
Dietary glycine and taurine on bile acid conjugation in man.
Proc. Soc. Exp. Biol. Med., 100:676.

Sjovall,J., 1960.
Bile acids in man under normal and pathological conditions. Bile acids and steroids, 73.
Clin. Chim. Acta 5:33.

Small,D.M., Dowling,R.H., and Redinger,R.N., 1972.
The enterohepatic circulation of bile salts.
Arch. Intern. Med., 130:551.

Stanley,M.M., and Nemchausky,B., 1967.
Fecal C^{14}-bile acid excretion in normal subjects and patients with steroid-wasting syndromes secondary to ileal dysfunction.
J. Lab. Clin. Med., 70:627.

Stewart,J.S., Pollock,D.J., Hoffbrand,A.V., Mollin,D.L., and Booth,C.C., 1967.
A study of proximal and distal intestinal structure and absorptive function in idiopathic steatorrhea.
Q. J. Med., 36:425.

Tabaqchali,S., Hatzioannou,J., and Booth,C.C., 1968.
Bile-salt deconjugation and steatorrhea in patients with the stagnant-loop syndrome.
Lancet, 2:12.

Tyor,M., Garbutt,J.T., and Lack,L., 1972.
Metabolism and transport of bile salts in the intestine.
Am. J. Med., 51:614.

VanDeest,B.W., Fordtran,J.S., Morawski,S.G., and Wilson,J.D., 1968.
Bile salt and micellar fat concentration in proximal small bowel contents of ileectomised patients.
J. Clin. Invest., 47:1314.

Van der Linden,W., 1971.
Bile acid pattern of patients with and without gallstones.
Gastroenterology, 60:1144.

Vlahcevic,Z.R., Bell,C.C., Buha,I., Farrar,J.T., and Swell,L., 1970.
Diminished bile acid pool size in patients with gallstones.
Gastroenterology, 59:165.

Vlahcevic,Z.R., Buhac,I., Farrar,J.T., Bell,C.C., and Swell,L., 1971.
Bile acid metabolism in patients with cirrhosis. I. Kinetic aspects of cholic acid metabolism.
Gastroenterology, 60:491.

Vlahcevic,Z.R., Miller,J.R., Farrar,J.T., and Swell,L., 1971.
Kinetics and pool size of primary bile acids in man.
Gastroenterology, 61:85.

Vlahcevic,Z.R., Yoshida,T., Juttijudata,P., Bell,C.C., and Swell,L., 1973.
Bile acid metabolism in cirrhosis. III. Biliary lipid secretion in patients with cirrhosis and its relevance to gallstone formation.
Gastroenterology, 64:298.

Williams,C.N., Kaye,R., Bkaer,L., Hurwitz,R., and Senior,J.R., 1972.
Progressive familial cholestatic cirrhosis and bile acid metabolism.
Pediatrics, 81:493.

Wingate,D.L., Phillips,S.F., and Hofmann,A.F., 1973.
Effect of glycine-conjugated bile acids with and without lecithin on water and glucose absorption in perfused human jejunum.
J. Clin. Invest., 52:1230.

Woodbury,J.F., and Kern,F., 1971.
Fecal excretion of bile acids: a new technique for studying bile acid kinetics in patients with ileal resection.
J. Clin. Invest., 50:2531.

Yousef,I.M., and Fisher,M.M., 1973.
The biliary secretion of cholyl arginine.
Gastroenterology, 65:577.

ABSORPTIVE FUNCTIONS OF GALLBLADDER

Richard C. Rose

INTRODUCTION

Electrolyte transport by gallbladder epithelium has been studied in several laboratories under a variety of conditions in vivo and in vitro. The gallbladders of all species studied are capable of absorbing water and salts. Thus, there is sufficient evidence to conclude that the function of the gallbladder in situ is to concentrate bile detained enroute to the small intestine. The active transport of certain salts, notably NaCl, from mucosa to serosa appears to be the primary driving force in absorption; water is thought to follow passively according to an osmotic gradient.

Many important similarities in the basic properties of transport and permeability appear to exist between gallbladder and other important transporting epithelia. When investigated in vitro the gallbladders from different species are found to develop a continum of transmural electrical potential differences (PD) from −1 to +7 mv (serosa with respect to mucosa). A systematic investigation of the gallbladder of each species is to be encouraged, with the goal of identifying the biologic property or event which differs between them to explain why gallbladders from some species develop transmural PDs whereas those from other species do not. Such information would be of special value because it might further our understanding of transport properties of related epithelia, such as intestine. Finally, a study of human gallbladder freshly acquired following cholecystectomy for the usual medical reasons might help us to better understand the physiology of the gallbladder in health and various stages of disease.

A common means of investigating the mechanism of the active transport of ions in epithelial tissues is to relate net movement of anions and cations to the electrical properties of the tissue under well defined conditions in vitro. Until recently the primary species used for gallbladder studies were rabbit, fish and guinea pig. Several investigators have reported that during absorption these tissues develop little or no transmural electrical PD when bathed on both sides with the same buffered electrolyte solution (Dietschy, 1966; Diamond, 1962b; Cremaschi et al., 1971); in this respect these gallbladders differed from the epithelia of intestine (Rose and Schultz, 1971), stomach (Rehm, 1950), kidney (Boulpaep, 1967), and other transporting organs. The conclusion was drawn that the active transport process in gallbladder is unique by having a coupled active transport of Na and Cl across the serosal and/or lateral aspects of the cell membrane (Diamond, 1962b; Wheeler, 1963; Dietschy, 1964).

Recently, information has been obtained on the gallbladders of several species (man, goose, and rhesus, stump tail and African green monkeys) which differ from those previously studied by developing a significant serosa-positive PD (Rose et al., 1973; Gelarden and Rose, 1973). Information on human gallbladder is the most complete, and will be presented in the greatest detail.

METHODS OF STUDY

Cholecystectomies were performed in the Department of Surgery for the usual medical indications. All patients were symptomatic and gallstones were present in all patients except one patient in whom cholecystectomy was performed to relieve recurrent upper-right-quadlant pain not associated with cholelithiasis. Our research procedures were performed on the fundus of the gallbladder; the remainder of the organ was sent to the Department of Pathology for histologic examination. The section of tissue to be used by us was immediately placed in control Ringer solution at $0^{o}C$ and brought to the laboratory. Bile was removed from the mucosal surface by repeatedly washing the tissue in Ringer solution. The serosa was removed by blunt dissection before mounting the tissue.

The lucite bathing chamber and apparatus for measuring the transmural electrical potential difference (PD) and short circuit current (Isc) have been described elsewhere (Rose et al., 1973). Briefly, 1.13 cm^2 of tissue was held between the halves of the bathing chamber and exposed on each surface to 15 ml of Ringer solution 38°C. The composition of the Ringer solution was (in mM); NaCl, 142; $MgCl_2$, 1.2; $CaCl_2$, 0.9; K_2HPO_4, 4.2; KH_2PO_4, 1.5; and glucose, 5.5.

The bathing solution was perfused across each surface of the tissue by means of a gas-lift circulating system driven by water-saturated 100% O_2. The reservoirs were capped with glass condensers to minimize water loss by evaporation. In instances where Ringer solution containing HCO_3 was used, the solutions were bubbled with 95% O_2–5% CO_2.

The tips of Ringer-agar bridges were located close to each membrane surface and the PD was measured using a pair of matched calomel electrodes leading to a high-impedance electrometer (Keithley, model 602). Electrical asymmetry, measured prior to mounting the tissue and again at the end of each experiment, did not exceed 0.4 mv and corrections were made for this asymmetry during electrical measurements.

The tissue was short-circuited by applying external current through Ag-AgCl electrodes connected to a variable electromotive force. Current was passed to the extreme ends of the bathing chamber through Ringer-agar bridges; the magnitude of the applied current was measured on a Simpson microammeter. The Isc was corrected for fluid resistance so that the PD across the tissue was completely nulled during ion flux determinations. Tissue resistance was determined by recording the PD deflection in response to 50 ua of direct current from the external battery source.

Unidirectional transmural fluxes of Na and Cl were determined using ^{22}Na and ^{36}Cl. Because the tissues maintained a reasonably constant Isc for 3 to 5 hrs, it was usually practical to determine the oppositely directed unidirectional fluxes of an ion on each piece of tissue. The determination of the mucosa to serosa Na flux, for example, was made by adding a tracer quantity of ^{22}Na to 15 ml of Ringer solution in the mucosal reservoir. Aliquots of 1.0 ml were withdrawn from the serosal reservoir at 15 min intervals. Following sample removal, 1.0 ml of Ringer solution was added to the reservoir

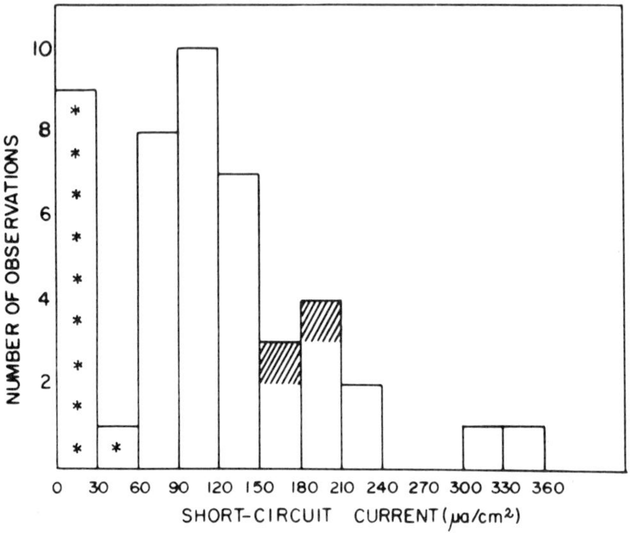

Fig. 1. A histogram of maximum short-circuit current of 46 samples of human gallbladder in control Ringer solution. Asterisks indicate tissue samples from inflamed gallbladders. Crosshatched areas represent I_{SC} values of two samples from a gallbladder removed for upper-right-quadrant pain not associated with cholelithiasis (From Rose et al., 1973).

to maintain constant volume. A 0.1 ml aliquot was withdrawn from the mucosal reservoir at the beginning and end of each experiment to use in determining specific activity. Radioisotopes were assayed in 10 ml of Aquasol using a well-type liquid scintillation counter. Net fluxes of Na and Cl were calculated as the difference between oppositely directed unidirectional fluxes determined sequentially on the same piece of tissue.

ELECTRICAL PROPERTIES OF GALLBLADDER

Transmural Electrical Potentials

Measurements of transmural PD were made on 46 samples of human gallbladder (table 1); in each instance the serosal surface was electropositive with respect to the mucosal surface with the maximum PD of the individual samples ranging from 0.8 to 13.1 mv. A histogram of the maximum Isc values is shown in figure 1. An asterisk indicates tissue samples from gallbladders which were

Table 1

Electrical Properties of Gallbladders (38°)

Species	PD (mv)	P_{Cl}/P_{Na}	R (Ω–cm^2)
Rabbit	–0.4	.32	23
Dog	0.2	.63	46
Stump tail monkey	1.5	.16	35
Rhesus monkey	2.5	.32	27
African green monkey	2.7	.29	35
Goose	3.6	.30	30
Human	7.6	.76	52

The sign of the spontaneous PD refers to the serosal surface. P_{Cl}/P_{Na} was calculated on the basis of diffusion potentials as discussed in the text.

reported by the pathologist to be acutely or chronically imflamed on the basis of light microscopy. The cross-hatched areas represent two samples of tissue from a gallbladder removed for recurrent right-upper-quadrant pain not associated with cholelithiasis; its epithelium was reported to be histologically normal. The remaining 34 tissue samples came from gallbladders which did not have stones, but which were reported to be histologically indistinguishable from normal gallbladder epithelium. There is clearly a greater electrical activity generated by the histologically normal samples of gallbladder tissue than by the diseased samples. Some possible clinical implications of these observations will be discussed toward the end of this presentation.

The significant observation from figure 1 is that normal human gallbladder epithelium developes an average serosa-positive transmural PD of 7.6 mv and an average short-circuit current of 136 ua/cm^2.

Serosa positive PDs were also consistently measured across the gallbladder wall of several other species. In these studies, gallbladders were removed immediately after sacrifice by pentobarbital

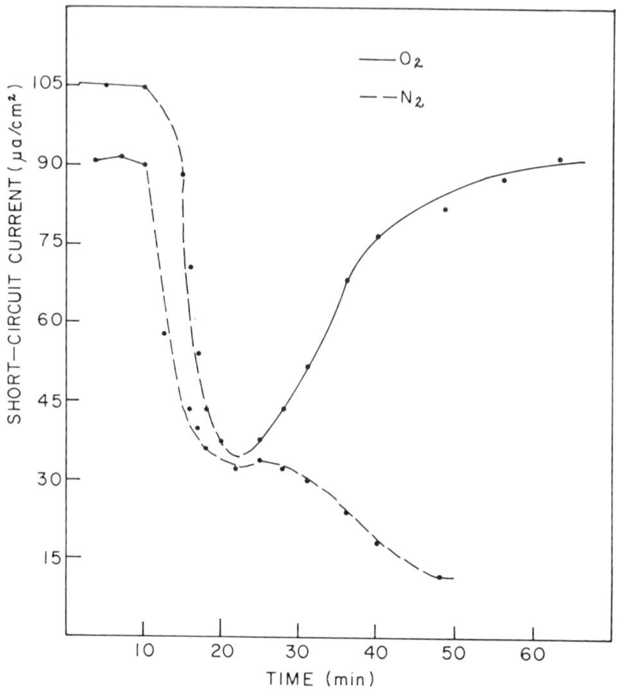

Fig. 2. Effect of anaerobiosis on I_{sc} of two paired tissues of human gallbladder. Effect is reversible if depletion of O_2 lasts no longer than 10 min. Solid lines represent time when O_2 is supplied; dashed lines represent time of O_2 depletion (From Rose et al., 1973).

injection. The serosa-positive PDs developed by the gallbladders of goose, rhesus monkey, African green monkey and stump tail monkey are reported in table 1. Also shown is the average PD across dog gallbladder (essentially zero) and the small serosa-negative PD of rabbit gallbladder. The PD of rabbit gallbladder was more serosa-negative and closer to the value reported by Machen and Diamond (1969) when the tissue was bathed in Ringer solution which contained HCO_3.

Effect of Anaerobiosis

Elimination of O_2 from the bathing solution resulted in a prompt reduction of Isc as shown in figure 2. By the end of 40–50 minutes of anaerobic conditions the Isc was usually eliminated. If the O_2 supply was restored after no longer than 10 minutes of anaerobic

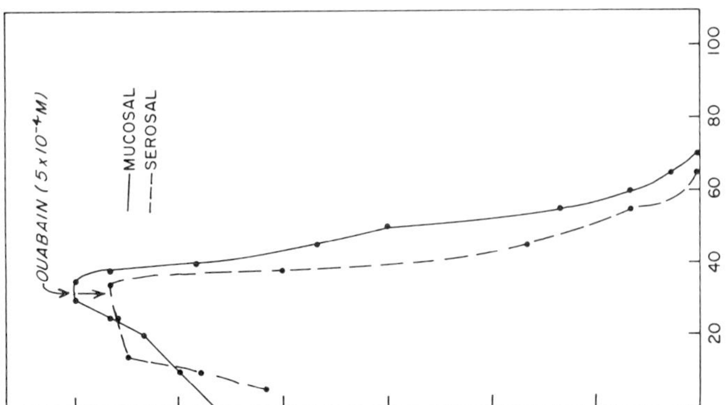

Figure 3

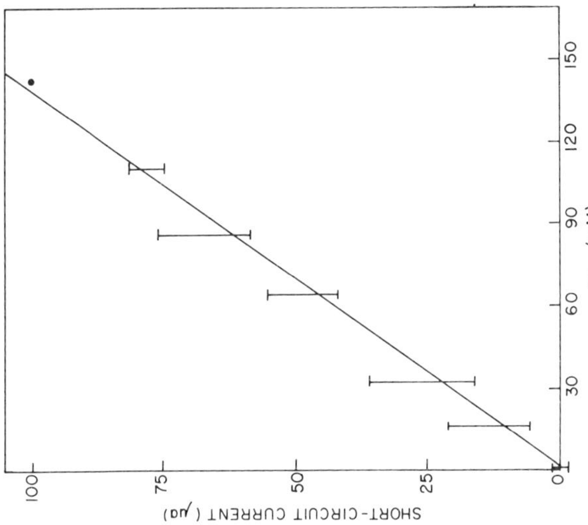

Figure 4

Fig. 3. Effect of ouabain in mucosal or serosal bathing solution on I_{sc} of two paired tissues of human gallbladder (From Rose et al., 1973).

Fig. 4. Effect of I_{sc} of reducing Na concentration in mucosal and serosal bathing solutions. Average initial I_{sc} was 104 u a at Na = 142 mM. Na replaced by choline. Human gallbladder. (From Rose et al., 1973).

---

conditions the electrical activity would usually return to its original value. Tissue resistance increased by approximately 20% during treatment with N_2, which may be attributed to swelling of the epithelial cells which would restrict passive diffusion of ions through extracellular channels of the tissue. The gallbladders of geese and monkey responded similarily to anaerobic conditions except that the resistance of these tissues did not change significantly.

Effect of Ouabain

Cardiac glycosides in low concentrations have been shown to inhibit active transport in several epithelial tissues. The effect of ouabain (5×10^{-4}M) on the Isc of human gallbladder is shown in figure 3. It is seen that ouabain is as effective in inhibiting the Isc when present in the mucosal solution as when present in the serosal solution. In contrast, ouabain in the serosal solution is much more effective in inhibiting the electrical activity of gallbladders from fish, monkeys and geese. A ouabain-sensitive Na-K stimulated ATPase system has been demonstrated in rabbit and guinea pig gallbladder epithelium (van Os and Slegers, 1971), but apparently has not been looked for in other gallbladder epithelia.

Ion Substitution Experiments

Experiments were performed to determine which cations and anions were necessary in the bathing solution for maintaining the electrical activity of gallbladder epithelia. The Na concentration was sequentially reduced from 142 mEq/liter (control Ringer solution) to zero by replacing Na with choline in the mucosal and serosal bathing solutions. The Isc was allowed to decline to a new fairly stable level before each successive dilution was made. A liner relation between Isc and the Na concentration (figure 4) suggests that Na transport is responsible for the observed transmural PD.

Abrupt total replacement of NaCl in the mucosal and serosal bathing solutions by choline chloride or KCl resulted in a transitory reversal of the PD which may be due either to a greater permeability of one surface of the cell membrane to choline or K than the opposite cell surface (Schultz and Zalusky, 1964), or to an asymmetry of unstirred layers at the mucosal and serosal cell borders (Barry and Diamond, 1970). These conditions could also explain the transitory PDs as large as +25 mv observed upon return to control conditions. The PD of goose and monkey gallbladders was also dependent on the presence of Na in the bathing solution. Diamond (1962a) found that removal of Na from the bathing solution eliminated fluid absorption by the fish gallbladder.

The choice of anions in the bathing solution for maintaining the electrical activity of the gallbladder was not as critical. Replacement of Cl by Br in both the mucosal and serosal bathing solutions of gallbladders of goose, monkey and man reduced the Isc by no more than 15%. Replacement of Cl by SO_4 reduced the Isc of human gallbladder by 30%. In SO_4-substituted Ringer solution the human gallbladder maintained an Isc as high as 70 u a/cm^2 for four hours. However, in goose and monkey gallbladders replacement of SO_4 for Cl abolished the Isc. Replacement of isethionate for Cl abolished the Isc of all goose gallbladders tested, but under these conditions some monkey gallbladders were able to maintain 50–75% of the Isc they had in control Ringer. Diamond (1962a) found that replacement of Cl by Br had little effect on fluid absorption but replacement by SO_4 in the mucosal solution eliminated absorption. Maximal rates of fluid absorption in rabbit gallbladder depended on the presence of Na and Cl in the mucosal bathing solution (Wheeler, 1963).

The presence of a Na-K stimulated ATPase in rabbit gallbladder suggests that the presence of K might be necessary for maximal transport. Elimination of K from the bathing solution did reduce electrolyte transport by fish gallbladder (Diamond, 1962a) and by rabbit gallbladder in the hands of Frederiksen and Leyssac (1969) but not Diamond (1964)

ION TRANSPORT

Ion Flux Determinations

The finding that the serosa-positive PD of human gallbladder is highly dependent on the presence of Na but not Cl in the bathing solution suggests that the PD might result from active transport of Na from mucosa to serosa in the absence of simultaneous net Cl transport. Unidirectional fluxes of Na and Cl from mucosa to serosa (J_{ms}) and serosa to mucosa (J_{sm}) were measured under short-circuit conditions to test this possibility. It is seen (table 2) that net Na flux calculated from the average of all J_{ms}^{Na} and J_{sm}^{Na} determinations is not significantly different in magnitude from the average Isc determined simultaneously. The net Cl flux calculated from the average of all determinations of J_{ms}^{Cl} and J_{sm}^{Cl} is not significantly different from zero.

From the results of experiments described thus far we might reasonably conclude that the electrical properties of gallbladders are in some way related to active transport of ions, particularly Na, from mucosa to serosa by the tissue epithelium. One important theoretical question remains unanswered: Why do the gallbladders of man, goose and monkey develop serosa positive potentials whereas the dog gallbladder has a transmural PD of essentially zero and rabbit gallbladder has a slightly serosa-negative PD? It is possible, of course, that a species difference exists in the primary active transport mechanism. Thus, in gallbladders of rabbit and dog the carrier molecule might obligatorily transport Na and Cl, as originally proposed by Diamond, (1962b) whereas the gallbladders of the human, goose and monkey might actively transport only Na with Cl following according to the serosa-positive PD. Before we accept this major species difference in the primary transport mechanism, however, at least two other possible causes of different electrical potential profiles should be considered.

Machen and Diamond (1969) suggested that a coupled transport of NaCl at the lateral surface of the epithelial cell produces a slightly hypertonic solution of sodium chloride within the lateral intercellular space. Because the tight junction is cation selective (Diamond, 1962b) Na in this hypertonic solution tends to diffuse more rapidly than Cl back across the tight junction into the mucosal solution. According to this scheme a diffusion potential would result with the serosal solution becoming electronegative with respect to the mucosal solution, which would account for the PD actually measured across rabbit gallbladder (Wheeler, 1963; Machen and Diamond, 1969; present observations, table 1). Thus, the possibility seemed to exist that gallbladders of man, goose and monkey could have the same coupled NaCl transport mechanism as that proposed for rabbit gallbladder, but if the tight junctions of these gallbladders

Table 2

Ion Flux Determinations on Human Gallbladder

Ion	J_{ms}	J_{sm}	J_{net}	I_{sc}
Na	11.4 ± 0.8 (33)	7.0 ± 0.4 (28)	4.4 ± 0.3	3.8 ± 0.4
Cl	7.1 ± 0.3 (15)	6.7 ± 0.2 (18)	0.4 ± 0.2	4.6 ± 0.4

Values are u Eq/cm^2—hr ± SE with the number of 15 min observation period given in parentheses. Isc is reported as flux of a monovalent cation from mucosa to serosa. (From Rose et al., 1973).

were selectively permeable to anions rather than cations the faster back diffusion of Cl from the lateral intercellular space toward the mucosal solution would result in the observed serosa-positive PD. Therefore, experiments were performed to compare the anion-cation selectivity of each of the gallbladders in question.

Diffusion Potentials

After the spontaneous PDs of gallbladders from each species had reached a stable value as described above, diffusion potentials were artifically established across the tissue; preliminary results of these observations (Gelarden and Rose, unpublished observation) are presented. The mucosal and serosal solutions were changed from control Ringer to a buffered electrolyte solution of the following composition (in mM): NaCl, 142; $MgCl_2$, 1.2; $CaCl_2$, 0.9; and mannitol, 12. After the PD had stablized, the solution which bathed the mucosal surface was replaced with a solution containing one-half the NaCl concentration present in the serosal solution; equal osmolarities of the two bathing solutions were maintained by adding mannitol to the mucosal solution. The resulting diffusion potential was corrected for junction potentials between the NaCl-agar bridges and bathing solutions as discussed by Barry and Diamond (1970). The magnitude of the recorded potential changes with time, and the most easily interpreted information comes shortly after the gradient is established, i.e., before ion concentrations in the tissue and potential sensing bridge have had time to change.

An additional problem arises in interpreting artifically induced diffusion potentials across gallbladders which develop spontaneous

PDs. That is, that reduction of the Na concentration in the bathing solution decreases the spontaneous PD even in the absence of a concentration gradient (see figure 4). This is likely due to decreased amounts of Na available from the mucosal solution to the cellular ion pump mechanism for transport across the tissue. Thus, advantage was taken of the linear relationship between the Na concentration and spontaneous PD to calculate what the spontaneous transmural PD would have been without the imposed NaCl concentration gradient. This PD was then used as a baseline value for calculating the diffusion potential.

Serosa-negative diffusion potentials were established by all gallbladders tested. These values were used to calculate the Cl:Na permeability ratio by means of the appropriate equation (Hodgkin & Katz, 1949). The values for this ratio (table 1) vary from 0.76 for human gallbladder to 0.16 for stump tail monkey, which indicates that gallbladders of all five species studied are more permeable to Na than to Cl.

This cation selectivity of gallbladders of man, goose and monkeys indicates that diffusion potentials normally established across the tight junction subsequent to NaCl absorption are of the wrong polarity to be the cause of spontaneous serosa-positive PDs associated with active transport. It does seem likely, however, that regardless of the cellular mechanism by which a serosa-positive PD is produced, diffusion potentials normally established across the tight junction during absorption do tend to modify the PD by making it less serosa-positive.

In developing diffusion potentials the membrane behaves as though it has aqueous pores which contain fixed negative charges. Both Na and Cl diffuse down their concentration gradients across the membrane but anions are retarded slightly more than cations by the fixed negative charges. The origin of the diffusion potential seems to be localized at one single membrane rather than across two membranes in series (Barry and Diamond, 1970). This information, coupled with the finding that tight junctions are the site of the high conductance pathway across gallbladder (Fromter, 1972, Barry, Diamond and Wright, 1971), allows us to conclude that the cation/anion selectivity takes place at the tight junction.

Electrogenic Transport

A second possibility by which all gallbladder epithelia in question could have the same basic ion transport mechanism and yet develop different transmural PDs is if the epithelia differ in certain ways in their ion conductance properties. For the purposes of argument, let us assume for a moment that gallbladder epithelia of all species concentrate bile by virtue of an ion pump which transports Na out of cell into the lateral intercellular space; this pump moves only Na, not Cl. The coupling of Na and Cl movement in this case will be electrical in nature. Chloride will follow Na from mucosa to serosa because the serosal solution becomes electrically positive with respect to the mucosal solution. The magnitude of the transmural PD necessary to draw the appropriate amount of Cl from mucosa to serosa to maintain bulk electroneutrality will depend on the partial ionic conductance of the tissue to Cl. Thus, if Cl does not readily diffuse through the membrane a larger electrical gradient must build up to force Cl from mucosa to serosa than if Cl does easily diffuse across the membrane. If this line of reasoning in its simplest application is to be successful in explaining the variety of observed spontaneous transmural PDs across gallbladders we should find the highest Cl conductance in those gallbladders with low PDs. Since Cl carries a substantial amount of the ionic conductance across gall-gladder, we would expect to find that the electrical resistance of gallbladders from man, goose and monkey are greater than the resistance of rabbit and dog gallbladder.

In the final column of table 1 is shown the resistance per serosal surface area of tissue exposed in the lucite chamber. Although human gallbladder has the greatest serosa-positive PD and the greatest resistance, and rabbit gallbladder has the lowest PD and the lowest resistance, there is little correlation between PD and resistance of other tissues. This comparison overlooks one significant factor, however; differences may exist in the microanatomy of the mucosal surface of gallbladders from various species. The gallbladder epithelium is not a flat sheet but rather it has a convoluted surface; we have found that gallbladders from different species are convoluted to different extents (Rose, unpublished observations). Thus, the conductance that we have reported in table 1 does not give an accurate assessment of the ionic conductance per unit area of mucosal membrane. It will be important to estimate the true surface area of gallbladders from individual species and use these values to calculate electrical resistance per mucosal surface area which may then be more meaningfully compared with the transmural PDs. The small serosa-negative PD of rabbit gallbladder might be imagined to be the combined product of a very low tissue resistance and a diffusion potential as discussed above.

In the preceeding discussion we treated the epithelial cells electrically as a black box. Our ultimate understanding of the electrical properties associated with electrolyte transport will depend on the availability of information concerning the electrical events across the individual mucosal and serosal cell borders of the epithelial cells. Recently, van Os and Slegers (1971) have demonstrated a ouabain-sensitive (Na^+-K^+)-stimulated ATPase in rabbit gallbladder epithelium. The ATPase activity was not stimulated by Cl over the control conditions in SO_4. On the basis of these results van Os and Slegers postulated that active Na transport is the electrical driving force and Cl follows passively because of a developed electrical potential difference. We believe, however, that electrogenic transport will be convincingly demonstrated only by measuring the resulting transmembrane electrical potential differences and showing that these PDs are not the result of other biological electromotive forces. Such information must come from the application of intracellular recording electrodes.

If future experiments do verify that the active Na transport mechanism at the latter and/or serosal surfaces of the epithelial cell operates independent of chloride transport, certain well documented observations in the literature will have to be reinterpreted. For instance, the theory of electrogenic Na transport in its simplest form would predict that replacement of Cl in the bathing solution by less permeant anions, such as SO_4 or isethionate, would lead to a greater transmural PD. However, no increase in PD under these circumstances was observed in the gallbladders of goose, monkey, man and rabbit.

Similar observations have been made on intestine under identical conditions in vitro. One possible explanation of these findings is that Na and Cl transport are, in fact, coupled, but the coupling takes place at the site of entry from the mucosal solution to the cell interior rather than at the pump site on the serosal side of the cell. Evidence for coupled NaCl entry across the brush border of rabbit small intestine has been presented (Frizzell & Schultz, 1972). Evidence for exchange diffusion of Br (Diamond, 1962b) and Cl (Wheeler, 1963) across gallbladder has also been postulated. Thus, removal of Cl from the mucosal solution might decrease the rate at which Na can diffuse into the cell and thereby reduce the amount of Na available to the pump mechanism. The PD may be seen to decrease because the pump has less Na available to transport.

CLINICAL SIGNIFICANCE

Let us now focus our attention briefly on the clinical implications of the results obtained from experiments on human gallbladder. Tissues which were considered to be histologically normal effected a net flux of Na from mucosa to serosa as previously mentioned (table 2). Similar ion flux experiments performed on diseased tissue indicate that net Na flux in this case is very small or nonexistent. Thus, it appears that a human gallbladder may be able to actively absorb electrolytes, and have normal appearing epithelium, but yet have gallstones. Kyd and Bouchier (1971) found that rabbits fed a lithogenic diet develop gallstones, but the gallbladders of these rabbits examined in vitro showed no difference in the rate of water absorption as comparied with control tissues. These observations are consistent with the recently formulated concept that gallstones do not necessarily form as a result of disease, but rather they are precipitated as a result of insufficient concentrations of bile salt or phospholipid molecules in bile necessary to keep cholesterol solublized. It may be that the high incidence of disease in human gallbladders which contain stones is secondary to a mechanical erosion of the gallbladder epithelium due to the presence of stones in this fragile organ. Any attempt to correlate more precisely the absorptive function of individual human gallbladders with the pathologic state of the tissue and the patients pre-operative symptomatology will depend on the selection of some appropriate measure for each parameter which can be conveniently quantitated.

SUMMARY

The gallbladders of man, goose and monkey investigated in vitro develop a serosa-positive PD. This PD is reduced by conditions that inhibit fluid transport by gallbladder epithelia, i.e., anaerobiosis, the presence of ouabain, or elimination of Na from the bathing solutions. The short-circuit current of human gallbladder is adequately accounted for by net Na flux from mucosa to serosa.

A detailed mechanism of the active transport process of absorption by gallbladder has previously been presented on the basis of experiments performed on the gallbladders of fish, rabbit and guinea pig (Diamond 1962b; Machen and Diamond, 1969). This model features electrically neutral transport of NaCl from the cell fluid into the apical portion of the lateral intercellular space. The small serosa-negative potential difference measured across rabbit gallbladder during maximal fluid transport is thought to be the result of faster back diffusion of Na than Cl from the hypertonic solution in the lateral intercellular space toward the mucosal bathing solution. The tight junction is the site of cation selectivity of the tissue. The possibility must be considered, however, that the resulting diffusion potential might represent an electromotive force of sufficient magnitude to obscure the effect of electrogenic Na transport from mucosa to serosa.

An explaination of the serosa-positive PDs of gallbladders of man, goose and monkey cannot be based on diffusion potentials established across the tight junction because these structures are cation selective, in common with gallbladders of fish and rabbit. Although the mechanism of ion transport in gallbladders which develop serosa-positive PDs has not been determined, the occurance of electrogenic Na transport remains a possibility. Thus, the PD across the gallbladder of all species might be the net result of electrogenic Na transport tending to make the serosal surface become electropositive, and diffusion potentials established across the tight junction tending to make the serosal surface electronegative. Information on the electrical potential profile of the epithelial cells of gallbladder might help to resolve this issue.

Many of the human gallbladders removed for cholelithiasis develop a serosa-positive PD, actively transport Na in the direction of absorption, and have mucosa which is histologically indistinguishable from normal. This information is consistent with the theory that gallstones form as a result of insufficient concentrations of bile salts or phospholipid in bile, rather than as a result of diseased gallbladder mucosa.

REFERENCES

Barry,P.H., and Diamond,J.D., 1970.
Junction potentials, electrode standard potentials, and other problems in interpreting electrical properties.
J. Membr. Biol., 3:93.

Barry,P.H., Diamond,J.M., and Wright,E.M., 1971.
The mechanism of cation permeation in rabbit gallbladder, dilution potentials and biionic potentials.
J. Membr. Biol., 4:358.

Boulpaep,E.L., 1967.
Ion permeability of the peritubular and luminal membrane of the renal tubular cell, in symposium uber transport and funktion intracellular elektrolyte, (Edit. by F. Kruck).
Munich: Urban and Schwarzengerg, 98.

Cremaschi,D., Henin,S., and Calvi,M., 1971.
Transepithelial potential difference induced by amphotericin B and NaCl-$NaHCO_3$ pump localization in gallbladder.
Arch. Int. Physiol. Biochim., 79:889.

Diamond,J.M., 1964.
Transport of salt and water in rabbit and guinea pig gallbladder.
J. Gen. Physiol., 48:1.

Diamond,J.M., 1962a.
The reabsorption function of the gallbladder.
J. Physiol., 161:442.

Diamond,J.M., 1962b.
The mechanism of solute transport by the gallbladder.
J. Physiol., 161:474.

Dietschy,J.M., 1966.
Tecent developments in solute and water transport across the gallbladder epithelium.
Gastroenterology, 50:692.

Dietschy,J.M., 1964.
Water and solute movement across the wall of the everted rabbit gallbladder.
Gastroenterology, 47:395.

Frederiksen,O., and Leyssac,P.P., 1969.
Transcellular transport of isosmotic volumes by the rabbit gallbladder.
J. Physiol., 201:201.

Fromter,E., 1972.
The route of passive ion movement through the epithelium of necturus gallbladder.
J. Membr. Biol., 8:259.

Gelarden,R.T., and Rose,R.C., 1973.
Electrical properties and diffusion potentials of gallbladders from various species.
The Physiologist, 16:319.

Hodgkin,A.L., and Katz,B., 1949.
The effect of sodium ions on the electrical activity of the giant azon of the squid.
J. Physiol., (London), 108:37.

Kyd,P.A., and Bouchier,I.A.D., 1971.
Absorption of water, unconjugated bilirubin, and sodium glycodeoxycholate by the rabbit gallbladder with dietary-induced gallstones.
Gastroenterology, 61:723.

Machen,T.E., and Diamond,J.M., 1969.
An estimate of the salt concentration in the lateral intercellular spaces of rabbit gallbladder during maximal fluid transport.
J. Membr. Biol., 1:194.

Rehm,W.S., 1950.
A theory of the formation of hydrochloric acid by the stomach.
Gastroenterology, 14:401.

Rose,R.C., Gelarden,R.T., and Nahrwold,D.L., 1973.
Electrical properties of isolated human gallbladder.
Am. J. Physiol., 224:1320.

Rose,R.C., and Schultz,S.G., 1971.
Studies on the electrical potential profile across rabbit ileum, effects of sugars and amino acids on transmural and transmucosal electrical potential differences.
J. Gen. Physiol., 57:639.

Schultz,S.G., and Zalusky,R., 1964.
Ion transport in isolated ileum. I. Short-circuit current and Na fluxes.
J. Gen. Physiol., 47:567.
Wheeler,H.O., 1963.
Transport of electrolytes and water across wall of rabbit gallbladder.
Am. J. Physiol., 205:427.
Van Os,C.H., and Slegers,J.F.G., 1971.
Correlation between (Na+_K+)-activated ATPase activities and the rate of isotonic fluid transport of gallbladder epithelium.
Biochim. Biophys. Acta., 241:89.

DRUG INTERACTIONS IN THE GASTROINTESTINAL TRACT

Ruth R. Levine and Carol T. Walsh

INTRODUCTION

Although two drugs administered simultaneously or in close sequency may act independently, they may also interact to alter the duration, the intensity, or even the quality of the anticipated effect of one or both drugs. Some of the numerous drug interactions that have been observed clinically are trivial because of the wide margin of safety of the particular drugs being used, while other drug interactions have proved disasterous. Many occur only when sufficiently large doses of the drugs are used; these pose no problems to the alert physician who adjusts dosage appropriate to the patient's needs. However, drug interactions that lead to toxic manifestations as well as those that result in less than desired effectiveness are justly termed adverse effects, since they are not beneficial to the patient.

The effect of two (or more) interacting drugs may be classified on the basis of whether the combined effect of the drugs acting in concert is equal to, greater than, or less than, the sum of the effects of each agent acting in solo (fig. 1). When the combined effect of two drugs that elicit the same overt response is the algebraic sum of their individual effects, the effect is termed summation or additive effect. Synergism refers to the situation in which the joint effect of two drugs is greater, and antagonism to that in which the combined effect is less, than the sum of the effects of the drugs acting separately. The general phenomenon of antagonism may be subdivided on the basis of the mechanism by which one drug opposes

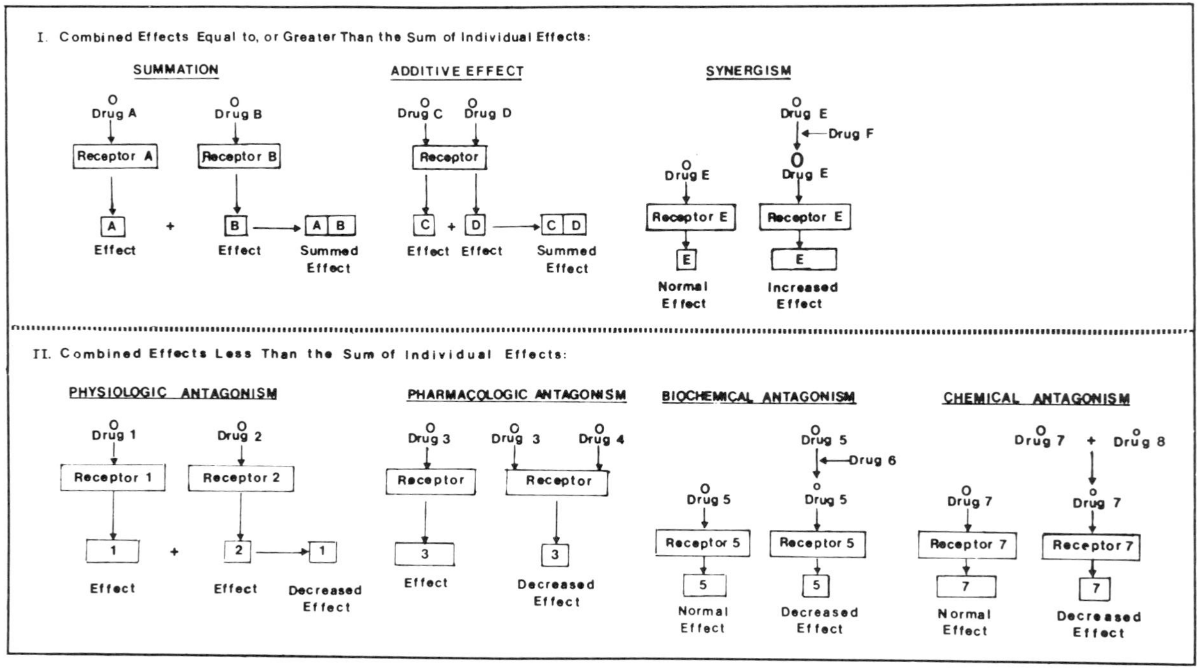

Fig. 1. Classification of drug interactions from Levine, R. R., 1973, Pharmacology: Drug Actions and Reactions. Little Brown Boston (by permission of the publisher).

the action of another, e.g.: physiologic, pharmacologic, biochemical, or chemical antagonism.

Ordinarily, adverse responses to combined medication are not the result of the summed effects of drugs that elicit the identical overt response by acting at the same or different receptors. Neither are they the consequency of pharmacologic or physiologic antagonism. The combined effects produced by such drug interactions are readily predictable from the known pharmacodynamics of the agents in question and can be taken into account before the conjoint administration of the several drugs. Moreover, in these four types of interaction, the alteration in drug response is brought about without affecting the drug concentration in plasma or at the site of action. Adverse reactions resulting from multiple-drug therapy are usually associated with drugs that act synergistically or are chemically or biochemically antagonistic, i.e., drug interactions that do produce changes in the concentration of drug available to a site of action. The concentration of drug at an active site is the net result of the rate and extent of its absorption, distribution, biotransformation and excretion. Thus the mechanisms commonly responsible for the clinically significant drug interactions are those by which one drug affects the pharmacokinetics of another drug. Interactions leading to alterations in absorption, distribution and elimination are relatively unpredictable; they usually influence only the duration and intensity of drug action.

Drug interactions influencing absorption are most likely to occur within the gut, since the oral route is the one most frequently used for drug administration. In general, one drug may increase or decrease the rate or extent of absorption of another drug by altering one or more of the determinants of the absorptive process, i.e.: 1) the physiocochemical state of the drug; 2) the nonabsorptive physiologic functions or state of the gut; 3) the metabolic activity and functions of the absorbing cell, and 4) the structure of the absorbing surface.

INTERACTIONS AFFECTING THE PHYSIOCOCHEMICAL STATE OF THE DRUG

Interactions Affecting Drug Solubility

For almost every therapeutic agent, absorption takes place from solution, the drug being a solute in the fluid at the site of absorption. Therefore, any chemical interaction which alters drug solubility may be expected to affect drug absorption; the usual result is a decrease in the rate or extent of the drug's availability to the absorbing surface.

Many of these undesirable interactions (incompatabilities) between agents coadministered or coexistent in the gut are well understood and relatively predictable (Felmeister, 1965). For example, some precipitation and drug inactivation may be anticipated in any mixture of an anionic and a cationic agent of fairly high molecular weight. Thus barbiturates and sulfonamides may form insoluble compounds with most alkaloids, antihistaminics or tranquilizers and, consequently, delay or reduce the therapeutic effectiveness of these agents. On this same basis, the insoluble anion exchange resins, cholestyramine and colestipol, might be expected to interfere with the absorption of a variety of anionic drugs, as, indeed has been demonstrated recently (table 1). However, these bile acid sequestering polymers are also capable of binding agents such as the cardiac glycosides (Bazzano and Bazzano, 1972) and inorganic iron (Greenberger, 1973). Since this binding has been shown to be pH-dependent, an anionic exchange resin can bind any drug with an appropriate charge at the pH at which the two coexist (table 1). It is highly likely, therefore, that such binding occurs with still other drugs as yet unreported. This interference with the absorption of other drugs has clinical relevance, since patients who are being treated with the anion exchange resins may also require digitalis glycosides, diuretics or anticoagulants. Proper timing of the administration of the resin and another medication, and strict adherence by the informed patient to the prescribed schedule, can minimize fluctuations in drug absorption. Adjustments in dosage and scheduling may not yield the desired results, however, when the anion exchange resins are used during clinical anticoagulation. By interfering with the absorption of both the coumarin anticoagulants and Vitamin K, the anion exchange resin can lower as well as enhance the effect on prothrombin formation.

Decrease in the quantity of drug available for absorption as a result of the formation of insoluble complexes has been shown to occur with agents other than the anion exchange resins. For example, although surface-active agents, such as polysorbate 80 (Tween 80),

Table 1

Decreased Drug Absorption in Man by Interactions with Cholestyramine or Colestipol

Drug Affected	Reference
Thyroxine	Northcutt et al., 1969
Acetylsalicylic acid	Hahn et al., 1972
Phenprocoumon	Hahn et al., 1972
Warfarin	Benjamin et al., 1970
Chlorothiazide	Kauffman and Azarnoff, 1973
Cardiac glycosides	Bazzano and Bazzano, 1972
$FeSO_4$	Greenberger, 1973
Vitamin K*	Gross and Brotman, 1970
Vitamin B_{12}**	Coronato and Glass, 1973

*Absorption decreased indirectly as a consequence of the binding of bile salts.

**Absorption decreased indirectly by competition of anion exchange resin for binding sites on intrinsic factor molecule.

dioctyl sodium sulfosuccinate and sorbitol, are frequently used as solubilizing adjuncts in drug preparations, and have been shown to increase the absorption of paracetamol and other drugs (Gwilt et al., 1963), the absorption of a variety of still other agents may be decreased by entrapment of the drug molecules within micelles of these same surfactants (Levine, 1971; Levine in press). Chemical interaction may also be responsible for the decreased absorption in man of anticoagulants and griseofulvin following pretreatment with barbiturates (O'Reilly and Aggelar, 1969; Riegelman et al., 1970); the increased fecal excretion of unchanged drug after oral administration of dicoumarol or griseofulvin cannot be attributed to the effect of the barbiturates on gut motility or enzyme induction in the gut.

Interactions with Adsorbents and Antacids

Alterations in absorption have frequently been associated with prescribed or self medication to treat gastrointestinal disorders caused by, or coincident with, the oral administration of other agents. Adsorption onto kaolin-pectin mixtures used to control diarrhea, for example, has been found to inhibit absorption of lincomycin (Wagner, 1968) and promazine (Sorby and Liu, 1966). An adsorption phenomenon may also account for the significantly decreased blood levels of chlorpromazine when given simultaneously with a magnesium trisilicate-aluminum hydroxide antacid (Fann et al., 1973), as has been shown to be the case for some anticholinergic drugs (Grote and Woods, 1953). Adsorption is, however, only one of several mechanisms by which antacids may influence drug absorption; depending on the type of antacid coadministered, absorption may be either increased or decreased by chelate formation or by changes in gut pH or motility. For example, the absorption of dicoumarol was found to be markedly increased in the presence of magnesium hydroxide but unaffected by aluminum hydroxide; neither antacid influenced warfarin absorption (Ambre and Fischer, 1973). These data suggest that the formation of a soluble magnesium-dicoumarol chelate may be involved in the enhanced absorption of the anticoagulant. In contrast, antacids containing magnesium, aluminum or calcium depress the absorption of tetracycline since this antibiotic forms insoluble chelates with polyvalent cations (Kunin and Finland, 1964). Although a monovalent cation cannot participate in chelate formation, sodium bicarbonate has also been found capable of reducing tetracycline absorption when the antibiotic is administered as a solid (Barr et al., 1971). The higher intragastric pH produced by sodium bicarbonate is not conducive to the dissolution of solid tetracycline; the pH of the duodenum is also unfavorable for dissolution of the considerable quantity of solid drug discharged into it. It follows that any antacid capable of raising intragastric pH may interfere with absorption of other drugs that are dependent on a low pH for dissolution prior to absorption.

It must be borne in mind that the acid-neutralizing capacity of antacids is different for different preparations. In addition, even though gastric emptying tends to become faster as gastric pH is raised, preparations containing aluminum or calcium are prone to retard, and those containing magnesium to promote, gastric emptying. Antacids are generally considered, particularly by the laity, to be free of serious side-effects. Yet it is obvious that these agents have the potential to interact with other orally administered drugs in so many ways that their ultimate effect on the efficacy or toxicity of other therapeutic agents in a given patient is hardly predictable.

The contradictory reports of the effect of antacids on the absorption of levadopa is a case in point. Levadopa is metabolized within the gastrointestinal tract. Since this degradation is more rapid in the stomach than in the intestine, the rate at which levadopa is emptied into the duodenum can markedly influence its bioavailability. Rivera-Calimlim et al. (1970) found a threefold increase in serum levadopa levels when an antacid was administered prior to levadopa; Leon and Spiegel (1972), using the same antacid, were able to confirm this finding in only an occasional parkinsonian patient among those they studied.

Relationship between Changes in pH and Absorption of Ionizable Drugs.

For drugs that are absorbed by passive diffusion the pH partition hypothesis predicts that decreasing the pH at the site of absorption would increase the absorption of weak acids and decrease that of weak bases, since the proportion of the more readily diffusable, nonionized moiety would increase for acids and decrease for bases. For example, when the pH of intestinal contents was significantly lowered by the systemic use of acetozolamide, the absorption of salicylic acid was correspondingly increased (Schnell and Miya, 1970). According to the pH partition hypothesis the absorption of weakly acidic drugs should also be: 1) more complete and more rapid from the gastric milieu than from the more alkaline medium of the intestine; 2) decreased by the administration of antacids, and 3) increased when gastric emptying is retarded. Such predictions have been made repeatedly in various reviews (Prescott, 1969; Rosenoer and Gill, 1972) and compendia of drug interactions (Anonymous, 1967; Hansten, 1972). Data obtained from studies in humans and in laboratory animals do not verify these predictions of gastric absorption of weak acids, however, as the following examples clearly indicate. Magnussen (1968), in studies comparing the absorption of phenobarbital and pentobarbital from rat stomach and small intestine, found that 50% of the dose of the agents in solution at pH 6.0 was absorbed from the intestine in 10 min, whereas only 20% in solution at pH 2.0 was absorbed from the stomach in 1 hr. The much greater surface area available for absorption within the intestine relative to that in the stomach more than compensates for the decrease in the relative proportion of nonionized drug and the decreased rate of absorption per unit of absorptive area. When acetylsalicylic acid (Levy, 1963) or warfarin (Ambre and Fischer, 1973) were administered with quantities of antacid sufficient to increase gastric pH, it was found that the overall rate of absorption of the analgesic and anticoagulant was not decreased compared to absorption in the absence of the antacid. These findings may be attributed to the fact that alkalinity increases the rate of drug passage into the small intestine, thereby offsetting the effect of increased pH on dissociation of the weak acids. In another study when human volunteers and rats were treated with diphenhydramine prior to the administration of p-aminosalicylate (PAS), the absorption of PAS was found to be significantly delayed (Lavigne and Marchand, 1973); the assumption that diphenhydramine inhibited stomach emptying was confirmed in the rats treated with the two drugs.

The results of the studies just cited are not irreconcilable with the general rules governing passive transport across biologic barriers. They are simply manifestations of the qualitative difference in the primary function of the stomach and intestine, and of the enormous quantitative difference in the absorptive surface available in these two regions of the gut. Thus the small intestine is the major site of absorption for all drugs regardless of whether they are weak acids or bases, or nonionized compounds.

INTERACTIONS WITH DRUGS AFFECTING THE FUNCTIONS AND STATE OF THE GUT

Interactions with Drugs That Alter Gut Motility

The foregoing discussion leads directly to the conclusion that the rate at which the stomach empties its content into the intestine can markedly affect the kinetics of drug absorption. Any delay in stomach emptying generally will delay absorption; any increase in gastric emptying rate will hasten absorption. Thus one could confidently predict that agents such as the narcotic analgesics and anticholinergic drugs would decrease the rate of drug absorption, whereas cholinergic stimulants would have the opposite effect (table 2). Considering these facts and the widespread use of some of these and other agents known to alter gastric motility, it seems rather surprising that their potential for influencing the absorption of

Table 2

Interactions with Drugs That Alter Rate of Gastric Emptying

Drug Affected	Affected by	Effect on Gastric Emptying And Absorption	Reference
In Man:			
Paracetamol	Propantheline		Nimmo et al., 1973
Tetracycline	Atropine		Gothoni et al., 1972
Ampicillin			
Tetracycline	Metoclopramide		Gothoni et al., 1972
Ampicillin			
Paracetamol	Metoclopramide		Nimmo et al., 1973
p-Aminosalicylate	Diphenhydramine		Lavigne and Marchand, 1973
In Rodents:			
Sulfadimethoxine	Indomethacin		Inamura and Ichibagase, 1973
Phenylbutazone	Desipramine		Consolo, 1968
Oxyphenbutazone	Chlorpromazine		Consolo and Ladinsky, 1971
Phenobarbital	Amphetamine		Frey and Kampmann, 1966
Phenytoin			
Ethosuximide			

concomitantly administered drugs has hardly been assessed. Numerous studies in animals (dating back almost seventy years [Baas, 1904]) indicate that such drug interactions do occur as predicted and, furthermore, that they may have clinical significance. Up to the present, however, only a few anticholinergic agents and one cholinergic stimulant have been studied in man; these agents have been shown to inhibit the absorption of coadministered drugs by slowing, and to enhance absorption by increasing, gastric emptying rate, respectively (table 2).

When drugs are discharged from the stomach into the duodenum, they come into immediate contact with the region of the gut having the greatest capacity for absorption; the proximal quarter of the small intestine has almost half of the total mucosal area of the gut and this surface area diminishes rapidly from proximal to distal segments. Given this distribution of absorptive surface, one would anticipate that the longer the residence time of an absorbable material within the more proximal segments of the intestine, the more rapid would be its overall rate of absorption. The same classes of drugs (the opiates and the anticholinergic agents) that retard the rate of gastric emptying also slow the rate of transit of material through the intestine. One might expect then, that drugs such as the anticholinergic agents would provide just the right conditions for rapid absorption from the intestine. Available experimental data indicate, however, that the administration of anticholinergic agents to human subjects slows the overall rate of absorption of coadministered drugs as measured by drug concentrations in plasma (table 2). One can only conclude that the motility of the stomach is the limiting factor in determining the overall rate of drug absorption when the motility of the entire gastrointestinal tract is reduced. This interpretation also places the apparently conflicting data of Manninen et al. (1973) into agreement with other reported data of the effect of decreased motility on absorption. Manninen et al. found that propantheline pretreatment increased and metoclopramide decreased the serum digoxin concentration when digoxin was administered in tablet form to human subjects; propantheline pretreatment has no effect on absorption of digoxin administered as a solution (metoclopramide was not tested with digoxin solutions). Disintegration and dissolution under gastric conditions are crucial to the bioavailability of digoxin. Slowing of gastric emptying by propantheline favors solubilization before digoxin is presented to the intestine, whereas metochlopramide decreases the fraction of soluble digoxin entering the duodenum.

All drugs that are absorbed to any extent can be absorbed in any region of the gut, since passive diffusion along electrochemical gradients plays some part in all absorption phenomena. Absorption of a drug will continue during its entire sojourn in the gut, unless fluid removal and increase in density of intraluminal contents prevent drug diffusion to the mucosa. Thus, the major factor determining how much of a drug is absorbed is not the rate of absorption but how long the agent has contact with an absorbing surface. Considering the many hours normally involved in transit through the gut, a decrease in gastric or intestinal motility has little or no effect on the total amount of drug absorbed. For example, the total 24-hr urinary excretion of paracetamol was not influenced by either propantheline or metoclopramide, even though these agents affected the initial absorption rate of the analgesic (Nimmo et al., 1973). However, agents or conditions inducing marked increases in motility have been shown to depress the total amount of drug absorbed, particularly of those agents whose absorption is ordinarily slow and incomplete. Hypermotility caused by excessive use of laxatives (an all-too-common drug misuse), for example, has been found to impair the absorption of the incompletely absorbed cardiac glycoside, digoxin, and to produce a lower than normal steady state of digoxin blood levels (Heizer et al., 1971). If a higher maintenance dosage were instituted to produce the desired therapeutic effect and the laxatives were subsequently discontinued, absorption would increase as the hypermotility subsided and digitalis toxicity would develop. One would predict that digitalized patients who require oral antibiotics which produce hypermotility states would also need careful supervision and adjustment of their digitalis dosage during the course, and after discontinuation of the antibiotic therapy (Bigger and Strauss, 1972).

Although generalizations based on few data are always suspect, it appears that the rate of drug absorption tends to be decreased by coadministered drugs which decrease both gastric and intestinal motility and increased only by agents which increase gastric emptying rate. Total drug absorption is affected only by marked increase in intestinal motility.

Microbial Flora

Comparative studies of conventional and gnotobiotic animals have suggested that the microbial flora of the gut influences the intestinal absorption of a variety of dietary substances. Yet few attempts have been made to determine the effects on drug absorption of either the presence or drug-induced changes in the normal microbial population. We have recently completed the first of such studies and have determined the effect of a series of regimens of different antibiotics on the absorption of diphenylhydantoin, chlorpromazine, tetracycline and the quaternary ammonium anticholinergic agent, benzomethamine (Walsh and Levine, in press). The bacterial changes induced by these antibiotic regimens apparently did not produce intraluminal or intramucosal alterations that were significant to the process of absorption of these drugs. The results of these experiments, if applicable to man, suggest that, in general, no adjustment of drug dosage is required for agents such as the chronically used chlorpromazine and diphenylhydantoin upon coadministration with certain antibiotics.

Alteration of the microbial population of the gut induced by antibiotics may, however, produce profound effects on the activity of oral anticoagulants; these effects are secondary to changes in the intestinal flora. Orally administered broad spectrum antibiotics may decrease vitamin K production by gut bacteria and cause excessive hypoprothrombinemia in patients receiving coumarin anticoagulants (Klippel and Pitsinger, 1968).

The metabolic activities of the microflora may also affect directly the quantity of drug available for absorption. Scheline (1968) has shown that the intestinal microflora are capable of biotransforming many different types of drugs. By analogy with enzyme activity at other sites, it is certainly possible that the activity of the intestinal microbial enzymes may be altered with respect to a given drug substrate by the presence of a second agent which may either inhibit or enhance enzyme activity.

The deconjugating enzyme systems of the microflora may be important factors in the enterohepatic cycling of drugs. Conjugates of many drugs, in particular the glucuronide conjugates, are actively secreted into the intestine in the bile. The microbial enzymes can remove the glucuronic acid from the parent compound and, if the latter is lipid soluble, it will be reabsorbed. We have recently begun an investigation to determine the effect of the bacterial composition of gut contents on this glucuronide hydrolysis, using ^{14}C-morphine as a specimen drug. The effect of reduction in the bacterial population produced by antibiotic pretreatment is shown in figure 2. Lincomycin was chosen as the antibiotic since it has been reported to markedly reduce β-glucuronidase activity of intestinal contents. A larger percentage of the dose of morphine was eliminated in the feces and less in the urine of antibiotic-treated animals compared to controls; a much higher percentage of the fecally excreted radioactivity was attributable to the conjugated form. These data clearly indicate that changes in the composition of intestinal bacteria affect the disposition of morphine and suggest that the morphine glucuronide is bacterially deconjugated prior to reabsorption of morphine from the gut.

Although less of the total dose of morphine appeared in the urine of lincomycin-treated animals, the percentage of the total excreted as free morphine was higher than that excreted by control animals. Subsequent studies, to determine the reason for this unanticipated urinary distribution of free and conjugated drug, indicated that the pH of the urine of lincomycin-treated animals was significantly lower than that of the untreated controls. For weak bases such as morphine, the more acid the urine, the greater the fraction of drug present as the ionized, less lipid soluble form, and the greater the urinary elimination. Such drug-induced changes in urinary pH can profoundly affect the duration of action of drugs; a decreased rate of excretion may permit drug concentrations to rise to toxic levels, whereas an increased rate may prevent the attainment of effective drug levels. We are continuing these investigations with other antibiotic regimens and in other species.

EFFECT OF INTERACTING DRUGS ON THE METABOLIC ACTIVITY OF THE EPITHELIAL CELL

The intestine is particularly susceptible to alterations in functional capacity brought about by changes in the biochemical activities of its constituent cells, since it is one of the most metabolically active organs. A variety of drugs such as aspirin and indomethacin have been shown, for example, to decrease the absorption of drugs as well as nutrients by interfering with reactions which normally supply

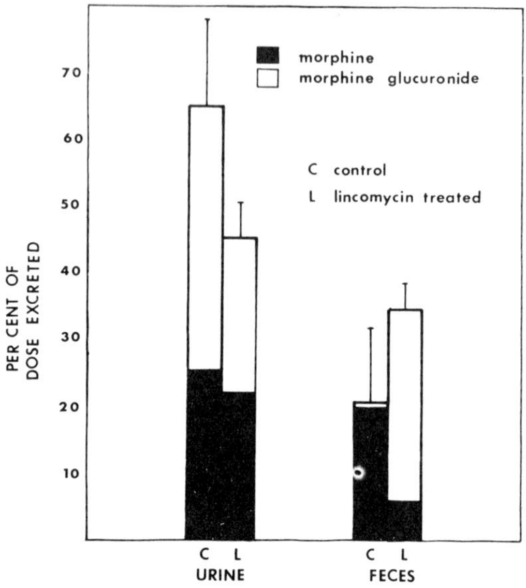

Fig. 2. Cumulative excretion of morphine and morphine glucuronide in the urine and feces of rats pretreated with lincomycin for four days. The bars represent the mean cumulative excretion of total radioactivity by each route as the per cent ± S.D. of the total radioactivity administered. The solid portion of each bar represents the per cent of dose excreted as free morphine (determined by selective extractions). Six female Sprague-Dawley rats were given 25 mg of lincomycin hydrochloride twice daily by gastric intubation. During these four days, and for two additional days their drinking water contained 500 mg/l lincomycin-HCl. At the end of the fourth day, lincomycin treated and untreated rats were given, s.c., ^{14}C-morphine-HCl, 5mg/kg. From each rat urine and feces were collected separately.

cellular energy (Levine, 1971). The drugs that are affected are those which bear close structural resemblence to, and share the same transport systems as, the nutrients, e.g., fluorouracil. So far such reactions have been found to have some clinical significance, but only with respect to the decreased bioavailability of nutrients. Specialized or active transport of various ions, sugars, amino acids, pyrimidines and vitamins may also be specifically inhibited by drugs; some of these interactions, such as the inhibition of folic acid absorption by diphenylhydantoin, are therapeutically important (Levine, 1971).

Alterations in the cellular biochemical activity would not be expected to produce changes in the absorption of drugs passively transferred unless such alterations lead to structural damage; in passive diffusion there is no requirement for energy over and above that needed to maintain cellular organization (Levine, 1971). Moreover, examples of drug interactions involving inhibition of the active transport of one drug by another are limited in number simply because so little attention has been directed toward obtaining the kinds of data that would delineate the mechanisms of absorption of specific drugs. That some specialized transport process may be involved in the absorption of some cardiac glycosides is evidenced by the findings that the absorption of convallatoxin is inhibited hydrocortisone (Lauterbach, 1967) and that the digitoxin transport rate is reduced by nitrogen, dinitrophenol and probenecid (Damm and Braun, 1973).

Detailed studies of absorption in our laboratory have yielded kinetic data which permit the inference that more than passive diffusion is involved in the absorption of benzomethamine (Bz), tetracycline (TET), and chlorpromazine (Levine, 1971; Levine et al., 1970). We have also found that the normal metabolic activities of the intestinal epithelium involved in the bidirectional fluxes of electrolytes influence the absorption of Bz and TET (table 3). The absorption of Bz was found to be depressed in the presence of isotonic NaCl and further depressed by prior treatment with ouabain. In contrast, TET absorption was significantly increased by the intraluminal presence of isotonic NaCl, an increase that could be inhibited by pretreatment either with ouabain or chlorothiazide. Ouabain significantly decreased the rate of absorption of TET from both water and isotonic NaCl but has no effect on the increased rate of absorption seen in the presence of KCl. The continued elucidation of a possible role of sodium ion in the absorption of specific drugs would not only be important for the drugs concerned but also for many therapeutic situations, since a number of agents in widespread clinical use have been shown to inhibit the transport of sodium ion, e.g.: the cardiac glycosides, various diuretics, hormones and carthartics.

The capacity of the intestinal epithelial cell to carry out a wide variety of drug biotransformations also offers opportunities for drug interactions that could alter drug bioavailability. For example, the duration of measurable blood levels of leucomycin, after ingestion, was prolonged by coadministration of sulfa drugs; other data

Table 3

Effect of Pretreatment with Ouabain or Chlorothiazide on the Absorption of Benzomethamine and Tetracycline from Rat Duodenum

Solvent for Drug	Pretreatment[b]	% Absorbed[a] Benzomethamine[c]	Tetracycline[d]
Water	None	20.4 ± 1.6	31.0 ± 2.2
	Ouabain	7.4 ± 1.0*	19.3 ± 1.7*
	Chlorothiazide	—	32.0 ± 3.8
0.154M NaCl	None	14.5 ± 0.9	47.0 ± 2.0
	Ouabain	6.9 ± 1.6*	24.0 ± 2.6*
	Chlorothiazide	—	32.6 ± 3.9*
0.154M KCl	None	—	42.7 ± 3.0
	Ouabain	—	46.0 ± 4.0
	Chlorothiazide	—	31.8 ± 2.5*

a. Values are means of 4–12 rats ± S.E.
b. Pretreatment: Ouabain, 10 mg/kg administered i.v. 2 hrs. before start of absorption studies; chlorothiazide, 20 mg/kg administered i.v. just before start of absorption studies.
c. Dose of benzomethamine: 0.5 mg/0.5 ml injected into ligated duodenal segment; absorption period, 1hr.
d. Dose of tetracyline: 1 mg/1.0 ml injected into ligated duodenal segment; absorption period, 2 hrs.
* $P < 0.05$.

suggested an inhibitory action of the latter on the intestinal biotransformation of leucomycin (Hoshino, 1967). On the other hand, the activity of several drug-metabolizing systems of the intestine has been shown to be increased by agents that act as enzyme inducers (Wattenberg and Leong, 1967; Hartiala, 1968). Although the therapeutic significance of such changes in intestinal drug-metabolizing activity has not been evaluated, the potential for such interactions warrants further investigation,particularly for agents slowly absorbed or slowly released from drug formulations, or for drugs given in small doses.

INTERACTIONS OF DRUGS INDUCING CHANGES IN GUT MORPHOLOGY

That the absorptive capacity and function of the gut is dependent on its morphology is well documented by studies of various malabsorption states. Some agents, such as anionic and nonionic surfactants (Short and Rhodes, 1972), can apparently enhance the absorption of other drugs by producing transitory structural alterations. In contrast, the effects on drug absorption produced by agents such as neomycin and p-aminosalicylic acid (PAS) are part of the total malabsorption syndromes induced by these drugs. Prolonged therapy with neomycin and other oral aminoglycosides has been shown to affect the absorption of penicillin G, vitamin B_{12} and a number of other nutrients (Kabins, 1972). The absorption of digoxin was shown to be impaired, however, by a single dose of neomycin, suggesting that prolonged neomycin therapy may require higher doses of digoxin for adequate digitalization (Lindenbaum et. al., 1972). The interference by PAS with the absorption of the potent, new tuberculostatic agent, rifampicin, is also a clinically important interaction, since these two agents are used concomitantly in the treatment of severe cases of tuberculosis (Boman et al., 1972). The effect of orally administered PAS on the absorption of rifampicin appears to be different from other PAS-induced malabsorptions, however (Halsted and McIntyre, 1972); when PAS and rifampicin are given 8 to 12 hrs apart, there is no adverse effect of PAS on the absorption of rifampicin. It appears obvious, nevertheless, that the influence on absorption produced by drug-induced changes in the morphology of the absorbing cell or surface are mainly associated with abnormal or pathologic conditions, whereas drug-induced changes in the physiologic function or state of the gut may affect drug absorption as a consequence of completely normal conditions.

CONCLUDING REMARKS

Although drug interactions present an increasing hazard in modern therapeutics, the great majority of adverse reactions are preventable. The physician, the dentist or the pharmacist can go far toward ensuring the safety and effectiveness of rational multiple-drug therapy through his awareness of reported interactions and his understanding of the general mechanisms responsible for drug interactions. However, adverse drug interactions are not always of iatrogenic origin. Self-medication with preparations that are available without prescription, pharmacologically active compounds present in common foodstuffs as normal constituents or as additives or contaminants, and exposure to household chemicals or environmental pollutants, can also be factors contributing to unwanted reactions to therapeutic agents. Thus there is need also to educate the general public to the risks of interactions. Otherwise, therapeutic catastrophies may become insurmountable obstacles in the path of progress toward the development and use of chemicals.

REFERENCES

Ambre,J.J., and Fischer,L.J., 1973.
Effect of coadministration of aluminum and magnesium hydroxides on absorption of anticoagulants in man.
Clin. Pharm. Therap., 14:231.

Anonymous, 1967.
Drug interactions that can affect your patients.
Patient Care, 1:32.

Baas,K.H., 1904
Ueber die Resorption von Jodkalium im Menschlichen und Tierischen Magen und ueger den Hemmenden Einfluss des Morphius auf die Magen entleerung.
Deutch. Arch. Klin. Med., 81:455.

Barr,W.H., Adir,J., and Garrettson,L., 1971.
Decrease of tetracycline absorption in man by sodium bicarbonate.
Lin. Pharm. Therap., 12:779.

Bazzano,G., and Bazzano,G.S., 1972.
Digitalis intoxication treatment with a new steroid-binding resin.
J.A.M.A., 220:828.

Benjamin,D., Robinson,D.S., and McCormack,J., 1970.
Cholestyramine binding of warfarin in man and in vitro.
Clin. Res., 18:336.

Bigger,J.T., Jr., and Strauss,H.C., 1972.
Digitalis toxicity: drug interactions promoting toxicity and the management of toxicity.
Semin. Drug Treat., 2:147.

Boman,G., Hanngren,A., Malmborg,A., Borga,O., and Sjoqvist,F., 1971.
Drug interaction: decreased serum concentration of refampicin when given with P.A.S.
Lancet, 1:800.

Braun,W., and Damm,K.H., 1973.
The effect of probenecid on the intestinal absorption of cardiac glycosides.
Naunyn-Schmiedeberg's Arch. Pharm., 277: Suppl. R11.

Consolo,S., 1968.
An interaction between desipramine and phenylbutazone.
J. Pharm. Pharmacol., 20:574.
Consolo,S., and Ladinsky,J., 1971.
Delayed oxyphenbutazone absorption by some tricyclic compounds in the rat.
Arch. Int. Pharmacodyn., 192:265.
Coronato,A., and Glass,G.B.J., 1973.
Depression of the intestinal uptake of radiovitamin B_{12} by cholestyramine.
Proc. Soc. Exptl. Biol. Med., 142:1341.
Fann,W.E., Davis,J.M., Janowski,D.S., and Schmidt,D., 1973.
The effects of antacids on the blood levels of chlorpromazine.
Clin. Pharm. Therap., 14:135.
Felmeister,A., 1965.
The prescription, in Martin,E.W., (Ed. in chief).
Mack Pub. Co., Easton, Pa., pp. 1688-1699.
Frey,H.H., and Kampmann,E., 1966.
Interaction of amphetamine with anticonvulsant drugs.
Acta Pharmacol., 24:310.
Gothoni,G., Pentikainen,P., Vapaatalo,H.I., Hackman, R., Bjorksten,K.A.F., 1972.
Absorption of antibiotics: influence of metoclopramide and atropine on serum levels of pivampicillin and tetracycline.
Ann. Clin. Res., 4:228.
Greenberger,N.J., 1973.
Effects of antibiotics and other agents on the intestinal transport of iron.
J. Clin. Nutr., 26:104.
Gross,L., and Brotman,M., 1970.
Hypoprothrombinemia and hemorrhage associated with cholestyramine therapy.
Ann. Intern. Med., 72:95.

Grote,I.W., and Woods,M., 1953.
Studies on antacids. IV. Adsorption effects of various aluminum antacids upon simultaneously administered anticholinergic drugs.
J. Am. Pharm. Ass., Sci. Ed., 42:319.

Gwilt,J.R., Robertson,A., Goldman,L., and Blanchard, A.W., 1963.
The absorption characteristics of paracetamol tablets in man.
J. Pharm. Pharmacol., 15:445.

Hahn,K.-J., Eiden,W., Schettle.M., Hahn,M., Walter,E., and Weber,E., 1972.
Effect of cholestyramine on the gastrointestinal absorption of phenprocoumon and acetylsalicylic acid in man.
Eur. J. Clin. Pharm., 4:142.

Halsted,C.H., and McIntyre,P.A., 1972.
Intestinal malabsorption caused by aminosalicylic acid therapy.
Arch. Int. Med., 130:935.

Hansten,P.D., 1972.
Drug Interactions.
Lea and Febiger, Philadelphia, 437 pp.

Hartiala,K., 1968.
Active metabolism of the gastrointestinal wall.
Proc. Intl. Union. Physiol. Sci., XXIV Intl. Congress, 6:29.

Heizer,W.D., Smith,T.W., and Goldfinger,S.E., 1971.
Absorption of digoxin in patients with malabsorption syndromes.
New. Eng. J. Med., 285:257.

Hoshino,Y., 1967.
Studies on absorption of leucomycin from intestinal tract.
J. Antibiotics, Series A., 20:361.

Imamura,Y., and Ichibagase,H., 1973.
Effects of simultaneous administration of drugs on absorption and excretion. II. Effects of non-steroidal anti-inflammatory drugs on absorption and excretion of sulfadimethoxine in rabbits.
Chem. Pharm. Bull., 21:668.

Kabins,S.A., 1972.
Interactions among antibiotics and other drugs.
J.A.M.A., 219:206.
Kauffman,R.E., and Azarnoff,D.L., 1973.
Effect of colestipal on gastrointestinal absorption of chlorothiazide in man.
Clin. Pharm. Therap., 14:886.
Klippel,A.P., and Pitsinger,B., 1968.
Hypoprothrombinemia secondary to antibiotic therapy and manifested by massive gastrointestinal hemorrhage - Report of three cases.
Arch. Surg., 96:266.
Kunin,C.M., and Finland,M., 1964.
Clinical pharmacology of the tetracycline antibiotics.
Clin. Pharm. Therap., 2:51.
Lauterbach,F., 1967.
Uber Unterschiede im Mechanismus der Enteralen Resorption Kardiotoner Steroide und andere Pharmaka.
Naunyn Schmiedeberg's Arch. Pharmak. Exp. Path., 257:432.
Lavigne,J.-G., and Marchand,C., 1973.
Inhibition of the gastrointestinal absorption of p-aminosalicylate (PAS) in rats and humans by diphenhydramine.
Clin. Pharm. Therap., 14:404.
Leon,A.S., and Spiegel,H.E., 1972.
The effect of antacid administration on the absorption and metabolism of levodopa.
J. Clin. Pharmacol., 12:263.
Levine,R.R., 1971.
Intestinal Absorption, in Rabinowitz,J.L., and Meyerson,R.M., Absorption Phenomena.
John Wiley and Sons, pp. 27-95.
Levine,R.R.
Facilitation and Inhibition of Drug Absorption, in Rummel,W., International Encyclopedia of Pharmacology and Therapeutics.
Pergamon Press, (London), Sect. 39B, (In Press).

Levine,R.R., Squires,C., and Donovan,A.M., 1970.
Studies of the influence of ion and solute transport of drug absorption.
Amer. Pharm. Assn., Acad. Pharm. Sci. Abs., 74.

Levy, G., 1963.
Biopharmaceutical aspects of the gastrointestinal absorption of salicylates, in Dixon,A.St.J., Martin,B.K., Smith,M.J.H., and Wood,P.H.N., Salicylates an International Symposium.
J. and A. Churchill, Ltd., (London), pp. 9-17.

Lindenbaum,J., Maulitz,R.M., Saha,J.R., Shea,N., and Buttler,V.P., Jr., 1972.
Impairment of digoxin absorption by neomycin.
Clin. Res., 20:410.

Magnussen,M.P., 1968.
The effect of ethanol on the gastrointestinal absorption of drugs in the rat.
Acta Pharmacol. (Kbh.), 26:130.

Manninen,V., Apajalahti,A., Melin,J., and Karesoja,M., 1973.
Altered absorption of digoxin in patients given propantheline and metoclopramide.
Lancet, 1:398.

Nimmo,J., Heading,R.C., Tothill,P., and Prescott,L.F., 1973.
Pharmacological modification of gastric emptying: Effects of propantheline and metoclopromide on paracetamol absorption.
Brit. Med. J., 1:587.

Northcutt,R.C., Stiel,J.N., Hollifield,J.A., and Stant, E.G., Jr., 1969.
The influence of cholestyramine on thyroxine absorption.
J.A.M.A., 208:1857.

O'Reilly,R.A., and Aggeler,P.M., 1969.
Effect of barbiturates on oral anticoagulants in man.
Clin. Res., 17:153.

Prescott,L.F., 1969.
Pharmacokinetic drug interactions.
Lancet, 2:1239.

Riegelman,S., Rowtand,M., and Epstein,W.L., 1970.
Griseofulvinphenobarbital interaction in man.
J.A.M.A., 213:426.
Rivera-Calimlim,L., Dujoune,C.A., Morgan,J.P., Lasagna,L., and Bianchine,J.R., 1970.
L-Dopa treatment failure: Explanation and correction.
Brit. Med. J., 4:93.
Rosenoer,V.M., and Gill,G.M., 1972.
Drug interactions in clinical medicine.
Med. Clinics of No. Amer., 56:585.
Scheline,R.R., 1968.
Drug metabolism by intestinal microorganisma.
J. Pharm. Sci., 57:2022.
Schnell,R.C., and Miya,T.S., 1970.
Increased ileal absorption of salicylic acid induced by carbonic anhydrase inhibition.
Biochem. Pharm., 19:303.
Short,M.P., and Rhodes,C.T., 1972.
Effect of surfactants on diffusion of drugs across membranes.
Nature New Biology, 236:44.
Sorby,D.L., and Liv, G., 1966.
Effects of adsorbents on drug absorption. II. Effect of an antidiarrhea misture on promazine absorption.
J. Pharm. Sci., 55:504.
Wagner,J.G., 1968.
Pharmacokinetics I. Definitions, modelling and reasons for measuring blood levels and urinary excretion.
Drug Intelligence, 2:38.
Walsh,C.T., and Levine,R.R.
Drug absorption in rats pretreated with antibiotics.
J. Pharm. Exptl. Therap. (In Press).
Walsh,C.T., and Levine,R.R.
The role of the intestinal flora in the disposition of morphine following parenteral and enteral administration.
(Submitted For Publication).

Wattenberg,L.W., and Leong,J.L., 1965.
Effects of phenthiazines on protective systems against polycyclic hydrocarbons.
Cancer Res., 25:365.

SESSION IV.
PATHOLOGIC PHYSIOLOGY

DYSFUNCTION OF THE ESOPHAGOGASTRIC JUNCTION

Donald O. Castell

INTRODUCTION

The esophagogastric junctional area performs at least two critical functions in normal digestive physiology. The tonic smooth muscle at the distal end of the esophagus shown schematically in figure 1 as the lower esophageal sphincter normally relaxes completely with each swallow allowing passage of food from the esophagus into the stomach. With the completion of the swallow, this sphincteric mechanism returns to its high pressure state. In addition to this swallowing function, the lower esophageal sphincter serves a very crucial function as a barrier against the reflux of the highly acid gastric contents into the lower esophagus, and thus prevents the damaging effects of acid on the sensitive esophageal mucosa. It is the purpose of this report to review recent insights into pathophysiology of this lower esophageal sphincteric mechanism.

Figure 2 is a schematic representation of the factors considered to be important in control of the lower esophageal sphincter pressure. The smooth muscle comprising this sphincter has been shown to be unique from smooth muscle in the esophagus above or the stomach below in that it has a selective sensitivity to certain chemical agents, the most important of which being the hormone gastrin (Christensen, 1970). It should be recognized that although a definite sphincteric mechanism does exist at the esophagogastric junction, as shown both manometrically and radiographically, no anatomic demonstration of a specialized sphincteric muscle in this region has ever been made in

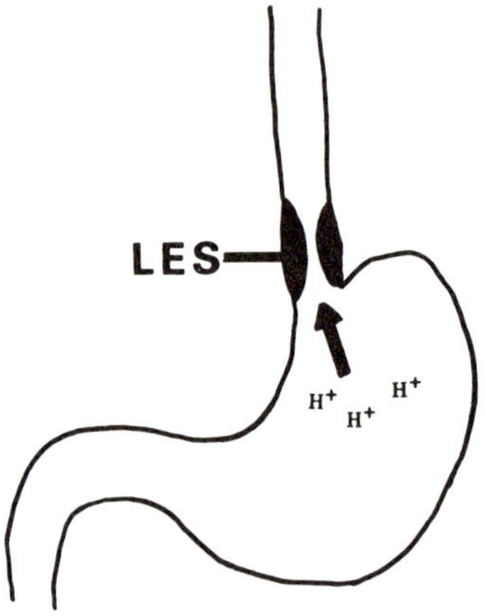

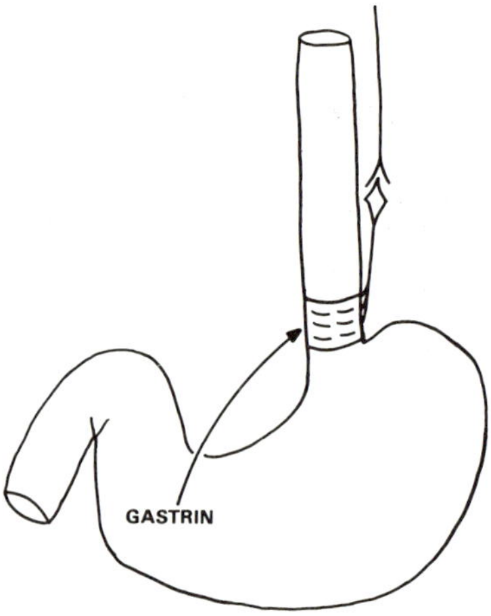

Fig. 1. Schematic representation of the lower esophageal sphincter (LES) and its physiologic function in prevention of acid gastroesophageal reflux.

Fig..2. Schematic representation of the 3 important factors controlling lower esophageal sphincter function; the neural supply to the sphincter, endogenous gastrin, and the circular smooth muscle.

human. Manometrically the lower esophageal sphincter is demonstrated as a zone of high pressure (usually about 20 mm Hg greater than intragastric pressure) which decreases transiently to the level of intragastric pressure in response to a swallow. It appears that the lower esophageal sphincter represents a region of esophageal smooth muscle which has specific characteristics and probably specific receptor sites for response to chemical and neural stimulation. The hormone gastrin from the gastrin antrum has been shown to dramatically increase pressure in this sphincter, and to be of major importance in physiologic control of lower esophageal sphincter pressure (Castell and Harris, 1970). In fact, elegant studies using antigastrin antibodies in the opossum indicate that endogenous gastrin may account for up to 80% of resting lower esophageal sphincter tone (Lipshutz and Cohen, 1972).

Finally, the neural supply to this sphincteric region, shown schematically in figure 2 as the pre- and postganglionic segments of the cholinergic system, plays a role in control of lower esophageal sphincter pressure. Cholinergic stimulation has been shown to result in marked increases in sphincter pressure, with this effect being at least partially dependent on the presence of endogenous gastrin (Roling et al., 1972). In fact, the hormone gastrin has been shown pharmacologically to act on the postganglionic segment of the cholinergic system (Lipshurz et al., 1971). Apparently an interaction between these nerves and gastrin is important in the maintenance of normal resting sphincter pressure. Furthermore, it has been shown quite recently that the alpha adrenergic component of the sympathetic nervous system exerts an important effect in maintenance of normal lower esophageal sphincter pressure (DiMarino and Cohen, 1973).

Thus, an abnormality in any of these three interrelated components, neural hormonal, or muscular could result in a defect in lower esophageal function. The subsequent discussion will be directed to those disease states and clinical syndromes in which dysfunction of the lower esophageal sphincter has been demonstrated.

ACHALASIA

Achalasia is a classic abnormality in esophageal function, characterized clinically by dysphagia, with progressive difficulty in transport of food from mouth to stomach. The pathologic abnormality in this condition has been shown to be a relative absence of ganglion cells in the myenteric plexus throughout the esophagus (Trounce et al., 1957). The manometric defect in achalasia is characterized by absent peristalsis in the body of the esophagus, marked elevation in resting lower esophageal sphincter pressure, and an imcomplete relaxation of the lower esophageal sphincter with swallowing (Cohen and Lipshutz, 1971). In addition, hyper-responsiveness of the esophagus and lower esophageal sphincter to cholinergic stimulation has been demonstrated, consistent with Cannon's law of denervation supersensitivity (Cohen and Guelrad, 1971). Comparison of resting lower esophageal sphincter pressures in achalasia patients with that found in normal subjects is shown in table 1. The marked elevation in resting lower esophageal sphincter pressure in achalasia is evident by the mean pressure level of 50.5 mm Hg. In the normal esophagus

Table 1

Comparison of Resting Lower Esophageal Sphincter (LES) Pressure Reported for Normals and for Conditions with Sphincter Dysfunction

Condition	LES Pressure (mm Hg) (Mean $\pm$ 1 SE)
Normal	17.2 $\pm$ 0.9 (18)*
Achalasia	50.5 $\pm$ 4.6 (10)
Scleroderma	5.8 $\pm$ 0.6 (14)
Gastroesophageal Reflux	7.3 $\pm$ 0.5 (16)
Zollinger-Ellison Syndrome	27.2 $\pm$ 2.1 (17)
Pernicious Anemia	9.9 $\pm$ 1.4 (18)

*Reference source from text

the lower esophageal sphincter relaxes with a swallow to a pressure level which is almost identical with the pressure existing in the stomach below the sphincter. By contrast, sphincter relaxation in the achalasia patient is incomplete. From the already elevated resting lower esophageal sphincter pressure partial relaxation with swallowing still leaves a significant pressure differential with the pressure in the stomach below the sphincter. This persistent zone of high pressure, even during swallowing, helps to explain the level of fluid accumulation in the esophagus in these patients.

An exciting aspect of the pathophysiology of achalasia has recently been elucidated. Cohen, Lipshutz, and Hughes (1971) have shown that the response of the lower esophageal sphincter to gastrin in achalasia patients is much greater than that found in normal subjects (Cohen et al., 1971). The lower esophageal sphincter pressure response curve of achalasia patients to intravenous gastrin is shifted to the left, showing greater sensitivity to submaximal doses of gastrin, but with the same maximal response. These observations are consistent with those occurring in a denervated structure being stimulated by the appropriate chemical agent as demonstrated by Cannon (Cannon, 1939). If we recall that gastrin has been shown to work at the postganglionic segment of the cholinergic system to the lower esophageal sphincter, it seems reasonable that such supersensitivity to gastrin occurs in these denervated subjects (Lipshutz et al.,

1971). In fact, further studies on the site of the lesion in achalasia have shown pharmacologically that the denervation appears to be primarily preganglionic (Cohen et al., 1972). Thus, supersensitivity to the patient's own endogenous gastrin may explain the hypertonic lower esophageal sphincter in achalasia.

SCLERODERMA

Scleroderma is a connective tissue disease that frequently involves the gastrointestinal tract. The pathologic abnormality of this lesion in the esophagus has been shown to involve atrophy of smooth muscle, with the muscle involvement occurring in areas showing manometric abnormality (Treacy et al., 1963). The resulting motility defects are characterized by weak to absent peristalsis and low to absent lower esophageal sphincter pressure. These manometric defects are found only in the lower two-thirds or smooth muscle portion of the human esophagus, with normal peristaltic activity usually occurring in the upper striated muscle portion of the esophagus.

Recent studies into the pathophysiology of esophageal dysfunction in scleroderma have revealed some interesting results (Cohen et al., 1972). Mean resting lower esophageal sphincter pressure in scleroderma patients having abnormal esophageal peristalsis was only 5.8 mm Hg. As shown in table 1, lower esophageal sphincter pressure in these patients was lower than that found in normal subjects. There is a striking similarity between the lower esophageal sphincter pressure in scleroderma patients and pressure levels occurring in patients with a clinically incompetent lower esophageal sphincter (i. e. patients with chronic gastroesophageal reflux). Decreased sphincter pressures combined with defective peristalsis in the lower esophagus explains the extreme heartburn often occurring in scleroderma patients.

The site of the lesion in scleroderma patients has been pharmacologically demonstrated (Cohen et al., 1972). Table 2 summarizes the responsiveness of the lower esophageal sphincter to pharmacologic stimulation in normal subjects and scleroderma patients. When methacholine (Mecholyl), acting as a direct stimulant to the smooth muscle, was utilized similar responses were obtained in all groups of subjects. These studies suggest that the sphincteric muscle in scleroderma patients is capable of functioning normally when an

Table 2

Approximate Average Response in Lower Esophageal Sphincter Pressure to Pharmacologic Stimulation for Normal Subjects and Scleroderma Patients*

	Methacholine (40 ug/kg Sub-Q)	Edrophonium (80 ug/kg IV)	Gastrin I (0.5 ug/kg IV)
Normals	200%	170%	450%
Scleroderma (with normal peristalsis)	200%	160%	190%
Scleroderma (with abnormal peristalsis)	220%	45%	40%

*From Cohen et. al., reference 4 from text

appropriate stimulus is applied. It should be noted, that in that report there were two patients in the group with scleroderma and absent peristalsis, who showed decreased responsiveness to methacholine. When the anticholinesterase edorphonium (Tensilon) was administered, there was clear separation of the patients with scleroderma and abnormal peristalsis from the other patient groups. It would appear that these patients were unable to manufacture sufficient acetylcholine to respond normally to Tensilon. These studies are consistent with a defect in nerve function. Such a defect is further illustrated by the response to gastrin. As stated previously, gastrin has been shown to exert its effect on the postganglionic segment of the parasympathetic system. All scleroderma patients had a defective response to gastrin, but those with absent peristalsis were almost totally unresponsive to gastrin. The results of these studies have been interpreted to indicate a primary defect in neural function in patients with scleroderma, although the pathogenesis of this neural dysfunction has not been clarified. With further progression of the disease, subsequent muscle abnormality may develop, as indicated by the two patients that failed to show a response in lower esophageal sphincter pressure to methacholine (Cohen et al., 1972).

GASTROESOPHAGEAL REFLUX

Patients with clinical incompetence of the lower esophageal sphincter as manifested by chronic symptoms of heartburn have been characterized by having decreased resting sphincteric pressure (Winans and Harris, 1967). This is illustrated by the mean lower esophageal sphincter pressure of 7.3 mm Hg observed in a group of reflux patients (table 1). It has also been shown that the lower esophageal sphincter in these patients showed a response similar to normal subjects when stimulated by methacholine (Cohen et al., 1972). These observations, combined with the importance attributed to endogenous gastrin in maintaining resting lower esophageal sphincter pressure, have suggested that there might be a defect in circulating gastrin in reflux patients.

Simultaneous measurements of sphincter pressures and serum gastrin concentrations both under basal conditions and after ingestion of a 100 gm roast beef meal have provided some insight into this hypothesis (Farrell et al., 1973). Although mean fasting serum gastrin values of 88.0 ± 7.9 pg/ml (± SE) for reflux patients were less than mean fasting values for normal subjects (103.0 ± 18.2 pg/ml), the difference was not statistically significant. This is in striking contrast to marked differences in the resting lower esophageal sphincter pressures noted in these subjects. Mean resting lower esophageal sphincter pressure was 16.2 ± 0.9 mm Hg for normals and 7.3 ± 0.5 mm Hg for reflux patients ($p < 0.01$). After ingestion of the protein meal, gastrin release by the reflux patients appears to be somewhat deficient. Release of endogenous gastrin after protein ingestion was compared by integration of the curves obtained after feeding, expressed as percent increase over the integrated fasting gastrin concentration. The mean integrated response to feeding, determined by measurement of the area under the curve, for the controls was 114 ± 25%. The mean integrated response for reflux patients was only 57 ± 17%, which is significantly less ($p < 0.05$) than that occurring in normal controls. It would appear from these studies that there is deficient gastrin release in patients with chronic gastroesophageal reflux and suggest an important role for gastrin deficiency in gastroesophageal reflux. However, studies to date have not fully explained the striking differences in resting sphincter pressure. Perhaps the circulating fractions of serum gastrin in these patients are different. In other words, there may be less of an active fraction in the reflux patients as opposed to controls. A more likely possibility seems to be that the defect in the lower esophageal sphincter of reflux patients is a compound one, with abnormality of the muscle itself in addition to gastrin deficiency.

ZOLLINGER-ELLISON SYNDROME

Recent observations on lower esophageal sphincter pressure in patients with the Zollinger-Ellison syndrome are of interest (Isenberg et al., 1971). These patients are characterized by having extremely high levels of circulating endogenous gastrin. With the recent appreciation of the importance of gastrin in maintenance of lower esophageal sphincter pressure, the question arose whether resting pressures were, in fact, increased in patients with Zollinger-Ellison syndrome. Comparison of lower esophageal sphincter pressures of six patients with Zollinger-Ellison syndrome to normal subjects have revealed a significant increase in resting sphincter pressure in these six patients (table 1). In addition, the elevated lower esophageal sphincter pressure was felt to be related to the increases in endogenous gastrin concentrations in these patients since a good linear correlation was noted when lower esophageal sphincter pressures were compared to serum gastrin levels.

PERNICIOUS ANEMIA

Again, because of the demonstration of high fasting serum gastrin values in patients with pernicious anemia, the question of lower esophageal sphincter pressures in these subjects became important. When lower esophageal sphincter pressures were measured in control subjects, patients with pernicious anemia (having elevated serum gastrin) and patients age-matched for the pernicious anemia group, surprising results were obtained. Mean resting pressures were 17.2 ± 0.9 mm Hg for controls, 14.8 ± 0.9 mm Hg for age-matched subjects, and only 9.9 ± 1.4 mm Hg for the pernicious anemia patients. In contrast to the expected elevation of lower esophageal sphincter pressure in pernicious anemia patients, resting pressures were noted to be significantly lower ($p<0.01$) than both controls and age-matched subjects (Farrell et al., 1973). These patients were subsequently studied for their ability to respond to gastric alkalinization, injections of pentagastrin, and also stimulation of smooth muscle with edrophonium and with betazole.

A decreased responsiveness of the pernicious anemia patients was noted to all agents tested. It was concluded from these studies that although serum gastrin is elevated in pernicious anemia, the lower esophageal sphincter pressure is not increased. This was felt to be due to a primary defect in smooth muscle in these patients, possibly related to the smooth muscle atrophy that has been demonstrated in the body of the stomach in this disease. The absence of lower esophageal sphincter response to cholinergic stimulation via edrophonium, and more directly by betazole, was interpreted as evidence for a defect in the smooth muscle in permicious anemia.

Table 3 summarizes the clinical defects in function of the lower esophageal sphincter that have been studied recently. If we consider the three factors that are important in control of this sphincter; neural, muscle, and gastrin, both hypertonic and hypotonic dysfunction have been identified in most of these areas. Achalasia appears to be a manifestation of a hypertonic sphincter secondary to a neural defect. The hypotonic lower esophageal sphincter of scleroderma now would appear to be at least partially due to a neural defect. Although no clear-cut histologic evidence of abnormal muscle at the lower esophageal sphincter has been demonstrated, the pharmacologic studies suggest that pernicious anemia patients have a primary smooth muscle defect. Finally the Zollinger-Ellison syndrome would appear to illustrate the hypertonic lower esophageal sphincter secondary to increases in gastrin, with patients with gastroesophageal reflux demonstrating a sphincter defect secondary to deficient endogenous gastrin.

However, there would appear to be some areas of overlap in this scheme. The studies in patients with gastroesophageal reflux indicate a probable abnormality in smooth muscle function, in addition to gastrin deficiency. In addition, scleroderma patients having a primary defect in neural function may have subsequent abnormality in smooth muscle function. Thus, dysfunction of the esophagogastric junction involves complex interactions between muscular, nervous and hormonal components.

Table 3

Clinical Disorders of Lower Esophageal Sphincter Function and the Proposed Pathophysiologic Mechanism

Hypertonic LES	Defect	Hypotonic LES
Achalasia	Neural	Scleroderma
?	Muscle	Pernicious Anemia
Zollinger-Ellison Syndrome	Endogenous Gastrin	Gastroesophageal Reflux

REFERENCES

Cannon,W., 1939.
A law of denervation.
Am. J. Med. Sci. 198:739.

Castell,D.O., and Harris,L.D., 1970.
Hormonal control of gastroesophageal sphincter strength.
N. Engl. J. Med. 282:886.

Christensen,J., 1970.
Pharmacologic identification of the lower esophageal sphincter.
J. Clin. Invest. 49:681.

Cohen,S., Fisher,R., Lipshutz,W., Turner,R., Myers,A., and Schumacher,R., 1972.
The pathogenesis of esophageal dysfunction in scleroderma and Raynaud's disease.
J. Clin. Invest. 51:2663.

Cohen,S., Fisher,R., and Tuch,A., 1972.
The site of denervation in achalasia.
Gut 13:556.

Cohen,B.R., and Guelrad,M., 1971.
Cardiospasm in achalasia: Demonstration of supersensitivity of the lower esophageal sphincter.
Gastroenterology 60:769.

Cohen,S., and Lipshutz,W., 1971.
Lower esophageal sphincter dysfunction in achalasia.
Gastroenterology 61:814.

Cohen,S., Lipshutz,W., and Hughes,W., 1971.
Role of gastrin supersensitivity in the pathogenesis of lower esophageal sphincter hypertension in achalasia.
J. Clin. Invest. 50:1241.

DiMarino,A.J., and Cohen,S., 1973.
The adrenergic control of lower esophageal sphincter function.
J. Clin. Invest. 52:2264.

Farrell,R.L., Castell,D.O., and McGuigan,J.E., 1973.
Measurements of lower esophageal sphincter pressure and gastrin levels in patients with gastroesophageal reflux.
Clin. Res. 21:512.

Farrell,R.L., Nebel,O.T., McGuire,A.T., and Castell, D.O., 1973.
The abnormal lower esophageal sphinter in pernicious anemia.
Gut (In press).

Isenberg,J., Csendes,J., and Walsh,J., 1971.
Resting and pentagastrin-stimulated gastroesophageal sphincter pressure in patients with Zollinger-Ellison syndrome.
Gastroenterology 61:655.

Lipshutz,W., Hughes,W., and Cohen,S., 1972.
The genesis of lower esophageal sphincter pressure: Its identification through the use of gastrin antiserum.
J. Clin. Invest. 51:522.

Lipshutz,W., Tuch,A., and Cohen,S., 1971.
A comparison of the site of action of gastrin I on lower esophageal and antral circular smooth muscle.
Gastroenterology 61:454.

Roling,G.T., Farrell,R.L., and Castell,D.O., 1972.
Cholinergic response of the lower esophageal sphincter.
Am. J. Physiol. 222:870.

Treacy,W.L., Baggenstoss,A.H., Slocumb,C.H., and Code, C.F., 1963.
Scleroderma of the esophagus. A correlation of histalogic and physiologic findings.
Ann. Intern. Med. 59:351.

Trounce,J.R., Deuchar,D.C., Kauntze,R., and Thomas, G.A., 1957.
Studies in achalasia of the cardia.
Quart. J. Med. 26:433.

Winans,C.S., and Harris,L.D., 1967.
Quantitation of lower esophageal sphincter competence.
Gastroenterology, 52:773.

GASTROINTESTINAL MOTOR DYSFUNCTIONS

Alastair M. Connell

INTRODUCTION

The term "gastrointestinal motor dysfunction" covers a large range of alterations in the function of the gastrointestinal tract. It is to an extent a term of convenience in that it does little but draw attention to the fact that some abnormality of the behavior of the GI muscle is occurring. For the most part, the disturbances which occur have until recently remained unexplained and our descriptions of the dysfunction remain vague and imprecise. In clinical literature the terms "spasm, tone, peristalsis, segmentation" are often used erroneously and an understanding of the abnormalities is frequently lacking.

Motor function of the alimentary tract is defective in a variety of diseases. In some the dysfunction is primary while in others is almost certainly secondary to pathology elsewhere in the gastrointestinal tract. Motor disturbances, the nature of which are still poorly understood, occur in association with pancreatitis, cholecystitis and ulcer disease. It is not uncommon for patients with duodenal ulcer to have lower abdominal cramping pain with a tendency towards constipation. These symptoms are not always prominent and they may be masked by the more severe epigastric discomfort. Marked alterations in the tone of the alimentary tract are well recognized in ulcerative colitis and in certain malabsorptive states. The mechanisms which result in these changes are all poorly understood.

Another preliminary consideration is the frequent coincidence of motor disturbances of different areas of the alimentary tract. It is well recognized that a high proportion of patients with diverticular disease will also have gall bladder disease. There is also a high degree of coincidence between hiatus hernia and diverticular disease. The combination of diverticular disease, hiatus hernia and gall bladder disease (Saint's triangle) occurs in four per cent of patients who have colonic diverticula.

In our present discussion we will focus attention on the lower half of the alimentary tract. Disorders of the lower esophageal sphincter which result in reflux and esophageal discomfort have been considered in another presentation in this Symposium (Castell, 1974). Unfortunately, remarkably little is known about either the normal or the disordered function of the small intestine in man. A reasonably clear understanding of both the electrical basis for contraction and the effects of the contraction of the intestinal muscle has been developed in animals but in man, only the activity of the duodenum has been intensively studied (Ingelfinger and Abbott, 1940; Foulk et al., 1954; Kewenter and Koch, 1960). In view of the paucity of normal data about the small intestine, it is hardly surprising that reports on disturbed motor function in the small intestine are largely anecdotal and uncontrolled (Ingelfinger and Abbott, 1940; Farrar and Bernstein, 1958; Connell, 1961).

A different picture emerges at the lower colon. This has been intensively studied over the past 15 years and an understanding of the functional disorders which occur in this area is slowly but definitely emerging. The very common disturbances normally described as the irritable colon syndrome are now better understood and probable mechanisms of their occurrence have been presented. Diverticular disease, whose incidence has shown a dramatic increase, is also much better understood and possible mechanisms of its occurrence have been described.

There is now agreement among investigators about the general features of the motility of the sigmoid colon. Both from the radiological and manometric analogues it has become apparent that the main, if not the sole, activity of sigmoid colon is segmenting contraction (Connell, 1961a). Peristaltic movements can occur and are a feature of normal defecation. While they can also be stimulated by certain laxatives (Hardcastle and Mann, 1968), in the normal resting state they occur very rarely.

It seems likely that the sigmoid colon is a specialized area. The frequency of contraction increases in the lower part of the sigmoid colon and continues to increase into the upper rectum (Connell, 1961b). This effect has also been observed in relation to the electrical activity of this area where an increased frequency of the pacesetter potential has been observed in the lower sigmoid and upper rectum (Christensen et al., 1969). The likely result of this change in the gradient is that there will be a greater number of systoles distally with the effect of containing stool and other colonic content above the recto-sigmoid junction. It is certainly clear from transit studies that the stool is retained in the sigmoid for long periods of time and thus it may not be surprising that this area of the colon is particularly susceptible to malfunction. For example, diverticula occur in the sigmoid colon in 94% of persons with diverticular disease (Parks, 1968), the sigmoid is the most common site of carcinoma of the colon, and the radiological changes which are associated with the irritable colon syndrome when observed appear to be concentrated in the sigmoid.

THE IRRITABLE COLON SYNDROME

The term "irritable colon syndrome" is synonymous with spastic colon and functional lower bowel disease. "Mucus colitis" expresses only that particular aspect of the irritable colon syndrome which is associated with the excess passage of mucus. It is a bad term since, to many patients, it has the significance of a more serious type of colitis. Two distinct clinical histories are recorded under the term irritable colon (Chaudhary and Truelove, 1962). The first and, in terms of numbers, less common syndrome is illustrated by the patient who has morning diarrhea. Typically, such a patient, on awakening may have several watery stools in rapid succession either before or after breakfast. Normally the diarrhea declines as the day progresses and usually in the latter half of the day the patient is completely comfortable. Pain is not a prominent feature in this condition nor are abdominal distension, bloating or upper GI symptoms. Typically this condition is associated with a featureless tonically contracted left colon which shows few or no haustrations on x-ray. Manometrically very few contractions are seen and it is likely that this colon is functioning as a drain pipe along which the watery stool passes unimpeded. Mechanisms causing this syndrome are not understood.

More commonly and more typically, the term "irritable bowel syndrome" refers to that condition in which occur intermittent episodes of lower abdominal pain associated with a disturbance of bowel habit. The patient is often a young person, most often female, and usually in an upper social group. The abdominal pain is intermittent with varying frequency but typically may occur once or twice a month. The pain frequently is described as cramping, usually left sided although not exclusively so, and can at times be very severe. The patient will normally describe constipation by which is implied the passage of small hard stools, often with straining and with a lack of satisfactory defecation. Sometimes diarrhea will be described, by which is usually meant frequent bowel actions in which small amount of stool are passed, sometimes containing large amounts of mucus. Not uncommonly, the abdominal pain is accompanied by bloating and objective distension and the pain can be relieved by passing flatus or defecation. In one particular variety of this condition symptoms are precipitated by eating and at such time the distension and bloating can be very severe. Patients with the irritable colon syndrome not infrequently admit to certain emotional tensions; marital disturbances seem to occur rather more frequently in this group of patients than in control groups (Kasich, 1965; Feldman, 1965; Diamond, 1964; Ryle, 1928; White and Jones, 1940; Chaudhary and Truelove, 1962).

Increased knowledge of the factors involving the control of the sigmoid colon have increased our understanding of the causation of the symptoms of the irritable colon syndrome. It has been known for several years that the colon responds to prostigmine more vigorously in patients with the irritable colon syndrome than in normal subjects (Chaudhary and Truelove, 1961; Wangel and Deller, 1965).

It is well known that the sigmoid colon responds to eating by an increase in the pressure activity and this so-called gastrocolic reflex has been studied intensively. The pathways for this response still remain obscure. It is clear, however, that the reflex can persist after vagotomy (figure 1) (Connell and McKelvey, 1970) and also persist after longitudinal transection of the spinal cord (Connell et al., 1963). More recently it has become apparent that the sigmoid colon responds to humoral stimuli. In cross-circulation experiments in dogs the colon of the recepient dog responds to the placing of food in the stomach of the donor dog (Logan, 1967). Gastrin in large doses causes an increase in the motility of the colon (Connell and Logan, 1967) but as the doses required are out of physiological range and, furthermore, the response persists after antrectomy, it is unlikely that this is the physiological stimulus. The placing of food in the duodenum results in a prompt response and this has focused attention on the possible role of CCK/PZ in this response. CCK/PZ, given in doses which produce submaximal or maximal response of pancreatic secretion, increases the motor activity of the sigmoid colon (Dinoso et al., 1973). The effect of secretin on the motility of the sigmoid colon is less well established. Following injections of secretin (Boots) in doses which are submaximal for the stimulation of pancreatic secretion, we observed no effect on the motility of the sigmoid colon. The same dose of secretin was also found to be without effect on the motility of the sigmoid colon which had been stimulated by food (Connell, unpublished observations) (table 1).

Table 1

Patient	Basal	Secretin	Difference
		Fasting	
I.C.	0	4.3	+ 4.3
M.P.	0	2	+ 2
C.B.	30.0	13.3	−16.7
M.D.	31.2	56.8	+25.6
W.M.	20.6	16.6	− 4.0
R.L.	16.4	18.5	+1.9
	Mean Difference = +2.18 cm^2		
		Fed	
W.S.	18.1	32.3	+14.2
D.M.	21.0	6.5	−14.5
E.M.	13.5	13.9	+0.4
F.M.	0	0	0
M.J.	8.5	16.7	+8.2
	Mean Difference = +1.66 cm^2		

Effect of secretin on motor response of sigmoid colon in fasting and fed patient as measured from area described by the trace above base line levels. Secretin dose: 1 unit/kg body wt.

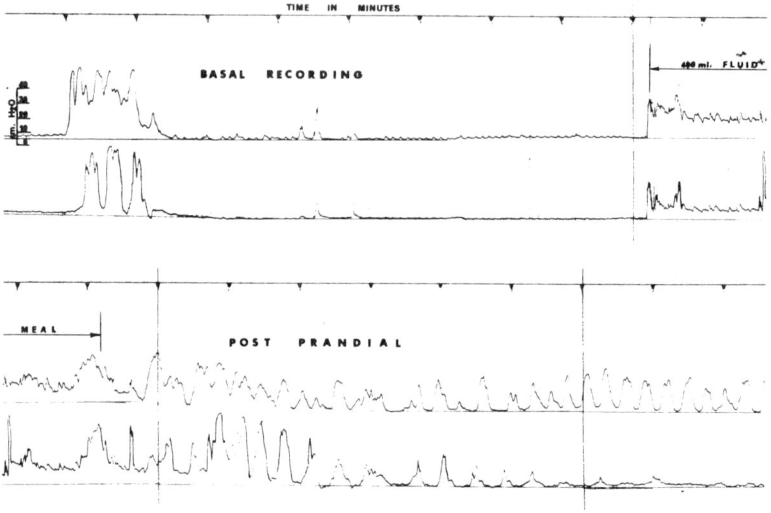

Fig. 1. The effect of feeding a fluid meal on the motility of the sigmoid colon in a patient who has a vagotomy and pyloroplasty. A vigorous gastro-colonic response is observed in the post-prandial period. (Two-minute recording between vertical lines omitted).

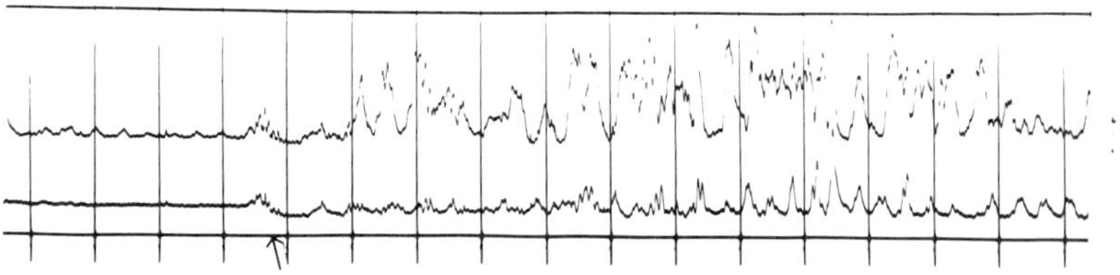

Fig. 2. The effect of eating (marked by the arrow) on the sigmoid motor activity of a patient with the irritable colon syndrome at a time when symptoms were active. A vigorous and exaggerated post-prandial response is observed, particularly in the upper channel (recording from the sigmoid colon).

Similarly, Dinoso et al., (1973) obtained unequivocal effects of secretin on spontaneous sigmoid colon motor activity. These workers also noted that the motor activity of the sigmoid which was induced by cholecystokinin was influenced by secretin (GIH–Karolinska Institute) only in doses of 2 units/kg. It is not yet certain whether levels produced by this dose are in the physiological range or are supraphysiological.

Certain patients with the irritable colon syndrome have an exaggerated response to prostigmine (Chaudhary and Truelove, 1961). If studied at a time when the symptoms are active such patients have also been shown to have an exaggerated response to eating (figure 2) and it has been postulated for some time that this response may be mediated by a humoral mechanism (Connell et al., 1965). The exaggerated segmenting activity of the sigmoid colon which occurs at this time results in a delayed forward movement with a tendency to distension proximally. It is likely that it is this distension which is the cause of the symptoms experienced by the patient and that the effector substance for this response is CCK/PZ. When patients who have the irritable colon syndrome are studied during a phase of symptoms, they can be shown to have an exaggerated response to CCK/PZ (Harvey et al., 1973).

At the present time it is not clear whether the exaggerated sigmoid response is due to excessive release of the hormone or to an undue sensitivity of the muscle but the latter is more likely. It may be that the exaggerated responses occur at a time where there is an increased cholenergic background for muscle contraction, possibly as a result of emotional factors.

RELATIONSHIP BETWEEN IRRITABLE COLON SYNDROME AND DIVERTICULAR DISEASE

It remains unsettled whether a prolonged history of the irritable colon syndrome finally gives rise to the presence of diverticula in the colon and diverticular disease. The natural history of the irritable colon syndrome is for continuation of the intermittent symptoms to persist over prolonged periods of time, often several years, and it has seemed reasonable to postulate that the persistent occurrence of high pressures in this area might give rise to pulsion diverticula. However, hard evidence remains lacking. Indeed, one

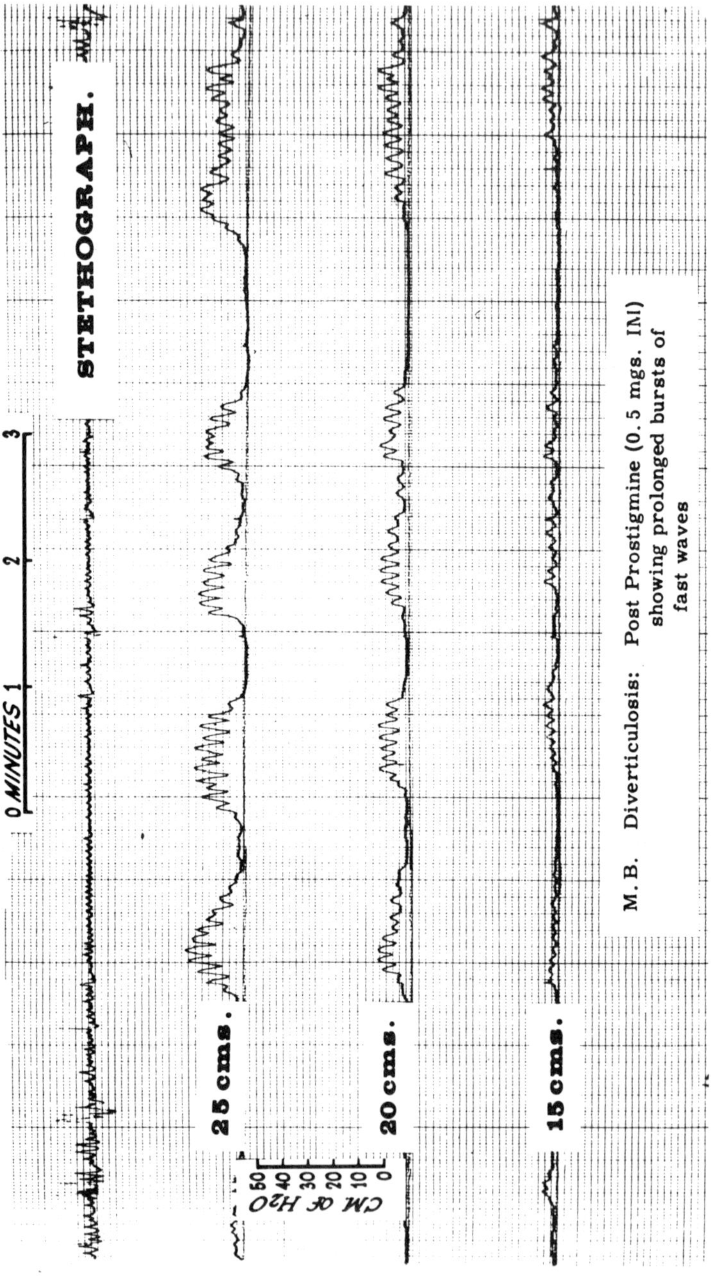

Fig. 3. An illustration of fast wave activity in the sigmoid and upper rectum of a patient with diverticular disease.

survey showed that more than half the patients admitted to hospital with acute diverticular disease had a history of less than one month (Parks and Connell, 1970). It is possible, therefore, that a number of routes exist for the production of diverticula and diverticular disease. The evidence for an association rests on radiological anecdotes, the fact that on occasion sigmoid muscle thickening occurs in the absence of diverticula and that in both of the conditions of irritable colon and established diverticular disease the sigmoid colon responds in an exaggerated way to pharmacological stimuli (Painter and Truelove, 1964; Arfwidsson, 1964; Chaudhary and Truelove, 1961). In addition, in both diseases the sigmoid colon can overreact to food as studied by measurement of intraluminal pressures using open-ended tubes (Parks and Connell, 1969; Arfwidsson, 1964). One other interesting similarity is the presence in both conditions of waves of greater frequency than occur normally. It is unusual in recordings from the normal colon to find waves of greater than 2 per minute. However, in a proportion of patients with the irritable colon syndrome and patients with diverticular disease a considerable proportion of the activity consists of waves at a frequency of 5 per minute or more (figure 3). The significance of these waves has not been explored and their occurrence in the two conditions may be coincidental.

The postulate that diverticula result from the existence of high pressures in the sigmoid colon is an attractive one. High pressures are more likely to occur in the colon when that organ is narrowed. For a pressure to be recorded from a tube such as the colon two conditions are required: not only should there be some alteration in the caliber of the organ resulting from a muscular contraction, but there also must be a resistence to the escape of content from the contracting segment. This is illustrated in figure 4. In the upper illustration where no resistence occurs muscular contraction does not result in any increased pressure in the recording point. In the lowest channel where there is a closure of the contracting segment a high pressure is measured. Where the closure is incomplete, as in the middle channel, only a modest pressure is recorded. Clearly the narrower the lumen of the bowel the more likely it is that complete segmental occlusion may occur and therefore the possibility of the occurrence of high pressures is enhanced. It is postulated that such high pressures result in pulsion diverticula. Diverticula do occur at

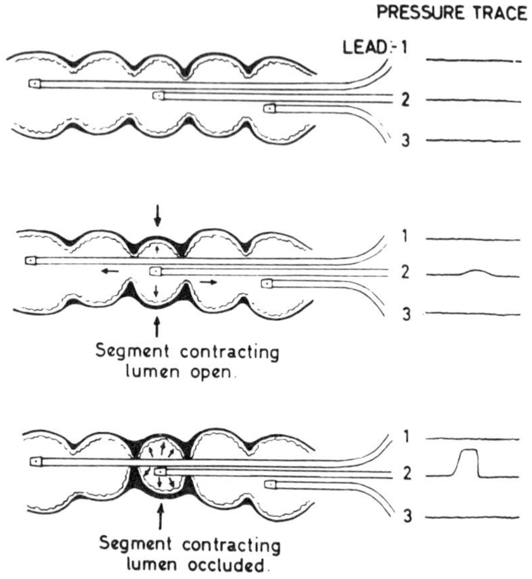

Fig. 4. The mechanism of production of pressure waves (See text for explanation) (After Painter et al., 1965).

areas of weakness in the muscle wall usually at the entry point of blood vessels on the mesenteric side of the bowel.

These pathological considerations are of interest in relation to current epidemiological studies in diverticular disease.

The incidence of diverticular disease has increased greatly in the western world in recent years. In 1930 Mayo thought that the disease affected 5% of the population over 40 (Mayo, 1930). In Great Britain the current incidence is very high. A 1967 study showed that, in the Oxford area of England, one-third of persons over the age of 60 and 40 per cent of those over 70 had the disease (Manousos et al., 1967). In Belfast, Northern Ireland, the incidence also rises markedly with age, reaching more than 40 per cent in persons 70 years and over (Parks, 1968).

There are also marked variations in incidence in different group of people. In non-Europeans the condition is rare. It is almost unknown in rural Africa and has a small incidence in the urban Africans of Johannesburg and Ibadan (Burkitt); however, its incidence and complications are as frequent in black Americans as in white. The disease is rare in the Japanese in Japan, but is seen in the Japanese living in Hawaii.

The common factor which seems to emerge from these observations is that in areas of the world where the diet contains large quantities of natural fibre the incidence of diverticular disease is low or nil, whereas in areas where the diet is highly refined and contains only small amounts of natural fibre the incidence of diverticular disease is high. There is no doubt that dietary fibre results in a large increase in the volume of the stool (table 2). In normal subjects the volume of the stool is doubled by increases in the intake of dietary fibre. It is likely that the presence of these large quantities of stool will result in time in a wider calibre in the bowel with the decreased likelihood of the existence of complete occlusion by muscular contractions of the sigmoid colon.

Table 2

Patient	Corn Flakes	Bran	Patient	Corn Flakes	Bran
A	145	291	E	148	394
B	76	130	F	98	180
C	149	211	G	127	235
D	136	282	H	104	195

Comparison of average daily total weight of stools from patients maintained on a corn flakes diet and a bran diet.

Whether or not an increase in the intake of dietary fibre will help patients with established diverticular disease is not established. A considerable number of physicians are now treating patients with diverticular disease with dietary fibre and enthusiastic reports are appearing in the literature. However, at this time no good controlled trial has emerged to establish the value of this treatment. It is conceivable too that once the diverticula are established, especially if fibrosis has occurred following infective complications of diverticula, that no dietary changes will affect the condition.

It should not be assumed that all functional bowel disease results from similar mechanisms. Other mechanisms clearly exist. For example, in patients who have dificiency of lactase, absolutely or partially, the ingestion of lactose results in an osmotic diarrhea due to the failure of the small bowel to split the lactose. On arrival in the colon the lactose is split by colonic bacteria with lactic acid production lowering the pH and diarrheal symptoms. In other situations patients who have had vagotomy and pyloroplasty have a condition symptomatically somewhat similar to that spontaneous irritable colon. The mechanism here, however, is almost certainly related to the rapid emptying to the stomach into the small intestine (McKelvey, 1970). In some of these patients symptoms become much worse following the ingestion of osmotic materials and the mechanism almost certainly is the failure of the food to achieve isotonicity before entering the small intestine. Individuals at certain times are unable to cope with this osmotic load which results in decompensation of the small and large intestine and resulting in frequency of defecation and diarrhea.

However, mechanisms are being established which account for a considerable proportion of the patients classed as functional bowel disorders and more encouragingly, rational means of therapy are beginning to emerge. It is probably time that new names develop for these conditions and clearly the existing umbrella term, colonic motor dysfunction, is unsatisfactory. It is not descriptive and retains overtones of a purely emotional disturbance. Now that the mechanisms become better understood more appropriate descriptive terms will no doubt be proposed.

REFERENCES

Arfwidsson,S., 1964.
Pathogenesis of multiple diverticula of the sigmoid colon in diverticular disease.
Acta Chir. Scand. (Suppl.), 342.

Burkitt,D., (Personal communication).

Chaudhary,N.A., and Truelove,S.C., 1961.
Human colonic motility: a comparative study of normal subjects, patients with ulcerative colitis and patients with the irritable colon syndrome.
Gastroenterology, 40:1.

Chaudhary,N.A., and Truelove,S.C., 1962.
The irritable colon syndrome.
Q. J. Med., 31:307.

Christensen,J., Caprilli,R., and Lund,G.F., 1969.
Electric slow waves in circular muscle of cat colon.
Am. J. Physiol., 217:771.

Connell,A., 1969a.
The motility of the small intestine.
Postgrad. Med. J., 37:703.

Connell,A., 1969b.
The motility of the pelvic colon. I. Motility in normals and in patients with asymptomatic duodenal ulcer.
Gut, 2:175.

Connell,A., Frankel,H., and Guttman,L., 1963.
The motility of the pelvic colon following complete lesion of the spinal cord.
Paraplegia, 1:98.

Connell,A., Avery-Jones,F., and Rowlands,E.N., 1965.
Motility of the pelvic colon. IV. Abdominal pain associated with colonic hypermotility after meals.
Gut, 6:105.

Connell,A., and Logan,C.J.H., 1967.
The role of gastrin in gastro-ileocolic responses.
Am. J. Dig. Dis., 12:277.

Connell,A., and McKelvey,S., 1970.
The influence of vagotomy on the colon.
Proc. R. Soc. Med., 63: (Suppl.)7-9.
Connell,A., and Smith,C.L., (Unpublished observations).
Diamond,S., 1964.
Amitriptyline in the treatment of gastrointestinal disorders.
Psychomatics, 5:211.
Dinoso,V.P., Meshkinpour,H., Lorber,S.H., Gutierrez, J.G., and Chey,W.Y., 1973.
Motor responses of the sigmoid colon and rectum to exogenous cholecystokinin and secretin.
Gastroenterology, 65:438.
Farrar,J., and Bernstein,J.S., 1958.
Recording of intraluminal gastrointestinal presures by a radiotelemetering capsule.
Gastroenterology, 35:603.
Feldman,P.E., 1965.
The mask of depression.
J. Kans. Med. Soc., 66:6.
Foulk,W.T., Code,C.F., Morlock,C.G., and Bargen,J.A., 1954.
A study of the motility patterns and the basic ryhthm in the duodenum and upper part of the jujunum of human beings.
Gastroenterology, 26:601.
Hardcastle,J.O., and Mann,C.V., 1968.
Study of large bowel peristalsis.
Gut, 9:512.
Harvey,R.F., Pomare,E.W., and Heaton,K.W., 1973.
Effects of increased dietary fibre on intestinal transit.
Lancet., 1:1278.
Ingelfinger,F., and Abbott,W.O., 1940.
Intubation studies of the human small intestine. Diagnostic significance of motor disturbances.
Am. J. Dig. Dis. 7:468.
Kasich,A.M., 1965.
Management of emotional disorders, anxiety, and depression in patients with gastrointestinal disease.
Curr. Ther. Res., 7:542.

Kewenter,J., and Koch,N.G., 1960.
Motility of the small intestine. A method for the continuous recording of intraluminal pressure variations.
Acta Chir. Scand., 119:430.
Logan,C.J.H., 1967.
The role of gastrin in the control of intestinal motility.
M.Ch. Thesis, Queen's University of Belfast.
Manousos,O.N., Truelove,S.K., and Lumsden,K., 1967.
Prevalence of colonic diverticulosis in general population of Oxford area.
Br. Med. J., 3:762.
Mayo,W.J., 1930.
Diverticula of the sigmoid.
Ann. Surg., 92:739.
McKelvey,S., 1970.
Gastric incontinence in post-vagotomy diarrhea.
Br. J. Surg., 57:741.
Painter,N.S., and Truelove.S.C., 1964.
The intraluminal pressure patterns in diverticulosis of the colon. I. Resting patterns of pressure. II. The effect of morphine.
Gut, 5:201.
Parks,T.G., 1968.
Post mortem studies on the colon with special reference to diverticular disease.
Proc. R. Soc. Med., 61:30.
Parks,T.G., and Connell,A., 1969.
Motility studies in diverticular disease of the colon. I. basal activity and response to food assessed by open-ended tube and mineraturе balloon techniques. II. Effect of colonic and rectal distension.
Gut, 10:534.
Parks,T.G., and Connell,A., 1970.
The outcome in 455 patients admitted for treatment of diverticular disease of the colon.
Br. J. Surg., 57:775.
Ryle,J.A., 1928.
An address on chronic spasmatic effection of the colon and diseases which they stimulate.
Lancet., 2:1115.

Wangel,A.G., and Deller,D.J., 1965.
Intestinal motility in man. III. Mechanisms of constipation and diarrhea with particular reference to the irritable colon syndrome.
Gastroenterology, 48:69.
White,P.B., and Jones,C.M., 1940.
Mucus colitis: delineation of the syndrome with certain observations on its mechanism and the role of emotional stress as a precipitating factor.
Ann. Intern. Med., 14:854.

DYSFUNCTION OF GASTRIC SECRETION

S. P. Bralow

INTRODUCTION

Man has been interested in gastric function from the earliest of time. Undoubtedly, some Roman glutton described verbally or on waxed tablets the gastric contents he had forcefully evacuated after a recent debauch. However, it was not until the mid-18th Century that gastric digestion was considered to be a chemical action of acid gastric juice rather than bacterial fermentation. Although Beaumont (1833) passed a tube made of gum acacia through a gastric fistula and studied secretion during hunger and feeding it took 50 years more before Leube (1871) suggested that analysis of gastric contents aspirated via a stomach tube could be used for diagnostic purposes. During the next 100 years, well over 10,000 articles on gastric secretory function have been published making this scientific exercise probably the single most popular in the annals of medical history (Ingelfinger, 1973). Significant advances in our understanding of gastric secretion have resulted but clinical benefits are still limited.

Gastric juice contains a mixture of water, inorganic ions, hydrochloric acid, pepsinogen, mucus, polypeptides and intrinsic factor. Of these, the only essential component is intrinsic factor. The absence of acid or pepsin does not appear to influence body function significantly. The complexity of these electrolytic solutions was described in physico-chemical terms by Moore (1967). To achieve uniformity of terminology, it was suggested that terms such as clinical units, free acid, total acid, and combined acid be replaced by hydrogen ion concentration and titratable acidity. The electrolyte composition of gastric juice usually follows a fixed relationship to that of the hydrogen ion. When secretion is primarily from the parietal cells, acid and chloride outputs are increased and sodium concentration is decreased. High sodium concentration after maximal stimulation suggests either an increased non-parietal cell secretion or back diffusion of the hydrogen ion through an injured mucosa. With very few exceptions, the output of pepsin from the zymogen cells and the secretion of intrinsic factor from the parietal cells also parallel the acid output. Attempts at difining the characteristics of gastric mucus have been extensive but the results as yet have little clinical usefulness.

Gastric secretory studies are being used; to aid in the diagnosis of gastric and duodenal disease; as an indicator of the prognosis in peptic ulcer; to determine the completeness of surgically-induced vagotomy and for the selection of suitable surgical procedures. Maximal and peak acid output have been determined by using the "augmented histamine test" of Kay (1953) and the peak acid output of Baron (1963). The maximal acid output has been found to correlate well with the parietal cell mass (Card and Marks, 1960). Unfortunately, histamine produces many side effects which can be only partially blocked by the concomitant administration of an antihistaminic. An analogue of histamine, betazole hydrochloride has similar side effects though usually not as severe. Pentagastrin appears to be the safest of the gastric stimulants and has replaced the other agents in clinical practice in England.

The diagnostic value of gastric analysis has been limited by the degree of overlapping of values between normal populations and those with duodenal and gastric ulcerations. This has been especially true for basal acid secretion with a great variation from one study to the next in the same individual. Individual variations are less marked for maximal acid outputs. Blackman et al., (1970) established tables for peak acid output according to age, sex, and weight of the patients admitted to their hospital. The group with proven duodenal ulcer were clearly separable from non-ulcer patients when using their tables for expected values.

The responsiveness of the parietal cell mass to maximal stimulation varies under many conditions. Vagal stimulation may influence the oxyntic cells directly or via the antral release of gastrin. The degree of vagal influence may differ from one individual to another. Highly selective vagotomy of the parietal cell mass without concomitant drainage procedures decreases the sensitivity of the parietal cell mass to stimulation by shifting the dose response curve

Table 1

Range of Acid Secretion (mEq/hr.) in Various Diseases

	Basal	MAO
Control males	2.5(0 – 9.5)	22.4(10.1–34.5)
females	1.3(0 – 6.8)	14.8(0.1–31.3)
Duodenal ulcer		
males	6.0(0.1–23.1)	37.5(4.9–91.7)
females	3.3(0.1–14.9)	24.3(4.6–43.9)
Post-op dyspepsia	1.4(0 – 4.2)	4.3(0.8–14.7)
Stomal ulcers		
gastro-jej.	8.7(5.1–30.0)	43.5(26.6–60.7)
gastrectomy	7.7(0.6–19.8)	31.1(7.7–82.0)
vagotomy and drainage	3.1(0.1– 8.9)	19.3(6.8–39.0)
Gastric ulcers		
primary		15.7(0.5–48.0)
secondary to duod. ulcer		24.9(4.2–65.0)
Gastric cancer		
upper third		3.8(0 –15.5)
mid-third		3.7(0 –16.5)
lower third		11.7(0.5–47.3)

(Modified from: Baron, J. H., 1970)

Table 2

Dysfunction of Gastric Secretion—Clinical Situations

Diminished:	Increased:
Atrophic Gastritis	Duodenal Ulcer
Gastric Malignancy	Hypertrophic hypersecretory gastropathy
Pernicious Anemia	Zollinger-Ellison Syndrome
Adrenal Insufficiency	Short-bowel Syndrome
Hypophysectomy	Portocaval shunt
Menetrier's Disease	Hyperthyroidism
Post-vagotomy	Hyperparathyroidism (hypercalcemia)
	Renal dialysis and transplantation

for acid output to the right. The final maximal response appears to be the same, however. The release of hormones from the duodenal mucosa acts as a feedback mechanism for the control of acid secretion in man. Both secretin and cholecystokinin inhibit gastrin stimulated secretion.

Despite the limitations imposed by the clinical testing of gastric function, many disorders are associated with gastric dysfunction. Some conditions lead to secretory failure while others are associated with hypersecretion. Further clarification of the pathophysiology of these disorders may lead to improved diagnostic accuracy.

DECREASED GASTRIC FUNCTIONS

Gastritis

More than half of the random population have inflammatory changes in the gastric mucosa. These changes can be classified as follows:

1. Normal mucosa—slight infiltration of plasma cells and lymphocytes below the surface and above the muscularis mucosa. Lymphocytic aggregates can be present at the base of the mucosa.
2. Superficial gastritis—increased plasma cells and lymphocytes below the surface epithelium and lamina propria. The foveolar layer is thickened but the glandular layer and the body glands remain normal. Inflammatory cells can be seen between the gastric tubules (interstitial gastritis). Gastric secretion usually is normal.
3. Atrophic gastritis—loss of normal body glands but the foveolar layer is increased. Inflammatory cells may be present. Metaplasia or intestinalization may or may not be present. Associated with the decrease in the glandular mucosal thickness there is marked decrease in gastric secretion.

The presence of these inflammatory reactions increases with age in a linear fashion and Siurala et al., (1968) has calculated a yearly increased incidence of approximately 1.4% for the group of random population studied; 25% of the patients had superficial gastritis while 28% had atrophic gastritis. Sequential studies suggest that the transition from superficial to atrophic gastritis may require a period of 19 years or more and that acid secretion fails before pepsin secretion. The maximal acid output for patients with superficial gastritis showed marked overlap with the patients having normal gastric mucosa.

Table 3

Maximal Acid Secretion (mEq/hr.) in Gastritis

	Male	Female
Normal Mucosa	28.8 (10.7–72.4)	17.2 (2.6–46.8)
Superficial Gastritis	11.7 (1.9–21.6)	9.6 (0 –31.6)
Atrophic Gastritis	5.6 (0 –20.6)	3.2 (0 –18.6)

(Modified from J. H. Baron, 1970)

The responsiveness of the parietal cell mass also decreases with increasing gastritis and the dose response curve to histamine is shifted to the right. The ratio of basal acid output to maximal acid output is higher in atrophic gastritis because of a sustained gastrin release from the antrum in hypochlorhydric patients.

Studies correlating gastric mucosal histology with secretory function and the presence of auto-antibodies have demonstrated two distinct types of atrophic gastritis (Strickland et al., 1973). Patients with parietal cell antibodies in the serum usually have diffuse gastritis with markedly reduced acid secretion and raised serum gastrin level.

Table 4

Types of Atrophic Gastritis

	Type A	Type B
Parietal Cell Antibodies	+	0
Antral gastritis	–	+
Body gastritis		
diffuse	+	+/–
focal	+/–	+
Acid secretion	↓↓	↓
Raised gastrin	87%	10%
Intrinsic factor antibody	30%	0%
Pernicious anemia	16%	0%
Thyroid antibodies	66%	12%
Antinuclear antibodies	25%	25%

(Modified from R. G. Strickland and I. R. Mackay, Amer. J. Dig. Dis. 18:426, 1973).

Serum parietal cell auto-antibodies are detected in over 80% and intrinsic factor antibodies in 30% of the patients with Type A gastritis. Atrophic gastrits, Type A and pernicious anemia are frequently associated with other diseases of auto-immune mechanisms; Hashimoto's thyroiditis, hypoadrenalism, hypoparathyroidism, vitiligo, and diabetes mellitus. Non-organic specific antibodies; such as the antinuclear antibodies, occur in both Type A and Type B gastritis.

Gastrointestinal symptoms and complications are more frequently seen in the Type B gastritic group. Some degree of atrophic gastritis is invariably present in patients with chronic benign ulcer of the gastric corpus. The chronic gastritis persists after the ulcer has healed and this supports the view that the gastric ulcer originates from the chronic gastritis rather than vice versa. Experimental ulcers can be produced in transplanted atrophic gastric mucosa by irrigating with acid peptic juice. Type B patients who can still secrete some acid are more susceptible to gastric ulcer formation.

Type B gastritis occurs more frequently and is by far the most common type of inflammation associated with malignancy. In Japan, gastritis was equally severe in early and advanced gastric cancer and that antral gastritis was consistently present. Carcinomas of the gastric remnant are being reported more and more frequently following resections for previously benign lesions. The gastritis that develops after surgical resection resembles Type B.

Evidence of chronic recurring inflammation is often present in the Type B gastritic mucosa. Many irritants have been under suspect; tabacco, alcohol, and salicylates. In 80% of hospitalized alcoholics studied, evidence of antral gastritis returned to normal with abstinence. The maximum acid output in chronic alcoholics is dependent on the mucosal histology of the body of the stomach and is not influenced by concomitant pancreatic exocrine insufficiency or fatty liver. Chronic analgesic abuse may cause Type B gastritis, and the degree of damage is dependent upon the presence of acid in the lumen of the stomach. Reduction of acid by vagotomy, antacids or even radiation further protect the mucosa from aspirin damage. Achlorhydric patients have minimal blood loss after ingesting aspirin.

Type B gastritis may result from reflux of bile and duodenal contents through an incompetent pyloric sphincter into the antrum and body of the stomach. This mechanism may be the major cause of post-gastrectomy gastritis or antral gastritis secondary to duodenal ulceration. Bile destroys the gastric mucosal barrier with resultant back diffusion of hydrogen ion, increased pepsin secretion, and increased gastrin release. Similar bile reflux has been shown to occur following stress and may be the cause for stress ulceration especially when associated with ischemia due to shock.

Unexplained iron deficiency is found in 40–60% of patients with both Type A and Type B forms of atrophic gastritis. Possible mechanism include occult bleeding, loss of parietal cell mass, malabsorption of dietary iron due to the lack of gastric acid or other gastric factors that promote iron absorption. Correction of the iron deficiency anemia may result in improvement of gastric secretion and histology of the mucosa especially in young persons who do not have parietal cell antibodies in their serum.

Pernicious Anemia

Auto immune factors play a significant role in the eventual development of Type A atrophic gastritis and pernicious anemia. Auto antibodies to the microsomal components of gastric parietal cells as well as to intrinsic factor have been demonstrated in both serum and gastric juice. Complexes of intrinsic factor and its antibody in gastric juice suggest a causal relationship. Some patients with chronic atrophic gastritis have reduced intrinsic factor secretion but still are able to bind Vitamin B_{12} for small bowel absorption. The mucosa in these patients have the same appearance as in frank pernicious anemia but the sera do not contain IF antibodies. The presence of antibodies may determine which patients go on to develop pernicious anemia. Steroids by inhibiting IF antibody production may cause a partial regeneration of the body glands and aid Vitamin B_{12} absorption. Genetic factors have been implicated although the mode of inheritance remains unresolved. Combinations of atrophic gastritis, Vitamin B_{12} malabsorption and auto-antibodies to gastric antigens occur with greater frequency in first degree relatives of patients with pernicious anemia then in general population. Diseases associated with pernicious anemia also occur with increased frequency in relatives.

An inadequate production of intrinsic factor is present since birth in patients with juvenile pernicious anemia. Acid secretion may be normal during periods of remission secondary to Vitamin B_{12} therapy. In the absence of Vitamin B_{12}, histamine–fast achlorhydria will occur although the mucosa is still normal. Patients with

Carcinoma of the Stomach

Attempts to differentiate benign from malignant gastric lesion by gastric secretory function have not been successful. Patients with benign gastric ulcers have basal and maximal acid outputs corresponding to the residual parietal cell mass. Lesions involving the body of the stomach with destruction or involvement of the body glands have the lowest outputs, while lesions of the antrum with intact body glands have the highest and may be in the range of duodenal ulcerations. Acid may also diffuse back through the mucosa of the body or antrum when the barrier is broken by inflammatory changes. Only 20% of patients with malignant gastric ulcers have histamine-fast achlorhydria while 5% or more secrete more than control levels of acid. The combined criteria levels of anacidity and low intrinsic factor output reflect atrophy of the same parietal cells. The fasting serum gastrin levels vary inversely with the gastric acid output.

Table 5

Value of Gastric Secretory Studies in Cancer

	Benign Gastric Ulcer	Carcinoma
Anacidity (pH>7)	0%	18%
MAO>20 mEq/hr.	32%	5%
IF output<lower limits of normal	12%	67%
β-glucuronidase—units/mg. protein		
< lowest value of Ca (0.6)	50%	–
< lowest value of Ca (0.1)	0%	–
> highest value for non-Ca	–	9–24%

(Modified from J. H. Baron, 1970)

Various enzymes in the gastric juice have been studied in the hope of further defining patients with gastric malignancy from those with atrophy or benign lesions. β-glucuronidase activity is present at about 3 times the normal level in gastric tissue or juice of patients with gastric cancer, but the levels are better correlated with the severity of the surrounding gastritis than with the extent of malignant involvement or degree of differentiation. Considerable overlap between the normal and carcinoma ranges limits its clinical usefulness. A similar problem exists for lactic dehydrogenase and leucine aminopeptidase.

Imerslund Syndrome have adequate secretion of IF and acid but there is a specific small bowel malabsorption for the Vitamin B_{12}-IF complex due to blocking antibodies at the binding sites of the ileal mucosa.

Intrinsic factor secretion can be stimulated by histamine, insulin, gastrin and food in the normal stomach. Vagotomy causes a lesser reduction of IF secretion than acid secretion even though both are derived from parietal cells. Patients with gastric ulcer may have a normal or a low IF secretion and those with gastric cancer have levels as low as patients with PA. Gastric cancer develops in approximately 10% of patients with PA. This risk is 2 to 3 times greater than in the general Caucasian population.

Hypertrophic Gastropathy

Giant hypertrophy of the gastric mucosa is an uncommon lesion first described by Menetrier (1888). Confusion still exists about this disorder because of many variant manifestations. It may be classified as follows:

1. Benign hypertrophy—non-inflammatory enlargement of rugal folds and mucosal thickness.
2. Hypertrophic glandular gastritis—inflammatory changes present.
3. Hypertrophic hypersecretory gastritis—increased acid, pepsin and mucoprotein secretion but no excessive protein loss. It may be associated with:
   a. Intractable duodenal ulcer.
   b. Multiple endocrine adenopathies (Wermer syndrome).
   c. Zollinger-Ellison Syndrome.
4. Hypertrophic protein-losing gastropathy (Menetrier's disease)—hypoacidity or achlorhydria with marked loss of protein into the gastric lumen.

In Menetrier's disease the hyperplasia of the superficial epithelium is marked. The mucosa is edematous and infiltrated with chronic inflammatory cells. The glands are elongated and dilated and the chief cells are replaced by mucus producing cells. Atrophy of the duodenal bulb may be present. Sequential studies of Menetrier's disease have demonstrated cases in which progression to atrophic gastritis and to carcinoma have occurred. The diagnosis of Menetrier's disease depends upon full thickness biopsy obtained surgically rather than suction biopsy. Serum antibodies to parietal cells and intrinsic factor are not usually present.

dures should be based on the gastric acid output, post-operative levels of secretion can have prognostic significance. The completeness of a vagotomy can be ascertained by an insulin test or producing hypothalamic glycopenia by competitive inhibition with 2 deoxy-d-glucose. Studies have indicated that 20–30% of all truncal vagotomies are incomplete and the risk of recurrence of ulceration is 5 times greater in patients with incomplete vagotomies. Multiple criteria have been suggested for determining the completeness of vagotomy but none are adequate (Bachrach, 1962). The higher the rise in acid secretion the more parasympathetic fibers remain. In 50 % of cases a negative hypoglycemic response became positive within 6 months post-operative due to vagal regeneration (Smith, 1972). The definitive hypoglycemia ($<$30mg% blood sugar) test therefore should be deferred for 6 months.

Recently, highly selective gastric vagotomies have been performed in which only the parietal cell mass is denervated and no drainage procedure is required (E. Amdrup et al., 1970). This procedure reduces the maximal acid output by about 55% (D. Johnston et al., 1973). One week post-operatively the insulin test was negative in 97% of patients but one year later 51% were positive. Therefore, the results from this highly selective procedure are about the same as for truncal or bilateral selective vagotomies.

Following gastric resection, estimation of acid secretory capacity is technically more difficult (Marks, 1957). However, such studies may help in differentiating post-operative symptoms. Recurrent ulceration can be ruled out if the patient is achlorhydric after appropriate stimulation but anacidity in basal secretion is not diagnostic. A BAO greater than 5 mEq/hr. and a MAO between 15 and 22 mEq/hr. is highly suggestive of stomal ulcerations (Baron, 1970).

Coarse Duodenal Folds

Coarse duodenal folds may be associated with marked hypersecretion of gastric acid with or without concomitant duodenal ulcer disease. These large folds may start in the stomach and involve the entire duodenum and the proximal jejunum. The maximal acid output for patients with coarse duodenal folds may reach 44 mEq/hr. on the average even though no ulceration is present. Patients with ulceration plus coarse folds require gastric surgery three times more frequently as those with normal duodenal folds.

Partial or complete loss of ABH group specific isoantigen occurs in primary gastric epithelial malignancies and in metastatic lesions from such cancers (Sheahan et al., 1971). Since ABH and blood substances are glycoproteins in nature and have a common basic structure in their oligosaccharide component, this loss in malignant cells may represent a specific change in the oligosaccharide moiety due to altered or incomplete biosynthesis of blood group substances. However, the loss of these isoantigens bears no consistent relationship to the degree of histologic differentiation.

HYPERSECRETION

Duodenal Ulcer

On the average, patients with duodenal ulcer have a higher secretory volume, acid concentration and output then do normal individuals or patients with gastric ulcer. Similar results are noted for pepsin and intrinsic factor secretion. The acid secretory capacity was correlated with body weight but not with body habitus or blood group type in a prospective study by Novis et al., (1973). From a group of 176 medical students followed over a 10 year period, three students subsequently developed duodenal ulcer and all has preexistent high levels of basal (10 mEq/hr) and maximal acid output (40 mEq/hr). Students who later complained of dyspepsia had secretory values within the normal range.

Gastric secretory studies in the diagnosis of duodenal ulcer disease have been handicapped by a marked overlap between groups. The basal acid output discriminates only 20–30% of ulcer cases. Even basal anacidity does not rule out the possibility of duodenal ulcer. Maximum acid output will discriminate 30–50% of patients. According to Baron (1970), duodenal ulcer does not occur in patients with a maximum acid output less than 12 mEq/hr. or a peak acid output of less than 15 mEq/hr. Urinary and plasma pepsinogen are not helpful because of even greater overlapping of values. Although the risk of complications appears to be higher in patients with high acid outputs, it would appear that routine gastric function studies are not necessary in the management of medical patients with known gastric ulcer or duodenal ulcer.

Gastric Secretion Following Surgery

Although it has not been established what type of surgical proce-

Zollinger-Ellison Syndrome

The original description of the Zollinger-Ellison Syndrome reported cases of ulcer diathesis with a non-beta islet cell tumor of the pancreas. Subsequently, it has been proven that the tumor or its metastasis is capable of secreting gastrin. Approximately 90% of the cases have severe ulcer disease and half of these have associated severe diarrhea. Gastric hypersecretion may be present without ulceration or diarrhea and other patients have diarrhea without gastric hypersecretion or ulceration. Although radiographic criteria have been reported to be compatible with the diagnosis of Zollinger-Ellison Syndrome, the diagnosis is most depedent upon the findings of gastric hypersecretion and circulating hypergastrinemia. The diagnosis of an ulcerogenic tumor of the pancreas frequently remains unsuspected and 30% of cases are diagnosed at autopsy despite a history of recurrent ulcerations and multiple surgical procedures. Hyperplasia of the glandular mucosa occurs in ZE patients. Coupled with the marked hypersecretion of acid, hypersecretion of sialomucins frequently is present. Gastrin has trophic influence on the parietal cells and the parietal cell mass increases to a greater degree than the other mucosal cell types (Crean et al., 1969).

No single test of gastric secretion is capable of identifying all patients with Zollinger-Ellison Syndrome, and each of the listed criteria of gastric hypersecretion have been shown to be associated with false positive or false negative diagnoses.

Zollinger-Ellison Syndrome should be a clinical impression later confirmed by secretory studies as well as circulating gastrin levels. Radioimmunoassay for gastrin should be done on all patients with a history of intractable, recurrent ulcers or an ulcer at an atypical location. In duodenal ulcer patients the plasma gastrin level may increase three fold after a meal but falls to basal values during the interdigestive period. In the ZE patient, the serum gastrin levels after meals reach 50 times the normal mean and 30 times the upper limit for duodenal ulcer patients. Since the secretion of gastrin is more autonomous, it is not shut off by acidification of the antrum. Gastrin levels may still fluctuate however as the secretion by tumor and metastatic lesions may be irregular.

Other Causes for Gastric Hypersecretion

Patients may develop post-prandial gastric hypersecretion after massive small bowel resection. The mechanism is not known and

Table 6

Hypersecretory Levels in Zollinger-Ellison Syndrome

Volume	>100 to 200 ml/hr.
BAO	>15 mEq/hr.—unoperated
	>5 mEq/hr.—post-operatively
Nocturnal	>100 mEq/12hr.
Basal acidity	>100 mEq/1.—unoperated
	>70 mEq/1.—post-operatively
Ratio: BAO/MAO	>60%

Basal acidity/maximal acidity>60%

Disproportionate increase of acidity to pepsin conc. (K_{25} coefficient=peptic output/mEq acid output per 25 ml.<35)

(Modified from J. H. Baron, 1970)

vagotomy results only in a 47% reduction in acid output for the first six hours following a meal and the subsequent secretion rate for 24 hours may be greater than before vagotomy. Hypersecretion also has been reported following portocaval shunts. It has been postulated that short circuiting of gastrin away from the hepatic circulation was the mechanism but circulating serum gastrin is not elevated usually. Gastrointestinal bleeding due to peptic ulceration has been a recognized complication of renal failure, dialysis and transplantation. These patients appear to be more sensitive to gastrin and the circulating gastrin levels may be higher than normal because of failure of renal excretion. Patients who have received a cadaver donor kiendy have a five times greater risk of G. I. bleeding and ulcerations than when given a kidney from a living donor.

Changes in gastric secretion have also been demonstrated following stress or combat casualties. A prospective study demonstrated that on the day or injury the gastric acid outputs were very low and averaged 30 mEq/24 hrs. The mean acid outputs rose thereafter and in the patients who bled from stress ulcers there was a higher acid output than in those who did not bleed. Greater increases in acid output occurred in patients with central nervous system injury than those with abdominal trauma. Concomitant changes in ACTH or corticoid discharges were not demonstrated. The gastric juice contained increased amounts of plasma protein immediately following trauma suggesting that increased permeability and vascular congestion due to a damaged gastric mucosal epithelium occurred.

Histamine release secondary to back diffusion of hydrogen ion through the damaged gastric mucosa may explain these vascular and secretory changes.

Endocrine Influences

Marked decreases in gastric secretory function had been noted following hypophysectomy and adrenalectomy (Crean, 1968). After adrenalectomy, hyposecretion is not related to a concomitant decrease in the parietal cell population and has been attributed to intracellular inhibition or diminished metabolic function. Hypophysectomy places a severe limitation on the growth of stomach mucosa and the subsequent decrease in parietal cell mass and acid secretion could be partially related to the loss in body weight. Similarly, histamine response and parietal cell mass are increased in acromegalic patients. No correlation of acid secretion with the secretion of growth hormone was found, however (Hall, 1971). Posterior pituitary stimulation or pitressin inhibits gastric secretion for short periods but still may be of value in the management of gastric bleeding or stress ulcerations.

Clinical and experimental observations of the influence of thyroid disease on gastric secretory function have been confusing. Changes in gastric secretion appear to depend on the species studied, age, severity and duration of thyroid dysfunction. Achlorhydria, hyperchlorhydria, and hypochlorhydria are observed in patients with either hypo- or hyperthyroidism. Thyroxin may inhibit histamine activity and cause retention of body histamine. Tissue histamine is low in myxedema and elevated in hyperthyroidism. It is possible that the gastric secretory response to thyroid hormone depends on the antagonism or detoxification of histamine. Hyperthyroidism is frequently associated with gastritis and the status of the mucosa usually returns to normal as hyperthyroidism is controlled.

Pepsin Secretion

Much work has been done on the physiology of gastric proteases and protease inhibitors during the past decade. This subject was recently reviewed by Samloff (1971). Two groups of pepsin precursors in the fundic mucosa have been isolated from the fundic mucosa and one group from the antral and proximal dudoenum mucosa. The physiological significance of these proteases is not clear and no abnormal protease has been found in peptic ulcer patients. Pepsin secretion may be stimulated by gastrin, pentagastrin, cholinergic drugs and vagal stimulation. Histamine appears to have a weak effect which may be due to a wash-out of preformed pepsinogen. With continued stimulation, newly formed pepsinogen continues to be secreted making the maximal secretory capacity of the zymogen cell mass difficult to estimate (Hirschowitz, 1967).

CONCLUSIONS

Despite the great scientific attack on gastric secretory mechanisms waged over the past 100 years, clinical benefits gained from this information have been scant. Increasing knowledge of neurohumoral feedback mechanisms have suggested several therapeutic approaches to peptic ulcer and gastritic conditions. The refinement of these hormones, especially secretin, suggest another attempt may soon be forthcoming.

The diagnostic value of gastric secretory studies also appears to be limited to the two ends of a spectrum; suspected achlorhydria on one hand and Zollinger-Ellison Syndrome on the other. Overlapping of the amount of secretion in normal patients with those having peptic ulcer, gastritis, or malignancy, limits the usefulness of the present studies. New techniques and gastric secretory stimulants may help in separating these groups in the future. The choice of gastric stimulant should be based on a wide range of safety, comfort and availability. Pentagastrin appears to be the stimulant of choice at present even though it has not yet been cleared for clinical use in this country.

The future of gastric secretory studies will depend on further understanding of secretory patterns playing a diagnostic or prognostic value in clinical medicine. The role of maximal pepsin secretion in determining the rate of healing or recurrences in peptic ulcer and the therapeutic benefit of pepsin inhibitors still need to be determined. The components which protect the mucosal integrity in stress ulceration and drug induced erosions need to be clarified. The gastric secretory and enzymatic pattern that might lead to an earlier diagnosis of gastric malignancy should still be sought. Finally, therapeutic usefulness of various inhibitory mechanisms, such as secretin and H_2 receptor inhibitors needs to be demonstrated.

REFERENCES

Amdrup,E., and Jensen,H.E., 1970.
Selective vagotomy of the parietal cell mass preserving innervation of the undrained antrum.
Gastroenterology 59:522.

Baron,J.H., 1963.
Studies of basal and peak acid output with an augmented histamine test.
But 4:136.

Baron,J.H., 1970.
The clinical use of gastric function tests.
Scand. J. Gastroenterology 5, Suppl 6:9.

Beaumont,W., 1833.
Experiments and observations on the gastric juice and the physiology of digestion.
Dover Publications, New York, pp. 279.

Blackman,A.H., Lambert,D.L., Thayer,W.R., and Martin, H.F., 1970.
Computed normal values for peak acid output based on age, sex, and body weight.
Am. J. Dig. Dis. 15:783.

Card,W.I., and Marks,I.N., 1960.
The relationship between the acid output of the stomach following 'maximal' histamine stimulation and the parietal cell mass.
Clin. Sci. 19:147.

Crean,G.P., 1968.
A comparison between the effects of hypophysectomy and adrenalectomy on the gastric mucosa of the rat.
Gut 9:343.

Crean,G.P., Marshall,M.W., and Rumsey,R.D.E., 1969.
Parietal cell hyperplasia induced by the administration of pentagastrin to rats.
Gastroenterology 57:147.

Hall,W.H., 1971.
The parietal cell mass: growth hormone relationship in man.
Am. J. Dig. Dis. 16:139.

Hirschowitz,B.I., 1967.
Secretion of pepsinogens, in Handbook of Physiology. Edit by C.F. Code.
Am. Physiol. Soc., pp. 889.

Ingelfinger,F.J., 1973.
Gastric analysis: Ancient but going strong.
N.Eng. J. Med. 288:964.

Johnston,D., Wilkinson,A.R., Humphrey,C.S., Smith,R.B., Goligher,J.C., Dragelund,E., and Amdrup,E., 1973.
Serial studies of gastric secretion inppatients after highly selective (parietal cell) vagotomy without a drainage procedure for duodenal ulcer.
Gastroenterology 64:1.

Kay,A.W., 1953.
Effect of large doses of histamine on gastric secretion of HCL, an augmented histamine test.
Br. Med. J. 2:77.

Leube,W.O., from Ewald,C.A., 1882.
The diseases of the stomach.
D. Appleton and Co., New York.

Menetrier,P., 1888.
Des Polyadenomes gastriques et de leurs rapports avec le cancer de l'estomae.
Arch. Physiol. Norm. Pathol. 1:32.

Moore,E.W., 1967.
What is gastric acidity?
Ann. N.Y. Acad. Sci. 140:866.

Novis,B.H., Marks,I.N., Bank,S., and Sloan,A.W., 1973.
The relation between gastric acid secretion and body habitus, blood group, smoking, and the subsequent development of dyspepsia and duodenal ulcer.
Gut 14:107.

Samloff,I.M., 1971.
Pepsinogens, pepsins, and pepsin inhibitors.
Gastroenterology 60:586.

Sheahan,D.G., Horowitz,S.A. and Zamcheck,N., 1971.
Deletion of epithelial ABH isoantigens in primary gastric neoplasms and in metastatic cancer.
Am. J. Dig. Dis. 16:961.

Siurala,M., Isokoski,M., Varis,K., and Kekki,M., 1968.
Prevalence of gastritis in a rural population.
Scand. J. Gastroenterology 3:211.

Strickland,R.G., and Machay,I.R.
A reappraisal of the nature and significance of chronic atrophic gastritis.
Am. J. Dig. Dis. 18:426.

ENDOGENOUS INHIBITORS OF GASTRIC SECRETION

George B. Jerzy Glass

INTRODUCTION

The physiological inhibitors of gastric secretory function probably act as moderators which aim at the balancing, more or less successfully, the powerful secretory stimuli to which gastric mucosa is continuously exposed.

The main endogenous inhibitors, which reduce the secretory output of hydrochloric acid, are hormones originating in the duodenum (Johnson and Grossman, 1971), namely secretin (Greenlee et al., 1957; Wormsley and Grossman, 1964), cholecystokinin-pancreozymin (Gillespie and Grossman, 1964; Chey et al., 1970), and enterogastrone (Kosaka and Lim, 1930), which has been recently isolated and purified under the name of gastric inhibitory peptide, GIP (Brown et al., 1970; Pederson and Brown, 1972). We should also include vasoactive inhibitory peptide, VIP (Said and Mutt, 1970) which has a depressing action on the output of HCl by the stomach. The other known inhibitors of gastric secretion are glucagon (Cohen et al., 1960), anti-diuretic hormone (Schapiro et al., 1972) and prostaglandin E (Robert et al., 1968; Classen et al., 1971) and its methylated derivatives (Robert and Magerlein, 1973). It should be stated, however, that none of the various forms of gastric secretory failure is known to develop as result of the prolonged exposure of the gastric mucosa to the action of any of these physiological inhibitors.

Today I will discuss two other types of endogenous inhibitors of gastric secretion. These do not participate in physiological regulation of gastric secretory output but may gain significance under pathological conditions. These are gastrone and the circulating antibodies to parietal cells, and to intrinsic factor.

GASTRONE

Assay

About 30 years ago, Brunschwig and his co-workers (Brunschwig et al., 1939) reported the presence of a non-identified secretory depressant in anacid human gastric juice, for which, a few years later, Code suggested the name Gastrone (Code, 1958). Although this name presupposed a chalone-like nature of the inhibitor, no evidence has yet been adduced that this material indeed gets into the circulation. About 10 years ago, guided and supported by the bioassays in Dr. Code's laboratory, we, in association with Drs. K. Kubo and R. Fiasse, had separated on Sephadex G-100 column and partly purified this inhibitor from anacid gastric juices (Glass et al., 1956; Fiasse et al., 1968). The inhibitor was contained in so-called 'Fraction 7', later called 'Gastrone B' (Glass and Code, 1968) (figure 1). In rats with pyloric ligation this fraction reduced the output of HCl by 50% at an average dose of about 20 u g. This represented a 150-fold increase in inhibitory potency since 3 mg of the lyophilized anacid gastric juice is required to produce a similar inhibition.

More recently, with Dr. J. T. Balanzo, we have improved the bioassay of gastrone, using rats with chronic gastric fistula. Figure 2 and 3 show the inhibitory effect of gastrone B in this preparation on the volume of gastric secretion and hydrochloric acid output at 40 ug dose, as compared with saline controls. Both effects parallel each other, which indicates that the primary action of gastrone in rats is upon the volume of gastric secretion and not upon HCl concentration.

In order to evaluate, in more detail, the quantitative aspects of the inhibitory mechanism of gastrone, with Dr. Balanzo, we studied a Ghosh-Lai rat preparation, that was stimulated by low doses of histamine or pentagastrin. As shown in figure 4, 50 u g of gastrone produces as early as half an hour after its i.v. injection a 30% inhibition of the pentagastrin stimulated secretion. We have recorded

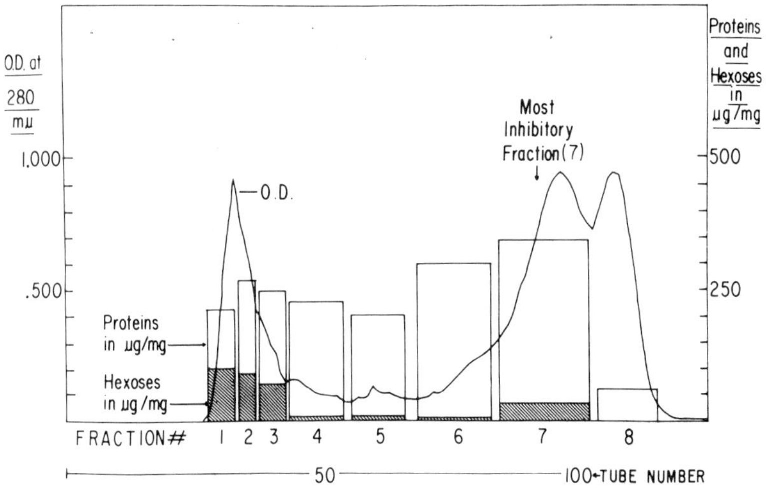

Fig. 1. Fractionation and partial purification of gastrone on Sephadex G-100 column. (From Fiasse et al., Gastroenterology 54: 1018–1031, 1968).

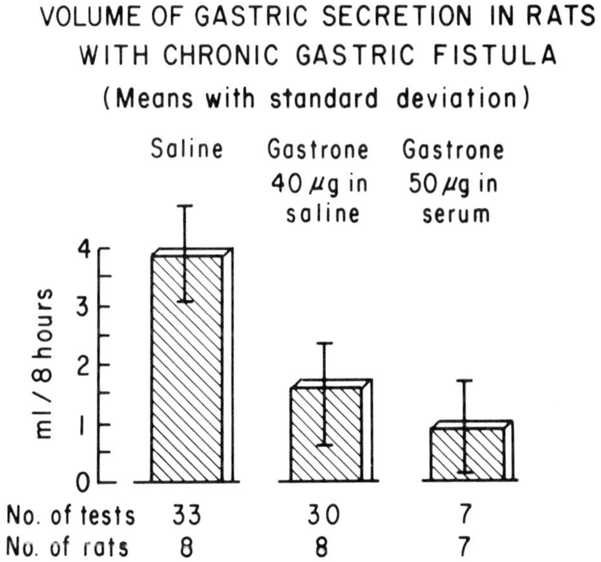

Fig. 2. Volume of gastric secretion in rats with chronic gastric fistula following i.v. administration of saline or gastrone. (Balanzo and Glass, unpublished).

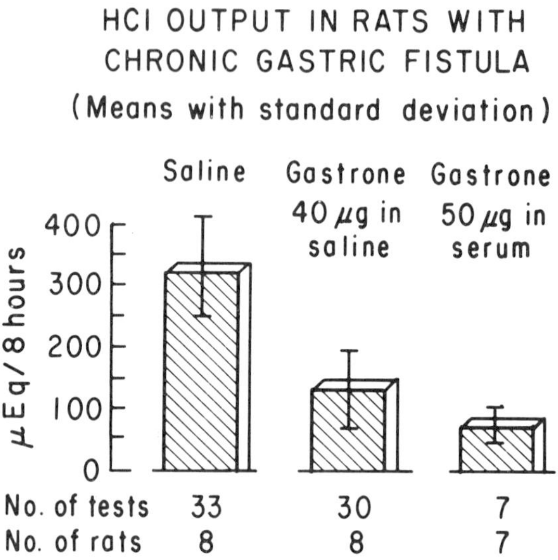

Fig. 3. HCl output in rats with chronic gastric fistula following i.v. administration of saline or gastrone. (Balanzo and Glass, unpublished).

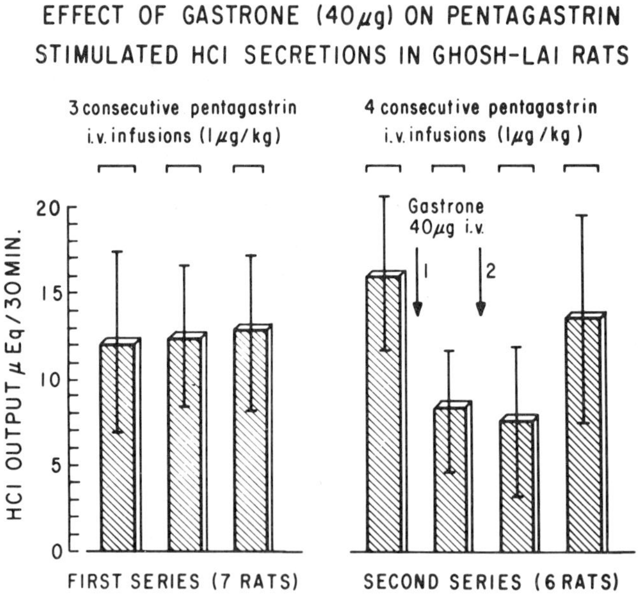

Fig. 4. Effect of gastrone (40 u g) on pentagastrin stimulated HCl secretion in Ghosh-Lai rats. (Balanzo and Glass, unpublished).

similar findings in regard to the histamine stimulated secretion (figure 5). where the effect of gastrone ensues also about half an hour after its i.v. administration, and where it also causes a 30% inhibition of the acid output.

Cellular Origins

Gastrone B, so-called 'fraction 7', is a glycopolypeptide that contains a large peptide moiety (nitrogen content of 10.1%), a small carbohydrate moiety (about 1/6 of gastrone total weight), and no lipids (negative Sudan black staining on electrophoresis). The estimated molecular weight of gastrone, recently determined by Lopes (Glass and Rosenthal, 1973) in our laboratory on Sephadex columns with the use of series of protein markers is below 12,000, as shown in figure 6.

In order to determine the homogeneity and the cellular origin of gastrone, with Drs. Rosenthal and Balanzo we raised anti-gastrone antibody by repeated injections to rabbits of 'fraction 7' (Rosenthal et al., 1973). The antibody obtained formed a single precipitin arc with 'fraction 7' indicating relative homogeneity of this material. We then used this antibody with a fluorescein labelled anti-IgG globulin in the indirect Coons' test for immunofluorescent localization of gastrone's origin in the gastroduodenal mucosa of man and dog (Glass et al., 1973). As shown in figure 7, gastrone's fluorescence was detected in pyloric glands and surface epithelium of the human antral mucosa, but not in the fundal portion of the stomach. A similar fluorescence was obtained in dog pyloric glands with anti-gastrone serum, as shown by figure 8, but not when the same mucosa was exposed to normal rabbit serum (figure 9). Definite fluorescence developed with the anti-gastrone serum also in the crypt epithelium of the dog duodenal bulb (figure 10).

Thus, in man and dog, the large mass of epithelial cells of pyloric glands and surface epithelium of the antrum, and in dog also the crypts of the duodenal bulb, represent the cellular source of gastrone B (Glass et al., 1973). Gastrone B is thus not derived from single endocrine cells scattered through the gastroduodenal mucosa, as it the case with gastrin, secretin, or glucagon. This makes it doubtful that gastrone belongs to the class of the inhibitory peptide hormones.

One of the important gastrone problems is whether gastrone, as secreted into the gastric lumen,exerts its inhibitory activity on gastric

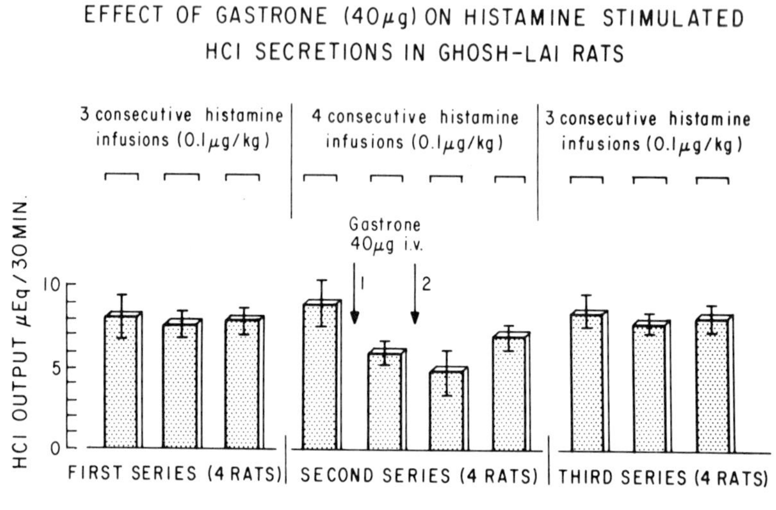

Fig. 5. Effect of gastrone (40 u g) on histamine stimulated HCl secretion in Ghosh-Lai rats. (Balanzo and Glass, unpublished).

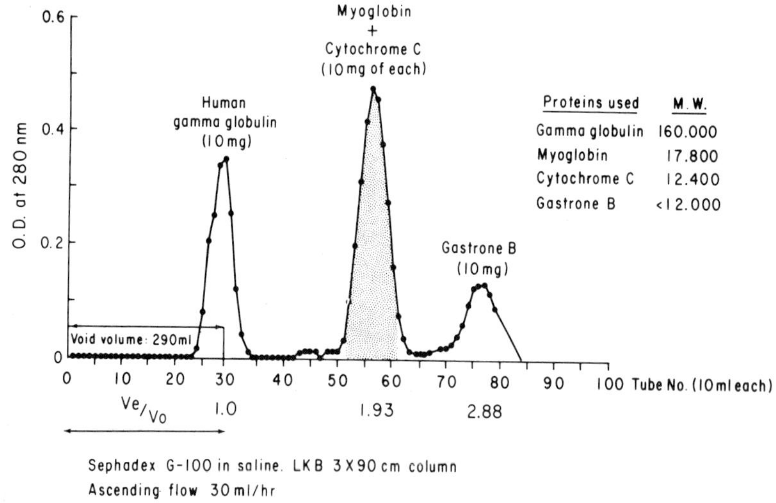

Fig. 6. Elution of gastrone with materials of known molecular size from G-100 column. (Lopes, unpublished).

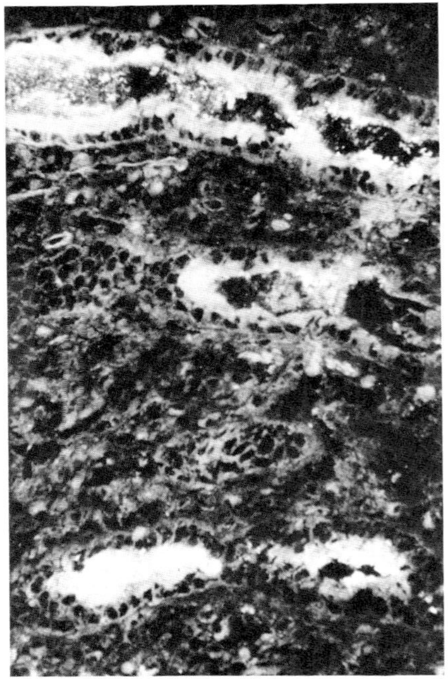

Fig. 7. Normal human antral mucosa exposed in indirect Coons' test to antigastrone B rabbit serum and fluoresceinated goat, antirabbit IgG (X250). Note fluorescence of pyloric glands. (From Glass et al., Am. J. Digest Dis. 18: 279–288, 1973).

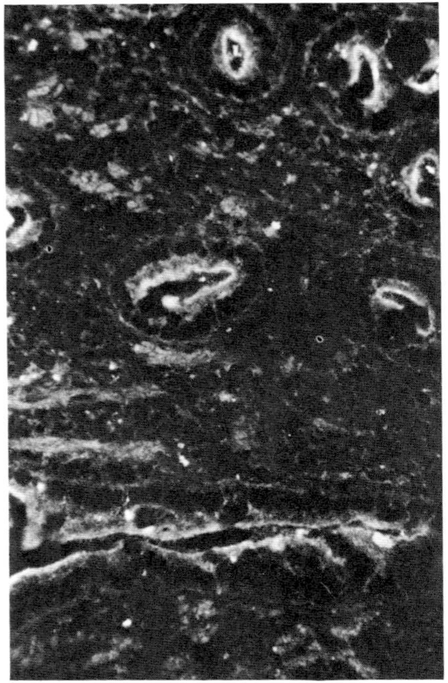

Fig. 8. Dog pyloric mucosa exposed in indirect Coons' test to antigastrone B rabbit serum and fluoresceinated goat antirabbit IgG (X250). Note fluorescence of pyloric glands. (From Glass et al., ibidem).

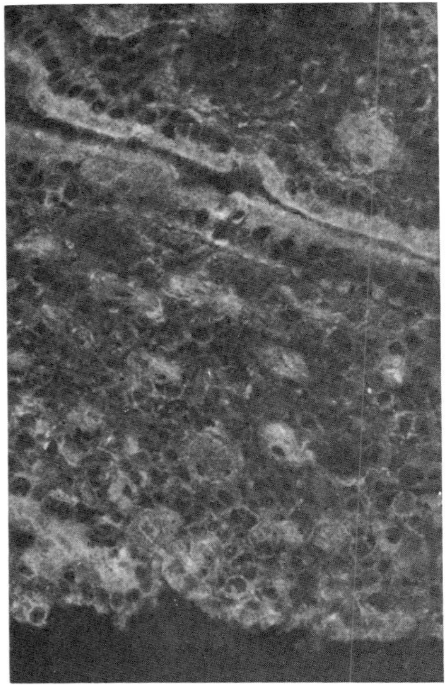

Fig. 9. Dog pyloric mucosa exposed in indirect Coons' test to normal rabbit serum and fluoresceinated goat antirabbit IgG (X 250). Note the staining, but no fluorescence in pyloric glands. (From Glass et al., ibidem).

secretion, and not only when it is injected into the circulation. To obtain some relevant information on this subject, with Dr. Lopes (Glass and Rosenthal, 1973), we have recently instilled gastrone intragastrically to our rats with chronic gastric fistula. As shown in figure 11, gastrone B introduced at the dose of 0.3 mg into the stomach caused a decrease of HCl output in 6 out of 7 rats within 4 hours. When measurements were continued into the 5th and 6th hours a highly significant decrease of gastric volume was noted ($P < .001$) (figure 12).

At this point, it is not clear whether this effect of gastrone is due to its absorption into the blood from the small intestine, or rather to its topical action upon the parietal cells. The fact that Rosenthal and Rudick (Rosenthal and Rudick, 1971) have detected a gastrone-like material in the lymph of fasting dogs may speak for the intestinal absorption of gastrone, but more studies on this subject are needed.

Unless new data are obtained to indicate that gastrone can be further fractionated, and that a highly active peptide is hidden somewhere in its protein moiety, one is left with the impression that gastrone does not belong to the class of gastrointestinal inhibitory peptide hormones such as secretin, cholecystokinin or glucagon. Yet, this does not necessarily rule out gastrone's role in the inhibition of gastric secretion. Gastrone is known to be destroyed by acid-pepsin digestion. However, gastrone may exert its inhibitory effect upon gastric mucosa, either topically or after reabsorption from the intestine during period of low gastric secretory activity or under pathological conditions associated with anacidity. Further research is badly needed to clarify the gastrone story.

ANTIBODIES

Parietal Cell Antibodies

Another class of endogenous inhibitors of gastric secretion includes circulating antibodies to the components of parietal cells in man, namely (1) antibodies to the microsomal component of the parietal cell cytoplasm, called "Parietal cell antibody" (PCA), and (2) antibodies to the intrinsic factor (IF), called "Intrinsic factor antibodies" (IFA). Until recently it was believed that the PCA and IFA in man are manifestations of the humoral response to the injury

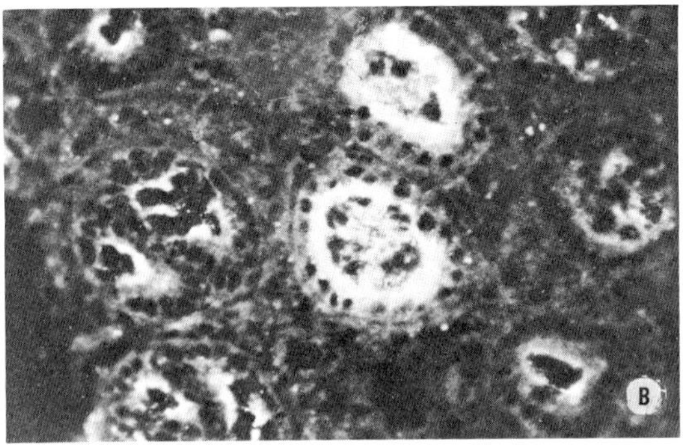

Fig. 10. Dog duodenal bulb mucosa exposed in indirect Coons test to antigastrone B rabbit IgG (X250). Note striking fluorescence of crypts and its epithelium. (From Glass et. al., Am. J. Digest. Dis. 18: 279–288, 1973).

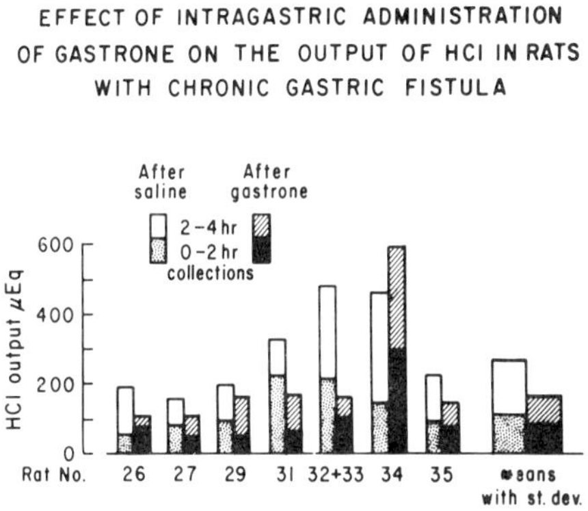

Fig. 11. Effect of intragastric administration of gastrone on the output of HCl in rats with chronic gastric fistula. (Lopes, unpublished).

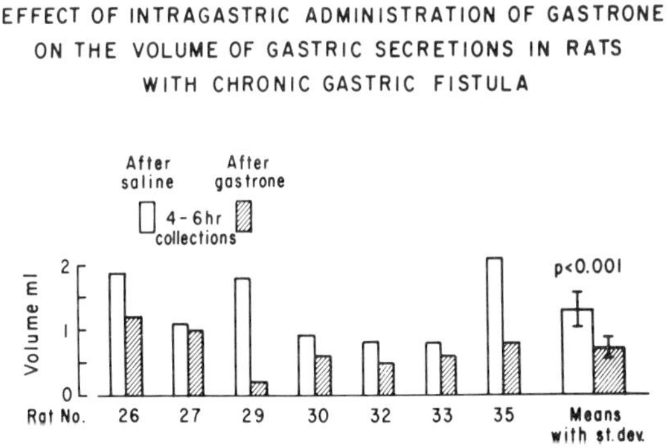

Fig. 12. Effect of intragastric administration of gastrone on the volume of gastric secre tion in rats with chronic gastric fistula. (Lopes, unpublished).

to parietal cells, and that they have no significance in the pathophysiology of the disorder. However, recent investigations from our laboratory have shown that both antibodies represent a significant factor in the dynamic evolution of the atrophic gastritis, and that they exert an important inhibitory effect upon the secretory activity of peptic and parietal cells.

The presence of PCA circulating in the serum can be best demonstrated with the use of the immunofluorescent technique and the indirect Coons' test (Taylor et al., 1962; Irvine, 1963) (figure 13). These antibodies have been found in over 90% of pernicious anemia patients below 60 years of age, and in a certain percent of cases of other conditions associated with gastric atrophy such as gastric cancer, "idiopathic" atrophic gastritis, iron deficiency anemia, Hashimoto thyroiditis, hyperthyroidism, adrenal insufficiency and insulin dependent diabetes (Irvine et al., 1965; Wright et al., 1966).

When we determined the incidence of the PCA in patients with gastric secretory failure and histamine-fast anacidity (Glass et al., 1968), we found it to be highest in pernicious anemia, lowest after subtotal gastrectomy and in gastric cancer (unless it was secondary to pernicious anemia), and intermediate in "idiopathic" atrophic gastritis (figure 14). The incidence of PCA does not correlate with the morphology of the gastric mucosa, but with etiology and physiopathology of the gastric secretory failure. This is demonstrated by differences in the incidence of PCA in patients with identical gastric mucosal lesion, namely in advanced atrophic gastritis with intestinal metaplasia (figure 15). Again, the highest incidence of PCA was found in pernicious anemia, lowest after subtotal gastrectomy and in gastric cancer, and intermediate in atrophic gastritis.

Intrinsic Factor Antibodies

The other types of antibodies directed against IF, namely IFA (see Glass, 1972), are found in the serum of patients with pernicious anemia, and also in some patients with hyperthyroidism and Hashimoto's struma, in which there is a cross-reactivity between gastric and thyroid antigens, IFA are of two types: One, called "blocking antibody", prevents the binding of vitamin B_{12} to IF, and is found in the sera of some 2/3 of pernicious anemia patients. The other, called "binding antibody", binds to IF-B_{12} complex, causes its precipitation from the solution and is found in about 1/3 of the

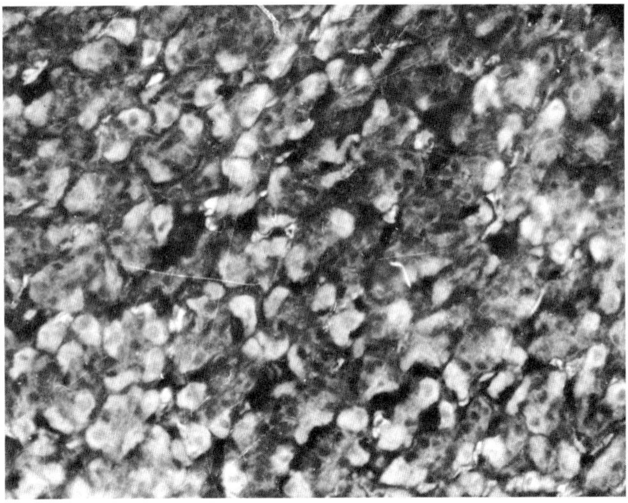

Fig. 13. Immuno-fluorescence of parietal cells in the human gastric mucosa in indirect Coons' test when exposed to PCA-containing human serum and fluorescein-labelled anti-IgG.

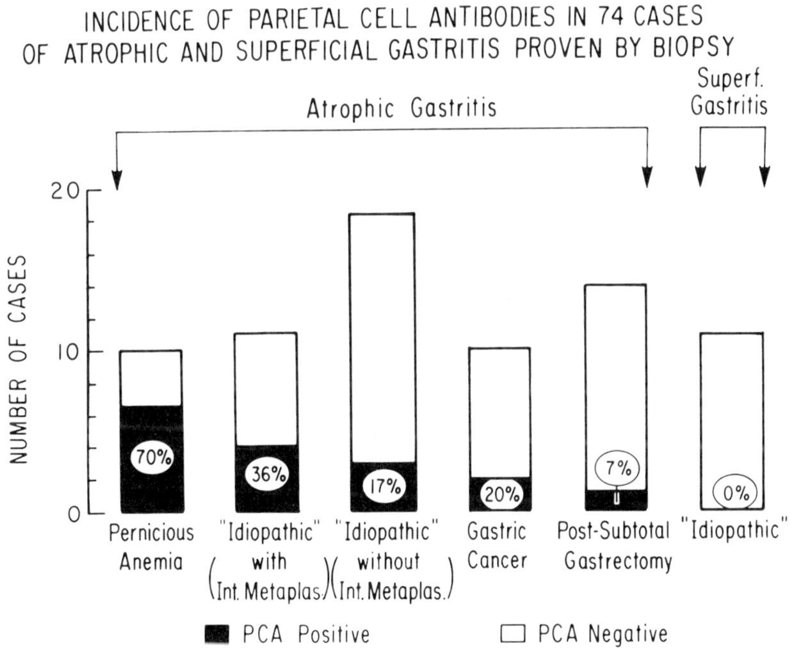

Fig. 14. Incidence of parietal cell antibodies in 74 cases of atrophic and superficial gastritis proven by biopsy. (From Glass et al., Trans. Assoc. Am. Phys. 81: 288–301, 1968).

sera of these patients. We have demonstrated, with Dr. Elisabeth Jacob, the presence of IFA in sera of PA patients by the indirect Coons' test on normal human gastric mucosa using fluorescein labelled anti-IgG (Jacob and Glass, 1971). As shown in figure 16, a striking immunofluorescence developed, under these conditions, on the periphery of the parietal cells under the cellular membrane where IF is located.

Until recently the only indirect evidence for the inhibitory effect of PCA and IFA on gastric secretion was the low output of HCl and IF in the stomach of patients with circulating antibodies. Only lately, with Drs. N. Tanaka and M. Inada, we have adduced indirect experimental evidence for the inhibitory activity of these antibodies on gastric secretion.

Modes of Secretory Depression

We have first studied the effects of prolonged administration of human PCA on parietal cell mass and HCl output in about 100 rats, by injecting PCA containing IgG i.v. daily for 4 to 8 weeks (Tanaka and Glass, 1970). The immunoglobulin G was separated on DEAE-cellulose column from PCA-containing sera of patients with atrophic gastritis and pernicious anemia, and also from normal controls (figure 17). At the end of the 4 to 8 weeks experimental period the rats were fasted for 48 hours, their pylorus was ligated under light anesthesia, 1 mg per kg weight of histamine was injected, and the 3-hour HCl and IF outputs were determined electrometrically and by the zirconium gel method, respectively.

Rats treated with PCA-containing IgG showed statistically significant decrease in thickness and volume of gastric mucosa, as compared to controls treated with normal IgG or saline (figure 18). This was due to a progressive and statistically significant decrease of parietal cell mass in these animals, which was not seen in rats treated with saline or IgG processed from normal individuals (figure 19).

The 3-hour HCl output showed a statistically significant decrease in animals treated for 6 to 8 weeks with PCA-containing IgG, which was not seen in controls, as shown in figure 20. The HCl reduction was significantly greater than the reduction of the parietal cell mass. When we had recalculated HCl output per unit of parietal cells, the hourly HCl output of the parietal cell was reduced by 1/2 of that of control rats after 8 weeks of PCA injections (figure 21).

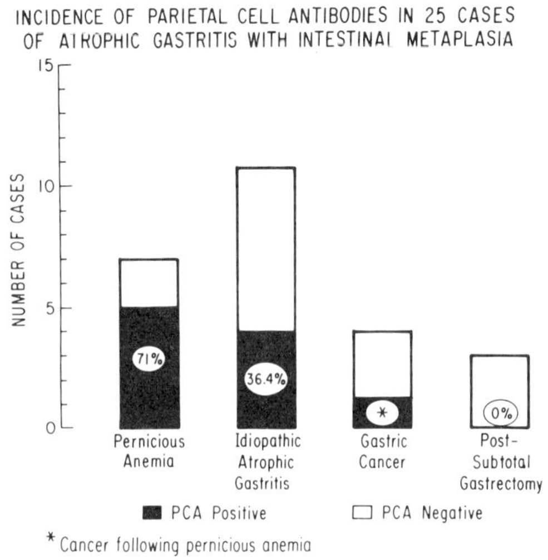

Fig. 15. Incidence of parietal cell antibodies in 25 cases of atrophic gastritis with intestinal metaplasia. (From Glass et al., Trans. Assoc. Am. Phys. 81: 288–301, 1968)

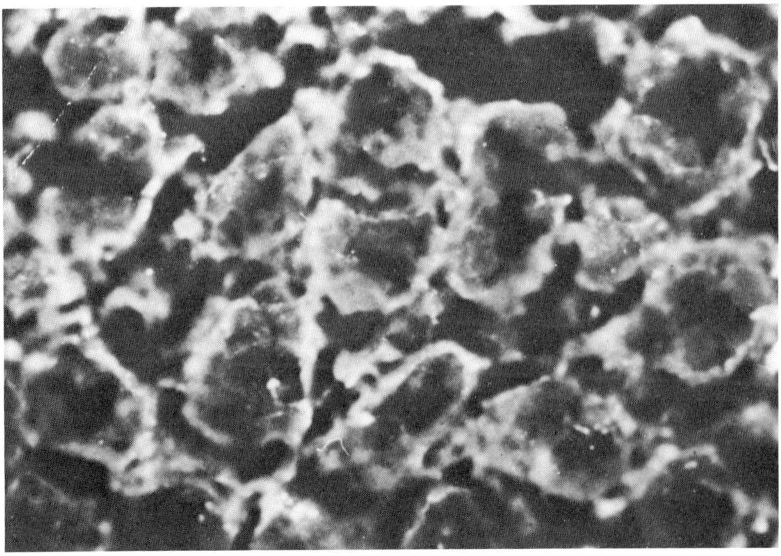

Fig. 16. Immunofluorescence of human parietal cell at its periphery under the membrane in indirect Coons' test when exposed to fluorescein labelled anti-rabbit IgG and rabbit serum containing antibodies to human IF. (From Jacob and Glass, Clin. Exp. Immunol. 8: 517–527, 1971).

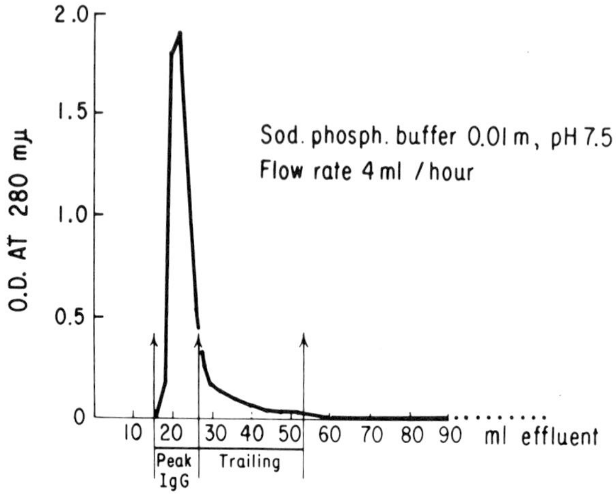

Fig. 17. Separation of IgG from PA serum on DEAE-cellulose column. (From Tanaka and Glass, Gastroenterology 58: 482–494, 1970).

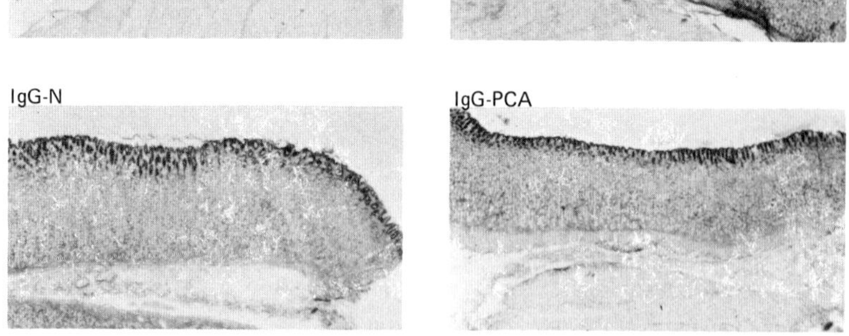

Fig. 18. Rat gastric mucosa after 8 weeks of treatment with saline, normal IgG (IgG_N) and PCA-containing IgG (IgG_{PCA}). Aurantia-and periodic acid Schiff stain, X100. (From Tanaka and Glass, ibidem).

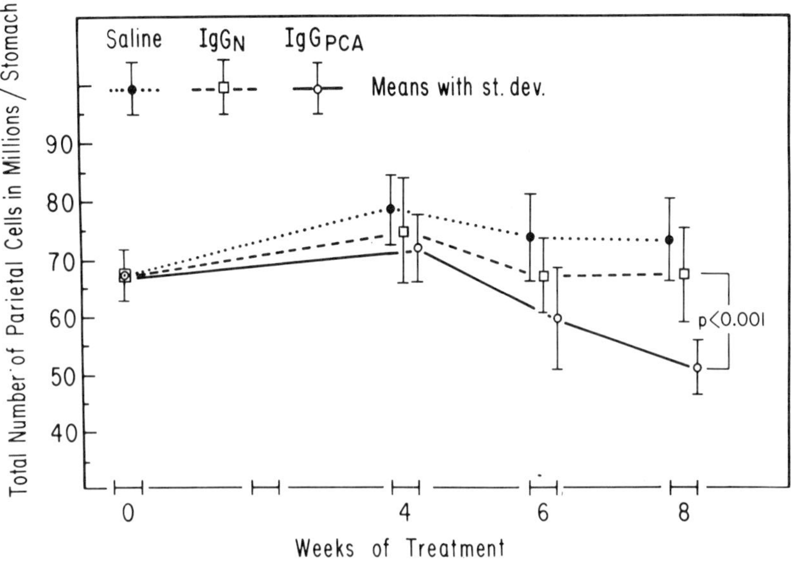

Fig. 19. Rat parietal cell mass before and during 8 weeks of treatment with saline, normal IgG (IgG_N) and PCA-containing IgG (IgG_{PCA}). (From Tanaka and Glass, Gastroenterology 58: 482–494, 1970).

HCL OUTPUT BEFORE AND DURING 8 WEEKS OF TREATMENT WITH SALINE, IgG_N AND IgG_{PCA}

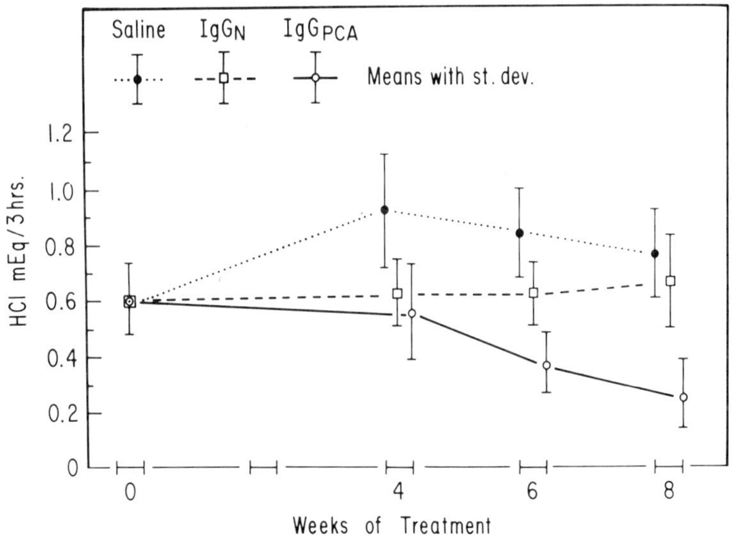

Fig. 20. HCl 3-hour output before and during 8 weeks of treatment of rats with normal IgG (IgG_N), saline, and PCA-containing IgG (IgG_{PCA}). (From Tanaka and Glass, ibidem).

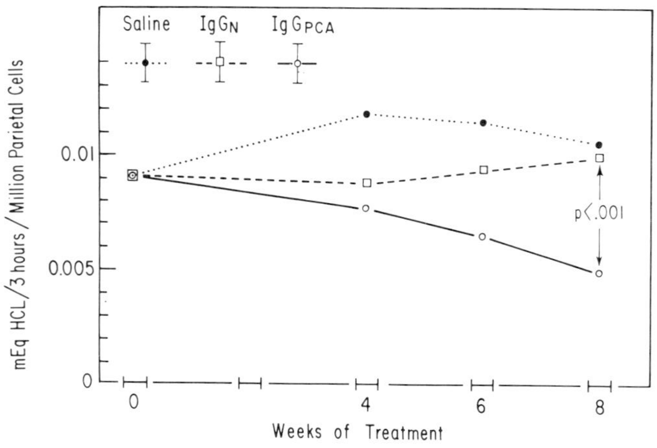

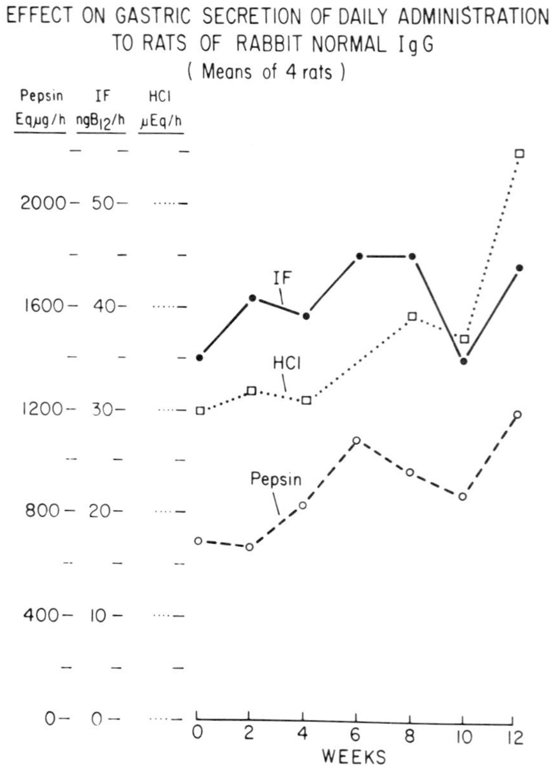

Fig. 21 (Left) HCl 3-hour output calculated per unit of rat parietal cells before and during 8 weeks of treatment with saline, normal IgG (IgG_N) and PCA-containing IgG (IgG_{PCA}). (From Tanaka and Glass, Gastroenterology 58: 482–494, 1970).

Fig. 22 (Right) Effect on gastric secretion of daily administration to rats of rabbit normal IgG. (Inada and Glass, unpublished).

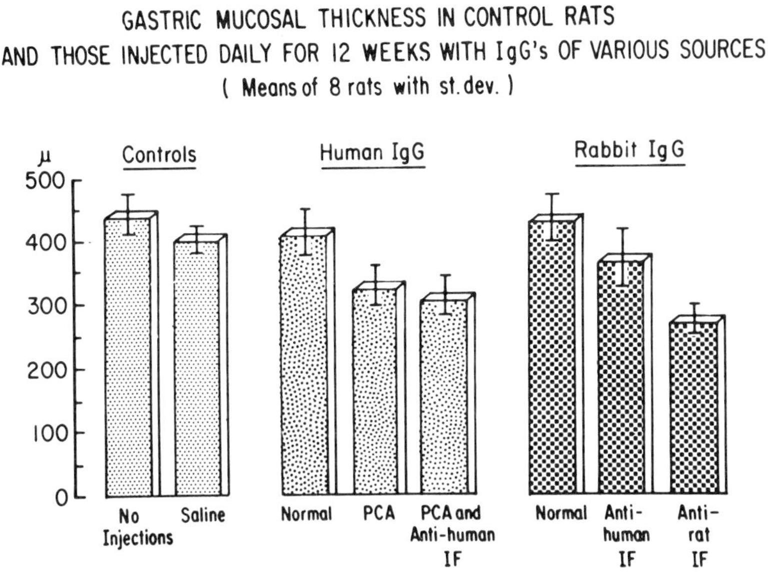

Fig. 23. Gastric mucosal thickness in control rats and those injected daily for 12 weeks with IgG's from various sources. (Inada and Glass, unpublished).

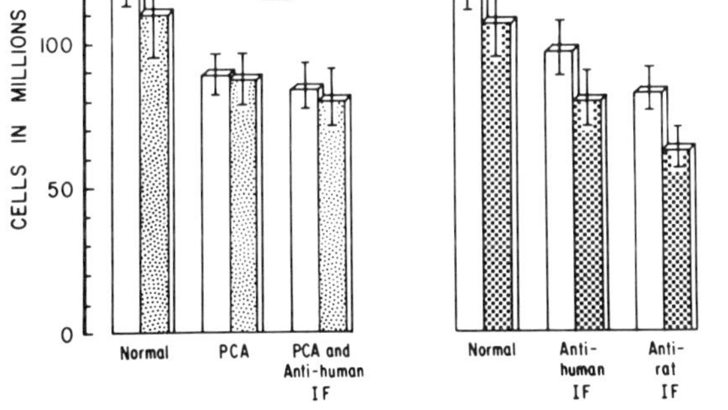

Fig. 24. Parietal cell and peptic cell masses in rats injected daily for 12 weeks with IgG's of various sources. (Inada and Glass, unpublished).

Thus, the circulating PCA causes not only the reduction of the parietal cell mass, (resulting thereby in a decrease of HCl output) but also produces an impairment of the function of the individual parietal cells and the decrease of their secretory output. These findings support the concept of an active role of the circulating PCA in the decrease of the parietal cell mass and in the depression of the HCl output seen in patients with circulating antibodies (Tanaka and Glass, 1970).

In another set of experiments on about 100 rats, we determined the effect of IFA on the gastric mucosa and secretion of HCl, pepsin and IF (Inada and Glass, 1972). Rats were divided into several groups, each of which had received daily i.v. injections of various IgG fractions for the duration of 10 to 12 weeks. The material injected included IgG fractions (separated on DEAE cellulose column from sera of rabbits immunized with human or rat IF and containing IFA to human or rat IF), IgG from PA sera (containing both IFA and PCA, or IFA alone after removal of the PCA by gel filtration), IgG from sera of patients with atrophic gastritis (which contained PCA only), control IgG fractions (separated from normal human or rabbit sera), and saline. Hourly outputs of HCl, pepsin and IF were measured at 2 weeks interval by intubation after injection of histamine, 1mg/kg body weight.

The control rats showed progressive increase in the parietal and peptic cells masses and HCl, pepsin and IF outputs, as result of animal growth during the intervening 12 weeks (figure 22). In contrast, rats injected with rabbit antibodies to human or rat IF showed marked thinning of the gastric mucosa (figure 23) and reduction of peptic cells (figure 24). These animals also demonstrated a corresponding decrease in pepsin and IF outputs (figures 25, 26 and 27), which amounted to about 50% of initial values, and represented a reduction by 62% or 75% respectively when compared to rats injected with normal human or rabbit IgG.

The mechanism of the inhibition of the gastric secretion and reduction of the parietal and peptic cell masses by the parietal cell and intrinsic factor antibodies is not yet understood. Various possibilities may be entertained, but none of them have been supported by adequate evidence. Nevertheless, our work has brought a strong support for the concept of an active role of circulating humoral antibodies in the reduction of the parietal and peptic cell secretion in the stomach.

Fig. 25. Effect on gastric secretion of daily administration to rats of rabbit IgG containing antibodies to human and rat IF. (Inada and Glass, unpublished).

Fig. 26. Pepsin output in rats injected daily for 12 weeks with IgG's of various sources or saline. (Inada and Glass, unpublished).

Fig. 27. IF output in rats injected daily for 12 weeks with IgG's of various sources or saline. (Inada and Glass, unpublished).

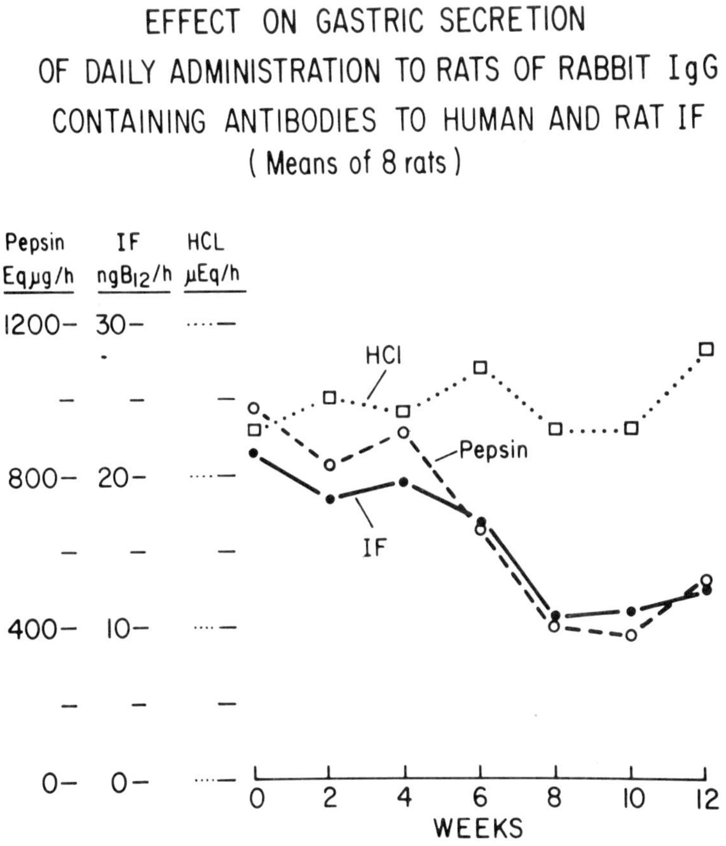

Figure 25

PEPSIN OUTPUT IN RATS INJECTED DAILY FOR 12 WEEKS WITH IgG's OF VARIOUS SOURCES OR SALINE

(Means of 4 rats with stand. error)

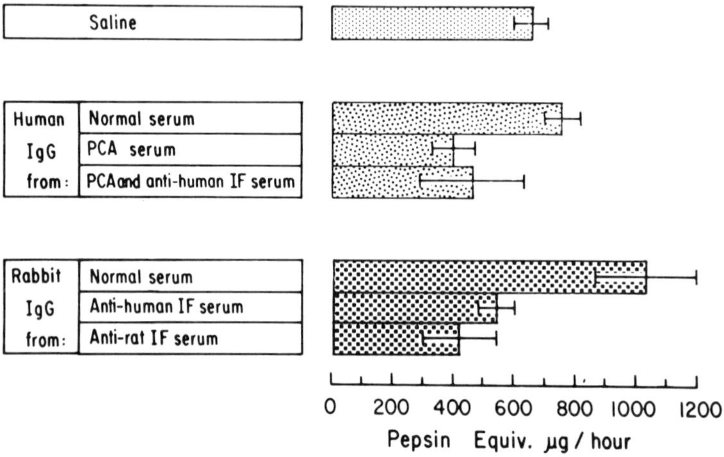

Figure 26

IF OUTPUT IN RATS INJECTED DAILY FOR 12 WEEKS WITH IgG's OF VARIOUS SOURCES OR SALINE

(Means of 4 rats with stand. error)

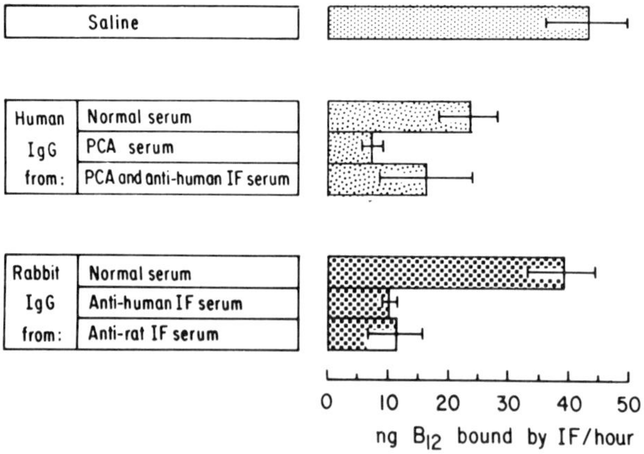

Figure 27

REFERENCES

Brown,J.C., Mutt,V., and Pederson,R.A., 1970.
Further purification of a polypetide demonstrating enterogastrone activity.
J. Physiol., 209:57.

Brunschwig,A., van Prohaska,J., and Clarke,T.H., 1937.
A secretory depressant in the gastric juice of patients with pernicious anemia.
J. Clin. Invest., 18:415.

Chey,W.Y., Hitanant,S., and Hendricks,J., et al, 1970.
Effect of secretin and cholecystokinin on gastric emptying and gastric secretion in man.
Gastroenterology, 58:820.

Classen,M., Koch,H., and Bickhardt,J., et al, 1971.
The effect of prostaglandin E_1 on the pentagastrin-stimulated gastric secretion in man.
Dig., 4:333.

Code,C.F., 1958.
Discussion.
Gastroenterology, 34:210.

Cohen,N., Mazure,P., and Dreiling,D.A., et al, 1960.
The effect of glucagon on histamine-stimulated gastric secretion in man.
Gastroenterology, 39:48.

Fiasse,R., Code,C.F., and Glass,G.B.J., 1968.
Fractionation and partial purification of gastrone.
Gastroenterology, 54:1018.

Gillespie,I.E., and Grossman,M.I., 1964.
Inhibitory effect of secretin and cholecystokinin on Heidenhain pouch responses to gastric extract and histamine.
Gut, 5:342.

Glass,G.B.J., 1972.
Gastric intrinsic factor and other vitamin B_{12} binding proteins in Biochemistry, physiology, pathology and relation to vitamin B_{12} metabolism.
Georg Theme, Stuttgart, (In Press).

Glass,G.B.J., Balanzo,J.T., and Rosenthal,W.S., 1973.
Cellular localization of gastrone, in gastro-duodenal mucosa by immunofluorescence.
Am. J. Dig. Dis., 18:279.
Glass,G.B.J., Brus,I., and Jacob,E., et al, 1968.
Immunological differentiation of etiologic types of atrophic gastritis.
Trans. Assoc. Am. Physicians, 81:288.
Glass,G.B.J., and Code,C.F., 1968.
Gastrone, endogenous inhibitor of gastric secretion, in Progress in Gastroenterology, Edit. by G.B.J. Glass.
Grune and Stratton, New York, p. 221.
Glass,G.B.J., Code,C.F., and Kubo,K., et al, 1967.
Fractionation of endogenous inhibitors of gastric secretion (Gastrone) by physio-chemical means, in Gastric secretion, mechanisms and controls, Edit. by T.K. Schnitka, J.A.L. Gilbert, and R.C. Harrison.
Pergamon Press, Oxford, New York, p. 405.
Glass,G.B.J., Inada,M., and Jacob,E., et al, 1972.
Immune complexes in gastric mucosa, and their role in the development of gastric atrophy and gastric secretory failure.
Arch. F. Mal. App. Dig., 61:93C, (abstr.).
Clin. Res., 20:V.
Glass,G.B.J., and Rosenthal,W.S., 1973.
Gastrone today, in Proc. Symposium on Recent Advances in Gastrointestinal Hormone Research, Edit. by W.Y. Chey, and F.P. Brooks.
Rochester, New York, p. 25, (In Press).
Greenlee,H.B., Longhi,E.H., and Guerrero,J.D., et al, 1957.
Inhibitory effect of pancreatic secretion on gastric secretion.
Am. J. Physiol., 190:396.
Inada,M., and Glass,G.B.J., 1972.
Effect of prolonged administration of intrinsic factor antibodies on gastric morphology and secretion in rats.
Fed. Proc., 31:299, (abstr.).

Irvine,W.J., 1963.
Gastric antibodies studied by fluorescence microscopy.
Exp. Physiol., 48:427.
Irvine,W.J., Davies,S.H., and Teirelbaum,S., et al, 1965.
The clinical and pathological significance of gastric parietal cell antibody.
Ann. New York Acad. Sci., 124:657.
Jacob,E., and Glass,G.B.J., 1971.
Localization of intrinsic factor and complement fixing intrinsic factor-intrinsic factor antibody comples in parietal cell of man.
Clin. Exp. Immunol., 8:517.
Johnson,L.R., and Grossman,M.I., 1971.
Intestinal hormones as inhibitors of gastric secretion.
Gastroenterology, 60:120.
Kosaka,T., and Lim,R.K.S., 1930.
Demonstration of the humoral agent in fat inhibition of gastric secretion.
Proc. Soc. Exp. Biol. Med., 27:890.
Pederson,R.A., and Brown,J.C., 1972.
Inhibition of histamine-, pentagastrin-, and insulin-stimulated canine gastric secretion by pure "gastric inhibitary polypeptide".
Gastroenterology, 62:393.
Robert,A., and Magerlein,B.J., 1973.
15-Methyl PGE_2 and 16, 16-Dimethyl PGE_2: Potent inhibitors of gastric secretion.
Adv. Biosci., 9:247.
Robert,A., Nezamis,J.E., and Phillips,J.P., 1968.
Effect of prostaglandin E_1 on gastric secretion and ulcer formation in the rat.
Gastroenterology, 55:481.
Rosenthal,W.S., Balanzo,J.T., and Glass,G.B.J., 1973.
Antibody to gastrone - endogenous inhibitor of gastric secretion.
Am. J. Dig. Dis., 18:349.
Rosenthal,W.S., and Rudick,J., 1971.
Chylogastrone: Gastric secretory inhibitor in thoracic duct lymph of man and dog.
Am. J. Physiol., 220:452.

Said,S.I., and Mutt,V., 1970.
Polypeptide with broad biological activity: Isolation from small intestine.
Sci., 169:1217.
Schapiro,H., Britt,L.G., and Lewis,M., et al, 1972.
The effect of antidiuretic hormone on gastric secretion in man.
Am. J. Dig. Dis., 17:519.
Tanaka,N., and Glass,G.B.J., 1970.
Effect of prolonged administration of parietal cell antibodies from patients with atrophic gastritis and pernicious anemia on the parietal cell mass and hydrochloric acid output in rats.
Gastroenterology, 58:482.
Taylor,K.B., Roitt,I.M., and Doniach,D., et al, 1962.
Autoimmune phenomena in pernicious anemia: gastric antibodies.
Br. Med. J., 2:1347.
Wormsley,K.G., and Grossman,M.I., 1964.
Inhibition of gastric acid secretion by secretin and by endogenous acid in the duodenum.
Gastroenterology, 47:72.
Wright,R., Whitehead,R., and Wangel,A.G., et al, 1966.
Auto-antibodies and microscopic appearance of gastric mucosa.
Lancet, 1:618.

INTESTINAL MALABSORPTION

O. Dhodanand Kowlessar

INTRODUCTION

Significant advances have been made in our understanding of the physiology and biochemistry of intestinal fat digestion and absorption. The information gained from these studies in both man and experimental animals has led to a clearer understanding of the pathophysiology of fat malabsorption in disease states. It has provided investigators and clinicians with an opportunity to characterize a disease process in terms of a specific event in fat absorption. Furthermore, it is now apparent that in some diseases more than one mechanism of fat malabsorption is applicable, while in others, in spite of detailed investigation, the mechanism remains undefined. Thus, the purposes of this review are two fold: (a) to outline current concepts of normal fat digestion and absorption and (b) to identify the defect in fat malabsorption as they apply to specific disease states.

NORMAL PHYSIOLOGY

Normal Fat Digestion and Absorption

Long chain triglycerides make up the bulk of food fats, the remainder consisting of phospholipids and cholesterol esters. The triglycerides contain saturated and unsaturated fatty acids of varying chain lengths ($>$ 14 carbon atoms) linked to glycerol via ester bonds at the 1, 2 and 3 positions. They are very non-polar and quite insoluble in water. The digestion and absorption of these ingested dietary lipids involve at least four phases: lipolysis, micellarization, cellular and delivery. After ingestion, partial hydrolysis of fat occurs in the stomach catalyzed by lingual and/or gastric lipase (Hamosh and Scow, 1973). However, the major portion of fat hydrolysis occurs in the proximal small intestine (Borgström et al., 1957).

Lipolysis

In the presence of pancreatic lipase (glycerol ester hydrolase), an alkaline pH (around 7), calcium ions and emulsification, significant lipolysis occurs. The glycerol ester hydrolase has absolute specificity for the outside positions (α and α') of the glycerol molecule, thus leading to the production of 1, 2-diglycerides, 2-monoglycerides and free fatty acids. Cholesterol esters are hydrolyzed by cholesterol esterase to free cholesterol and fatty acids, while phospholipase hydrolyzes lecithin to lysolecithin and fatty acid. These insoluble substances, namely fatty acids, cholesterol and monoglycerides, are rendered soluble by conjugated bile acids. These products of lipolysis are constantly removed to a different physicochemical state and the interior of the epithelial cell.

Micellerization

During a meal the gallbladder contracts in response to cholecystokinin-pancreozymin (CCK-PZ), resulting in the discharge of conjugated bile acids in a concentration of 3 to 6 mM into the proximal small intestine. This concentration of conjugated bile acids exceeds the average critical micellar concentration of 2.5 mM (VanDeest et al., 1968). The individual monomers of glycine-conjugated and taurine-conjugated primary bile acids (cholic and chenodeoxycholic) and the secondary (deoxycholic) bile acids aggregate to form pure micelles.

Monoglycerides and fatty acids, because they are both hydrophobic and hydrophilic are oriented at the oil-water interface and thus become incorporated in the water-soluble bile salt micelles to form "mixed micelles" accounting for 96 to 99 percent of long chain fatty acid or sterol in the bile acid micelle. A small amount of fatty acid and sterol dissolved in the aqueous phase is in equilibrium with the micellar lipids, resulting in a constant exchange between molecules in the micellar and aqueous phase. On the other hand, medium chain fatty acids (8 to 14 carbon atoms chain lengths) are predominantly solubilized in the aqueous phase of intestinal contents and do not require bile acid micelles for solubilization. It is critical that the proximal small intestine content reach an alkaline pH which is contributed by the bicarbonate concentration of bile and pancreatic juice. Thus, the prerequisites for micellerization are: (a) appropriate lipid substrates, (b) conjugated bile acids exceeding their critical micellar concentration and (c) an alkaline pH.

Cellular Stage

The process responsible for the uptake of fatty acids, monoglycerides and cholesterol by the intestinal epithelial cell appears to be one of passive diffusion. Recent evidence by Dietschy, Salee and Wilson (1971) suggests that the bile acid micelle acts as a carrier for fatty acids, monoglyceride and cholesterol overcoming the resistance of the unstirred water layer to the free diffusion of individual lipid molecules from the intestinal contents to the microvillus border of the intestinal epithelial cell. In some way, the bulk of conjugated bile acids is freed from the mixed micelle. Only insignificant quantities of conjugated bile acids are absorbed in the proximal small intestine, while the major absorption occurs in the distal ileum by active transport mechanisms.

Once within the epithelial cells, the long chain fatty acids are activated by fatty acid:CoA lipase to long chain fatty acid thioesters which are then esterified to form triglycerides principally by the monoglyceride pathway and to a small extent by the L-α-glycerophosphate pathway (Johnston, 1968). The enzymes necessary for the synthesis of triglycerides from β-monoglyceride and activated long chain fatty acids are localized in the microsomal fraction and are called "triglyceride synthetase". Glycolysis or monoglyceride lipase produces the glycerol for phosphorylation to form L-α-glycerophosphate which can then accept two activated long chain fatty acids to form phosphatidic acid for conversion into either phospholipids or triglycerides. Cholesterol is esterified by cholesterol esterase which is found in the soluble fraction of the epithelial cell.

The resynthesized triglycerides, phospholipids and cholesterol esters combine with free cholesterol and a small amount of specific protein to form the final products of fat absorption; namely, chylomicrons and very-low density lipoproteins (VLDL). The specific protein associated with the two lipoproteins are synthesized in the microsomes. The manner in which the proteins associate with the lipids remains unclear. Nevertheless, both protein synthesis and incorporation into the lipoprotein particle are essential for fat absorption. After the formation of chylomicrons and VLDL, they are transported out of the epithelial cell, by as yet unproved mechanism, although reversed pinocytosis has been suggested. They then diffuse into the central lacteals, for transport into the lymphatic system to the superior vena cava via the thoracic duct for distribution, storage and utilization to the liver, muscle and adipose tissue.

The above mechanisms do not apply to lipids of carbon chain length of 10 or less. They escape re-esterification and chylomicron formation and are absorbed unchanged, attached to albumin, into the portal system. Triglycerides of medium and short chain length can be hydrolyzed by a separate heat-labile microsomal lipase. Thus, in the absence of pancreatic lipase there is a cellular enzyme capable of hydrolyzing medium and short chain triglycerides.

PATHOPHYSIOLOGY

Fat Malabsorption

The maldigestion and malabsorption of fat occur in association with a number of disease states (Wilson and Dietschy, 1971). It is now possible to relate a specific disease process to one or more defects in terms of the phases of fat absorption; namely, lipolysis, micellerization, cellular and delivery. A broad classification of the disease states involved is shown in table 1. In some patients there will be single or multiple defects to explain the mechanism of fat malabsorption, while in others there may be no documented mechanism to explain the excess fat excretion ($>$6 gm fat per day).

Defective Lipolysis

The prototype of this defect is illustrated by any patient whose disease process leads to significant destruction of the pancreas or surgical removal of all or most of this gland. These diseases include: chronic pancreatitis with or without calcification, carcinoma of the head of the pancreas with obstruction of the main and accessory pancreatic ducts, diffuse carcinoma of the pancreas, cyctic fibrosis of the pancreas, primary pancreatic atrophy, 95% or total pancreat-

Table 1

Disorders of Fat Malabsorption and Associated Defects
in the Various Phases of Fat Absorption

I. Lipolysis
- A. Primary (decreased enzyme secretion)
  - Chronic pancreatitis (with or without calcification)
  - Carcinoma of pancreas
  - Cystic fibrosis
  - Primary pancreatic atrophy
  - Congenital absence of lipase
  - 95% or total pancreatectomy
- B. Secondary
  - Intraluminal destruction of lipase (Zollinger-Ellison Syndrome)
  - Diminished pancreatic secretion or asynchrony
    - Small bowel mucosal disease (celiac disease)
    - Gastric resection (Billroth II operation, vagotomy and pyloroplasty)

II. Micellerization
- Bacterial overgrowths
  - Afferent limb stasis, colejejunal fistulas, diabetes multiple jejunal diverticula, scleroderma
- Biliary tract disease (atresia, common duct obstruction)
- Chronic liver disease
- Cholestyramine and neomycin therapy
- Gastric resection
- Ileal resection ($>$100 cm), inflammation or bypass

Table 1 (continued)

III. Cellular Phase
- Abetalipoproteinemia
- Amyloidosis
- Celiac disease
- Congestive heart failure
- Dermatitis herpetiformis
- Ileojejunitis
- Intestinal resection
- Mast cell disease
- Small bowel ischemia

IV. Delivery Phase
- Chronic congestive heart failure
- Constrictive pericarditis
- Intestinal lymphangiectasia
- Lymphatic obstruction by lymphoma, carcinoma, fibrosis and inflammation
- Whipple's disease

V. Undefined Etiology
- Carcinoid syndrome
- Diabetes mellitus
- Hypoparathyroidism, myxedema, hyperthyroidism, Addison's disease
- Immunoglobulin deficiency syndromes

ectomy. The defect is related to poor or absent pancreatic lipase and striking reduction of bicarbonate. In patients with congenital absence of lipase the defect is primarily one of lipolysis, since the bicarbonate secretion is normal.

Intraluminal destruction of lipase is well documented in the Zollinger-Ellison Syndrome and contributes in part to fat malabsorption. The excessive gastric hypersecretion of acid secondary to a gastrin-producing pancreatic tumor produces an acid pH in the proximal small intestine which irreversibly destroys pancreatic lipase and precipitates glycine dihydroxy bile acids resulting in maldigestion of fat (Go et al., 1970).

The effect of vagotomy and gastric surgery on pancreatic secretion and secondary maldigestion has not been fully clarified. The disorders of motility, secretion and digestion are difficult to distinguish post-operatively, but fat malabsorption is a sequel to vagotomy and gastric surgery. This defect may be related to a disturbance of the neural and hormonal regulation of pancreatic secretion. Vagotomy with pyloroplasty induces delayed and diminished CCK-PZ secretion which in turn leads to maldigestion. Gastrojejunal anastomosis with vagotomy may increase incoordination between the passage of food through the proximal small intestine and the mixing of biliary and pancreatic secretions (Moreland and Johnson, 1971). Thus, the meal which stimulates CCK-PZ secretion passes distally before bile acids and enzymes are secreted.

In the presence of decreased lipase production or impaired lipase activity (vide supra) there is insufficient formation of monoglyceride and fatty acids to form mixed micelles.

In anomalies of fat lipolysis, steatorrhea involves fatty acids and, to a lesser extent, triglycerides. The fact that the fat excretion is not one of pure triglycerides suggests the possibility of a secondary hydrolysis, perhaps by intestinal bacteria, occurring too far along the intestinal tract for the fatty acids to be absorbed.

Defective Micellar Solubilization

The micellar phase defects may be due either to failure of conjugated bile acids to achieve critical micellar concentration ($>$2.5 mM) or insufficient lipid substrate for the formation of mixed micelles. Impaired critical micellar concentration secondary to decreased availability of bile salts is encountered in obstructive jaundice (extrahepatic or intrahepatic), and in gastric surgery with associated pancreatic-biliary-cibal asynchrony (vide supra). Decreased bile acid pool is encountered in patients with ileal resection ($>$100 cm), intestinal bypass, severe ileal inflammation or on cholestyramine therapy. In patients with impaired hepatic synthesis secondary to cirrhosis and hepatitis the bile acid pool is also reduced. In the presence of anaerobic bacterial deconjugation and dehydroxylation, the bile acids will be qualitatively altered, resulting in significant formation of unconjugated bile acids. These either precipitate or are rapidly absorbed in the proximal small intestine, resulting in a marked reduction in the effective concentration of bile acids in the lumen.

The bacterial overgrowth syndromes represent an expanding spectrum of diseases and include blind loop syndromes secondary to afferent loop stasis following gastric surgery, multiple small intestinal strictures and stenosis, multiple duodenal and jejunal diverticula, single large duodenal diverticulum and bowel hypotonia secondary to scleroderma, diabetes, amyloidosis and pseudo-obstruction of the small intestine. Gastrojejunocolic fistulas secondary to gastric carcinoma or stomal ulceration or other forms of enteroenteric fistulas will also lead to bacterial overgrowth with anaerobic flora.

Since micellerization is dependent on a neutral pH, patients with Zollinger-Ellison Syndrome or those with defective bicarbonate production secondary to pancreatic insufficiency may have significant duodenojejunal acidification with resultant failure of bile acids to reach a critical micellar concentration (Go et al., 1970).

Disorders of the Cellular Phase

These disorders include both decreased mucosal uptake and re-esterification. They are found in a wide variety of disease: celiac disease, tropical sprue, amyloidosis, non-specific jejunoileitis, abetalipoproteinemia, mast cell disease, massive small intestinal resection, small bowel ischemia, congestive heart failure, dermatitis herpetiformis, periarteritis nodosa, Dego's disease, radiation enteritis, etc. (Rogers, 1971). The prototype of significant abnormality in brush border and epithelial cells of the small intestine is celiac disease. It is of interest that in patients with celiac disease there is a varying degree of fat malabsorption including a group of patients with normal fat absorption. In this latter group, it is possible that the disease is limited to the proximal jejunum, thereby permitting the normal distal jejunum to take over fat absorption. In those cases with extensive disease including the distal ileum, one would anticipate a greater degree of steatorrhea and in such instances there will be defective micellerization and decreased cellular synthesis. It has been recently shown that CCK-PZ secretion is diminished and delayed in patients with celiac disease. In turn, there is an inertia of the gallbladder with delayed emptying and decreased lipase secretion. The meal passes through the proximal small intestine before adequate amounts of enzyme and bile acids are secreted. With excessive dilution and ineffective bile acid recirculation secondary to diminished small bowel motility and significant disease in the distal ileum (some patients), bile acid concentrations are decreased below the critical micellar concentration,resulting in poor fat solubilization and malabsorption. This appears to be more significant after a second meal (DiMagno, Go and Summerskill, 1972).

In patients with abetalipoproteinemia the defect is in chylomicron formation secondary to impaired synthesis of the protein moiety associated with the formation of chylomicron. This then results in accumulation of triglycerides in the intestinal epithelial cells.

Defective Delivery

Diseases characterized by defective delivery of chylomicrons to the intestinal lymphatics include intestinal lymphangiectasia, congestive heart failure, constrictive pericarditis, lymphatic obstruction by tumor or inflammation,and Whipple's disease. The defect in fat malabsorption in Whipple's disease may be related to both delivery and uptake, since it has been shown that small intestinal mucosa from patients with this disease have impaired capacity for fatty acid re-esterification (Wilson and Dietschy, 1971).

Unclassified Defects in Fat Malabsorption

There are a group of diseases in which the mechanisms of fat malabsorption are not well defined. These include patients with immunoglobulin deficiency states, endocrinopathies (hypoparathyroidism, hyperparathyroidism, myxedema, hyperthyroidism and Addison's disease), diabetes mellitus not related to bacterial overgrowth, some forms of parasitic infestations and malignant carcinoid syndrome. It would appear that in some patients with the malignant carcinoid syndrome secondary to ileal carcinoid the defect may reside in micellerization, because of the loss of ileal integrity and the extensive replacement of the liver by tumor. On the other hand, when the carcinoid replaces the pancreas with secondary pancreatic insufficiency, the defect resides in lipolysis.. If there is extensive retroperitoneal fibrosis or vascular insufficiency secondary to massive involvement with malignant carcinoid, the defect would be one of delivery or reduced metabolic function of the epithelial cells. Regardless of the mechanism, fat malabsorption in the carcinoid syndrome is relatively rare.

Further studies are needed to elucidate the mechanism of fat malabsorption in patients with immune deficiency states and endocrinopathies. In those cases where there is coexistence of selective IgA deficiency and celiac disease, the mechanisms of fat malabsorption are similar to those discussed under celiac disease. The role of giardiasis in association with nodular lymphoid hyperplasia and steatorrhea needs further research. It is possible that in many of these patients there is a combination of impaired micellerization and cellular defects. However, there is no hard evidence to validate this conjecture.

In summary, this review has outlined the phases of fat absorption and has attempted to place diseases with associated fat malabsorption in categories of lipolysis, micellerization, cellular and delivery. Furthermore, it is apparent that some diseases have more than one mechanism to explain the presence of steatorrhea, while in others there is no obvious explanation for the defect.

REFERENCES

Borgström, B., Dahlquist, A., Lundh, G., and Sjövall, J., 1957.
Studies of intestinal digestion and absorption in the human.
J. Clin. Invest., 36: 1536.

Dietschy, J. M., Sallee, V. L., and Wilson, F. A., 1971.
Unstirred water layers and absorption across the intestinal mucosa.
Gastroenterol., 61: 932.

DiMagno, E. P., Go, V. L. W., and Summerskill, W. H. J., 1972.
Impaired cholecystokinin-pancreozymin secretion, intraluminal dilution and maldigestion of fat in sprue.
Gastroenterol., 63: 25.

Go, V. L. W., Poley, J. R., Hoffman, A. F., et al., 1970.
Disturbance in fat digestion induced by acidic jejunal pH due to gastric hypersecretion in man.
Gastroenterol., 58: 638.

Hamosh, M. and Scow, R. O., 1973.
Lingual lipase and its role in the digestion of dietary lipid.
J. Clin. Invest., 52: 88.

Johnston, J. M., 1968.
Mechanism of fat absorption, p. 1353.
Handbook of Physiology, Section 6, Alimentary Canal, Vol. 3, Washington, American Physiological Society.

Moreland, H. J., and Johnson, L. R., 1971.
Effect of vagotomy on pancreatic secretin stimulated by endogenons and exogenons secretion.
Gastroenterol., 60: 425.

Rogers, A. I., 1971.
Steatorrhea.
Postgraduate Medicine, 50: 123.

VanDeest, B. W., Fordtran, J. S., Morawski, S. G., and Wilson, J. D., 1968.

Bile salt and micellar fat content in proximal small bowel contents of ileectomy patients.
J. Clin. Invest., 47: 1314.

Wilson, F. A., and Dietschy, J. M., 1971. Differential diagnostic approach to clinical problems of malabsorption. Gastroenterol., 61: 911.

INDEX TO CHARTS AND TABLES

Subject information contained in charts, graphs and tables, classified under broad general categories.

Absorption Processes
- Amino acids, molar ratios in food, jejunum and mesenteric vein, 264
- Bile, ion fluxes in gall bladder, 339
- Breath test, for bile acid malabsorption in ileal dysfunctions, 314
- Chylomicron components, 288
- Drug absorption, interaction with cholestyramine, 353
- Drug interaction affecting antibiotic absorption, 364
- Excretion of absorbed morphine and morphine glucuronide, 362
- Fatty acid uptake and release in intestinal mucosal cell, 286
- Glycochenodeoxycholic acid effect on colonic mucosa, 253
- Intestinal juice, total amino acid content, 260
- Lipid distribution in oil-water phase in intestinal lumen, 292
- Malabsorption of fat, classified by phases in absorption, 451, 452
- Mechanisms for net secretion, 251
- Net ion secretion, stimuli and conditions, 250
- Pathways controlling mucosal triglyceride synthesis, 288
- Triglyceride lipolysis requirements, 290

Bile and Biliary Duct System
- Bile, total free amino acids of, 260
  - ion fluxes in human gall bladder bile, 339
  - daily fractional tumore rates, 305
    - tumore of cholyl moiety of some bile acid, 304
  - pool size of conjugated bile acid moieties, 305
- Common bile duct, canine, cross section, 97, longitudinal section, 113
- Ductal sphincter (choledochoduodenal junction) opening pressures, 104
  - opening pressure, bile flow rate, intestinal motility and anterial pressure, 109
    - effects of histamine and norepinephrine, 111
    - vagotomy effect on, 104
    - vagus stimulation effects on, 106
    - relation to systemic anterial pressure, 108
  - effect of anaerobiosis on p.d., 334
- Gall bladder, electrical properties in different species, 333
  - maximum short-circuit current, 332
  - sodium reduction effect on p.d., 334

Blood Flow
- Mesenteric antery of dog, effects of epinephrine and norepinephrine, 198
- Mesenteric antery of baboon, effect of epinephrine infusion, 201

Colon Motor Activities
- Divertular disease, fast motor waves in sigmoid and upper rectum, 396
- Irritable colon syndrome, effect of meal on motor activity, 394
- Mechanism of production of colonic pressure waves, 398
- Secretin effect on sigmoid colon, 393
- Sigmoid colon response to meal after vagotomy, 394
- Stool weights of subjects on different diets, 399

Electrophysiology
Electrogenic pump for HCl secretion, 125
Gall bladder, electrical properties in various species, 333
potential differences in, 332
anaerobiosis effect on, 334
ouabain effect on, 335
sodium reduction effect on, 335
Mechanical and electrical activity in intestine, 21, 24, 25
Myoelectrical recordings following secretin, 42
Peristalsis and electrical activity in intestine, 22, 24
Slow electrical waves in intestine, 18
Vagus stimulation effect on electrical activity in small intestine, 27

Esophageal Sphincter, Lower (LES)
Clinical disorders and pathophysiological mechamisms, 386
Factors regulating function, 378
Response to pharmacologic stimulation, 382
Resting pressures in normal and dysfunction conditions, 380
Schema of mechanism preventing reflux, 378

Gastric Emptying
Caloric content of meal and gastric evacuation volume, 51
Drug interactions affecting rate of, 357
Half-life of various meals, 49
Relation between caloric value of meal and caloric content entering duodenum, 51
Volume of meal evacuated in 30 minutes, 49
Gastrointestinal Hormones
Actions, 180
Effects on secretions, 182
Gastrin-related heptopeptides, 184
Hormone release effects of hormones, 187
Hormone release, luminal factors for, 186
Hypersecretory effects of daily pentagastrin injections, 189
Secretin-related peptides, 185
Trophic actions of hormones, 188

Muscle, Striated
Sarcomere structure, 2
Three-dimensional view of fiber, 2

Muscle, Smooth
Active state, 10, 12, 13
Dose response curve, active tension, 35
, cholecystokinin, 37
, cholecystokinin plus secretin, 37
, gastrin, 33
, gastrin plus secretin, 35
, secretin, 35
Effect of Ca ion, 10, 12
Electrical activity and peristalsis, 22, 24
, effect of vagus stimulation, 27

Electrical and mechanical activity relations, 21, 24, 25
Force-velocity curve, 8, 39
Gastrin and gastrin agonists plus secretin, 37
Gastrin antiserum action on LES, 39
Length-tension curve, 8, 33
Myoelectric recording following secretin, 42
Pressure recording following secretin, 42
Slow electrical wave recording, 18

Secretory Processes: Gastric Secretion
Analogs of prostoglandin, effects on, 226
Antigastrone effects on, 428, 431
Atrophic effects of parietal cell antibodies, 439
gastritis, classification, 409
Basal acid output in disease conditions, 407
Carbachol effect on, 171
2-deoxy-d-glucose stimulation of gastric secretion;effects of brain stem transection,209
Denervation effects on secretory responses, 151
Drug interactions, classification, 350
Dysfunctions, clinical situations, 407
Gastrin antagonists, 224
Gastritis, maximum acid secretion in, 409
Gastrone effects, intragastric administration, 431
, intranervous administration, 425, 426, 428
, molecular size, 428
Histamine-atropine competitive inhibition, 152
HCl secretion by stomach, 125
: concept of elaboration by surface cells, 135
: effect of parietal cell antibodies, 437
Hypersecretion in Zollinger-Ellison syndrome, 417
Hypothalamic injections, effect on acid output, 209
Intrinsic factor antibodies, effect on gastric secretion, 441, 442
location and parietal cell, 435
Incidence of parietal cell antibodies, 433
Ion transport in gastric mucosa, 125
Maximum acid output in gastric disease, 407
Metiamide (H_2 block) effect on gastric secretion, 171, 173, 174
Mucus enhancers, 228
Parietal cells in human gastric mucosa, 433, 435
mass and peptic cell mass, 439
, influence of antibodies, 437
antibodies in atrophic gastritis, 435
Pentagastrin effects on gastric secretion, 171, 189
Pepsin antagonists, 229
Prostaglandin effects on gastric secretion, 226
Range of basal and maximal acid output in various diseases, 407
Regulatory modes for gastric secretion, 147
Secretory studies in cancer, 413
Stimuli for acid and pepsin secretion, 147

Small Intestine Motor Activities
Cold block of intestinal motility, 82
Duodeno-jejunal intraluminal pressures, 79
Entero-enteric reflex, 60, 65
Intraluminal pressure in spontaneous propulsive motility, 83
Intrinsic mucosal reflex, 82
Jejunal distension effect on gut motility, 65
Law of intestine, 60
Myenteric reflex, 60
Peristalsis and electrical activity, 22, 24, 27
Second law of intestine, 60
Soap and bicarbonate buffer effects on duodenojejunal motility, 82

SUBJECT INDEX

See also "Index to Charts and Tables" for additional subject matter.

A

Absorption in intestine
  amino acids, 264, 273–279
  antacids, 353–355
  bile salts, 306
  carbohydrate, 273–279
  drugs, 359, 363
  electrolyte, 247–249
  fats, 291, 447
  influence of antacids on, 354–355
    motility on, 357–359
    pH on, 355
  proteins, peptides, 262
  water, 247–249
Achalasia LES pressure in, 380
Alpha-beta-lipoproteinemeia, 293
Amino acid
  absorption, 264, 273–279
  homeostasis, 259–268
  in dietary imbalance, 266
  gut lumen, 265
  levels in plasma, 265
Amyl nitrite, action on gall bladder, 106
Anacidity
  in pernicious anemia, 411
  gastric malignancy, 413
Antibodies
  intrinsic factor, 432
  parietal cell, 430, 434
ATP
  in acid secretion, 126–129
  sugar transport, 279
Autodigestion of enzymes, 263

B

Basal electrical rhythm (BER)
  basis for peristalsis, 20
  frequency gradient, 25
  gastroduodenal junction, 26
  membrane properties, 19
  pacemaker, 23
  propagation of wave, 20–23
  recording, 18, 19
  w waves, 18–26
  spike potential, 20
Bile acid
  absorption mode, 301
    sites, 306
  bacterial transformation, 302
  conjugation, 304–306
  conservation, 303, 308
  effect on colon transport, 252
  enterohepatic circulation, 301–314
  metabolism, 301–307, 311
  micelles, 448
  pool, 302, 308, 311, 453
  solubilization action, 291
  turnover, 303
Bile duct
  blood flow, 157
  epithelium, 150
  innervation, 98
Bile salt
  (see bi le acid)
Biliary tract absorptive functions, 329–344
Bioelectric potentials
  gall bladder, 332
  intestinal muscle, 17–27
  stomach, 124
Biotransformation
  bacterial, 302
  by intestine, 363
Blood flow
  autoregulation, 198
  gastric mucosa, 159
  intestinal, 196
  mesenteric, 195
  bile duct, 105, 107
Brush border
  in active transport, 274
  plasma membrane, 277

C

Caerulin
  effect on gastric secretion,
  peptides, 184
  relation to gastin structure,183
Chloride
  in gastric juice, 123

transport, 123
Cholecystokine (CCK-PZ)
effect on colon, 393, 395
gastric secretion, 157
gastrin heptapeptide relations, 184
in coeliac disease, 454
pancreatic enzyme stimulus, 183
potentiation of secretion, 183
release by fat, 183
in sprue, 311
water-bicarbonate secretion, 183
Choledochoduodenal-junction, 93–115
Cholera, 251, 254
Choleresis, by secretion, 183
Cholesterol uptake, 449
Chylomicron, 289, 449, 455
Colon
contractions, 62
diverticuli, 395, 397–399
dysfunctions, 389-400
electrolyte transport in, 252
hormone action on, 393
irritable, syndrome, 391-395
intraluminal pressure, 397
motility inhibition, 59
stimulation, 64
Contraction process
electrical correlates, 20
energy requirement,
excitation coupling,
influence of hormones, 32, 41
in smooth muscle, 9, 11
striated muscle, 3
role of ions, 4, 7
spike potentials and, 21
Cyclic AMP in secretion, 249-252

D

Defecation
colon movements in, 390
diet effects on, 399
in irritable colon syndrome, 392
2-deoxyglucose stimulation
of gastric secretion, 149, 210
Digestion of fat, 447
Diverticular disease, 395, 397, 399
Drug interactions, 349–366
Duodenum
distension of, 61
mucosal DNA, RNA, 188
receptive relaxation of, 67
Dysphagia, 379

E

Eating reflex, 64, 392
Electrical p.d.
gall bladder, 333, 338, 341, 342
gastric mucosa, 123
muscle, 17, 20–23, 26, 27
Emptying of stomach
rate, 48, 52
relation to energy of meal, 50
composition of meal, 48
Endocrine adenopathy in gastric disease, 412
Energy
coupling, 278
for HCl secretion, 127
content of meal, 50
Entero-enteric reflexes, 57–68
Enterogastric reflex, 66
Enterohepatic circulation
bile acids, 301–314
enterectomy effect, 309
in ileal disease, 307
Enzyme
pepsin secretion, 419
secretion, effect of hormones, 180, 182
Epithelial cell fat uptake, 449
Esophageal sphincter (LES)
dysfunction, 379–384
hormonal control, 31
innervation, 379

F

Fat
absorption, 286–295, 447–450
cellular phase, 449
digestion, 447
impaired by bacteria, 454
pancreatic lipase, 290, 448
emulsification, 294
in intestinal mucosa, 294
malabsorption, 450–456
rate of lipolysis, 290
solubilization, 291
Fatty acid
absorption by diffusion, 287
concentration in lumen, 286
micellar formation, 286

uptake, 449
Feeding reflex
(see eating reflex)
Fiber content of food, 399
Fluid secretion by intestine, 249

G

Gall bladder
electrical potential, 333, 338, 341
electrolyte fluxes, 343
ion transport, 337
mucosa, 341, 342
sphincter mechanism, 150
stones in, 343
Gall stones
cholesterol, 310
formation, 343
Gastric emptying
(see stomach emptying)
Gastric inhibition hormones, 66, 423
Gastric inhibitor polypeptide (GIP), 7
Gastric motor activities
(see stomach emptying)
Gastric mucosa
barrier, 227
blood flow, 159
homeostasis, 166
Gastric pathophysiology
carcinoma, 413
gastritis, 408–411
hypertrophy, 412
ulcer, 415
pernicious anemia, 411
hyperplasia, 416
Zollinger-Ellison, 416
Gastric secretion
analysis in disease, 406
anticholinergics, 222
caerulein action, 156, 184
cholecystokinen, 156
control by brain, 207–214
drug effects on, 230–232
dysfunctions of, 405–419
gastrin effect, 155, 184
antagonists, 223
glucagon effec on, 157
hypersecretion, 412–415
hypoglycemia effect, 149, 158, 208–210
in gastritis, 408
intracranial injury, 211
pernicious anemia, 411
stress, 211
ulcer disease, 414
intrinsic factor, 411, 412
pharmacologic control, 411–432
regulation, 148
reversal of inhibition, 158
vagal stimulation, 146, 149
vagotomy, 415
Zollinger-Ellison syndrome, 416
Gastrin
antagonists, 233
antiserum, 40
effect in man, 146
effective dose, 181
effect on colon, 393
lower esophageal sphincter, 378,380
hypertrophic action, 188, 190
in Zollinger-Ellison syndrome, 416
release, 185, 186
serum concentration, 383
stimulus for acid secretion, 155, 156
structure, 183
Gastrointestinal hormones
actions, 180
activity relations, 183
assay, 181
dose-response, 32, 181
effect on absorption, 180
effect on enzyme secretion, 182
effect on sphincters, 40
effect on sphincter of Oddi, 100
effective doses, 181
inhibition of gastric secretion, 423
interactions, 34
motility control, 41, 42
pharmacologic effects, 181
release of, 185–187
species differences, 182
trophic actions, 187–190
(see also specific hormones)
Gastrointestinal sphincter, 26, 40, 41, 47
67
Gastritis
classification, 410
histology of mucosa, 409

parietal cell antibodies, 410
secretion in, 408
Gastrocolic reflexes, 63–65, 392
Gastrone, 424, 427
Glucagon
enteric, 179
effect on gastric secretion, 157
pancreatic, 179, 185
Glucose–Na absorption, 248

H

Histamine
block of H_2 receptors, 167
common mediator for acid secretion, 167
receptors, H_1 and H_2, 154
test of gastric secretory function, 406
Hormones, Gastrointestinal
actions, 180, 181
effects on motility, 34, 41, 180
regulation of
bile duct sphincter, 100
release of, regulation, 185–187
structure-activity relationships, 183–185
trophic effects, 187–190
HCl production mechanism, 123–137

I

Ileum
absorption after resection, 313
absorption and secretion from, 153
bile acid absorption from, 306, 307
fat absorption from, 292, 293
reflex effects from distension, 61
Immunofluorescent
location of antibodies, 432
Inhibitors of gastric secretion,
endogenous, 423–442
Insulin
effects on gastric secretion, 149, 158, 210
test for vagotomy, 414
Intrinsic factor
antibodies, 432, 440

J

Jejunum
atrophy of mucosa, 311
cholecystokinen release by, 311
distension effects on gastrointestinal motility, 63 , 66
fat absorption from, 292
Juice
gastric, composition, 405, 406
pancreatic, 290

L

Latent period, gastric inhibition, 66
Law of intestine
Bayliss and Starling, 58, 60
second law, 59, 60
Length-tension of muscle, 6
Lipase, pancreatic, 29
Lipemia, 289
Lipolyses, 448–450

M

Malabsorption, intestinal, 447-456
Meals
composition and gastric emptying, 47
effect on gut content, 261, 262
volume, 48
Membrane
of villus, 286, 287
potential, 19
Mesenteric blood flow
autoregulation, 198,
catecholamine effect, 197, 199
effect of histamine, 159
effects of nerve stimulation, 159
hyperemic overshoot, 199
ischemia, 200
species differences, 200
Mesenteric vasculature receptors, 199
Metabolism
bile acids, 312
intestinal mucosa, 263
proteins, 265
Micellerization of fat, 448
Microbial flora of intestine, 360
Monoglyceride absorption, 287
Motility
colon reflexes, 63, 64
dysfunctions, 384-400
esophagus, 380
small intestine, cold block, 81
effect of hormones, 41

effect of hormones on, 41, 42
vagus on, 26, 27
of gastroduodenal junction, 26
force-veolocity relations, 6
length tension, 6
mechanical activity and spike potential, 21
role of calcium in contraction, 7
ultrastructure, 5
Mucin secretion from stomach, 154
Muscle, smooth
contractile process, 9, 11
electrical activity, 17, 20
and peristalsis, 23
extrinsic reflexes of, 59
intrinsic reflexes of, 58
myenteric reflexes, 58
osmotic effects, 78
pH effects on, 78, 81
role of calcium in contraction, 7
splanchnics, 196
vagus, 195
Muscle, striated
ATP and ATPase in, 4
contractile process, 3
proteins of, 3
Mucosal cell
barrier, 227
turnover, 263
Mucus
colitis, 391
secretion, 227

N

Nerve, stimulation effects
on intestinal motility and blood flow, 195
on choledochoduodenal junction, 98,105
vagus, on gastric secretion, 149
Net flux secretion, 249

P

Pacemaker, electrical
in duodenum, 26
potentials and rhythmic contractions, 84
Parietal cell
antibodies, 410, 430
intracellular pH in, 129
mass, 130, 434, 406
membrane charge, 124, 125
site of acid formation, 129
Pentagastrin, 168, 174
Pepsin
antagonists, 229
pepsinogen, 145
secretion, 418
stimulation by gastrin, 84
Peptic ulcer
anticholinergic drugs in treatment of, 222
disease, 414
gastrin antagonists in, 223
mucus, enhancement of treatment, 227
Peristalsis
antiperistalsis, 61
electrical activity, 23
stretch receptors, 84
wave progression, 80
Pernicous anemia, gastric secretion, 411
Potential, electrical
smooth muscle, 17
vagus effect on, 26, 27
Prostaglandin effect on gastric secretion, 225
Pyloric sphincter, 26, 40, 41, 47, 67

R

Receptive relaxation, 67
Receptors
baro-, 63
block of H_2, 167, 168
chemoreceptor in intestinal mucosa, 63, 85
duodenal, control of gastric emptying, 52
histamine H_2, 154
inhibition in smooth muscle, 34
model for parietal cell, 156
osmo-, 63
peristaltic reflex, 63
stretch, intestinal, 63
Reflexes
distension effects, 59, 61
entero-enteric, 57-68
enterogastric, 66
gastro-colic, 63
intestino-intestinal inhibitory, 59
intrinsic mucosal, 75, 84
intrinsic muscular, 76
myenteric, 58
visceral, from intestine, 58
Reflux, gastroesophageal, 382

7

S

Sclerederma, 381
Secretin
  effect on gastric secretion, 157
    on lower esophageal sphincter, 34
  hormonal releasing action of, 186
  peptide structure, 185
  reciprocal effects with gastrin, 34
Secretion from stomach
  (see gastric secretion)
Sites of intestine for absorption, 291, 292
Slow electrical waves, 18–26
Small intestine
  amino acid homeostasis, 259–268
  bile acid absorption, 303
  cycles of activity/inactivity, 78
  electrical activity, 17–26
  intraluminal pressures, 80
  motility, effect of cold block, 81
      pH, 81
    reflexes for, 58
    mucosal reflexes, 78
Smooth muscle
  calcium action in, 7
  contractile processes, 9, 11
  effect of caffein on, 11
  force-velocity relations, 6
  hormone effects on, 34
  length-tension relations, 32
  ultrastructure, 5
Somatic reflexes from intestine, 59
Sodium ion
  in basal electrical rhythm, 19
  membrane repolarization, 19
  transport in gastric mucosal, 123
Sphincter
  choledochoduodenal, 93–115
    hormone regulation, 100
    innervation, 98
    nerve stimulation effect, 105
    opening pressures, 102–105
    resistance, 97
  esophageal, lower (LES), 32
    effect of gastrin on, 40
      secretion, 34
    pressures in, 38, 40
  pyloric, action of hormones, 40
    effect of cholecystokinen, 36
Spike potential
  calcium ion and, 20
  relation to mechanical contraction, 21
Splanchnic blood flow, 159
Sprue, enterohepatic circulation in, 311
Stomach emptying
  drug effects on, 359
  duodenal receptors for, 52
  dysfunctions, 389–100
  effect of drugs, 358
  enterogastric reflex, 66
  influence meal composition, 47–48
  inhibition, 62
    from bowel, 66
    rectum, 67
  rate and meal half-life, 48
  regulation of, 47
  reflex inhibition, 62, 66
Stomach mucosa
  barrier, 227
  hyperplasia, 416
  hypertrophy, 412
Stomach secretion
  (see gastric secretion)
Stones, biliary, 310, 343
Structure
  chemical, gastrointestinal hormones,183
  ultra, of intestinal mucosa, 293
    of smooth muscle, 5
Sugar transport, 279

T

Test of breath for bile acid conjugation,
  313
Transport
  across gall bladder mucosa, 331, 341
  of charge across parietal cell membrane,
    124
    ion in gastric mucosa, 123
    water in gastric mucosa, 123
  triglyceride, 287
Triglycerides
  absorption, 287
  accumulation in mucosa, 291
Trophic effects
  cholecystokinen (CCK-PZ), 190
  gastrin, 187–190
  gastric mucosa, 412
  pentagastrin, 188

U

Ulcer disease
(see peptic ulcer)
Ultrastructure
intestinal mucosa, 293
smooth muscle, 5

V

Vagotomy
effects on gastric secretion, 45
pancreatic secretion, 453
insulin test for, 415
in ulcer therapy, 415
malabsorption due to, 453
selective, 415
choledochoduodenal sphincter opening, 103
Vagus
effect on electrical activity of intestine, 26
gastric secretion, 149
vesceral blood flow, 159, 195–197
interactions, 150
regulator of gastric functions,68
Vasoactive inhibitor peptide, VIP, 179, 423
Vesicles, intestinal submucosa, 293
Villi, brush border in cells, 274, 277
Visceral blood flow regulation, 195–203

W

Water
transport in gastric mucosa, 123
unstirred layer and absorption, 286

Z

Zollinger-Ellison syndrome, 416, 452